Comprehensive Management of Headache for the Otolaryngologist

Editors

JONI K. DOHERTY
MICHAEL SETZEN

OTOLARYNGOLOGIC CLINICS OF NORTH AMERICA

www.oto.theclinics.com

Consulting Editor
SUJANA S. CHANDRASEKHAR

June 2022 • Volume 55 • Number 3

ELSEVIER

1600 John F. Kennedy Boulevard • Suite 1800 • Philadelphia, Pennsylvania, 19103-2899

http://www.oto.theclinics.com

OTOLARYNGOLOGIC CLINICS OF NORTH AMERICA Volume 55, Number 3
June 2022 ISSN 0030-6665, ISBN-13: 978-0-323-96175-2

Editor: Stacy Eastman
Developmental Editor: Diana Grace Ang

Otolaryngologic Clinics of North America (ISSN 0030-6665) is published bimonthly by Elsevier, Inc., 360 Park Avenue South, New York, NY 10010-1710. Months of issue are February, April, June, August, October, and December. Business and Editorial Offices: 1600 John F. Kennedy Blvd., Suite 1800, Philadelphia, PA 19103-2899. Customer Service Office: 6277 Sea Harbor Drive, Orlando, FL 32887-4800. Periodicals postage paid at New York, NY and additional mailing offices. Subscription prices are $450.00 per year (US individuals), $1336.00 per year (US institutions), $100.00 per year (US & Canadian student/resident), $576.00 per year (Canadian individuals), $1396.00 per year (Canadian institutions), $628.00 per year (international individuals), $1396.00 per year (international institutions), $270.00 per year (international student/resident). Foreign air speed delivery is included in all *Clinics'* subscription prices. All prices are subject to change without notice. **POSTMASTER:** Send address changes to *Otolaryngologic Clinics of North America*, Elsevier Health Sciences Division, Subscription Customer Service, 3251 Riverport Lane, Maryland Heights, MO 63043. **Telephone: 1-800-654-2452 (U.S. and Canada); 314-447-8871 (outside U.S. and Canada). Fax: 314-447-8029. E-mail: journalscustomerservice-usa@elsevier.com (for print support); journalsonlinesupport-usa@elsevier.com (for online support).**

Reprints. For copies of 100 or more of articles in this publication, please contact the Commercial Reprints Department, Elsevier Inc., 360 Park Avenue South, New York, NY 10010-1710. Tel.: 212-633-3874; Fax: 212-633-3820; E-mail: reprints@elsevier.com.

Otolaryngologic Clinics of North America is also published in Spanish by McGraw-Hill Interamericana Editores S.A., P.O. Box 5-237, 06500 Mexico D.F., Mexico.

Otolaryngologic Clinics of North America is covered in *MEDLINE/PubMed (Index Medicus), Current Contents/Clinical Medicine, Excerpta Medica, BIOSIS, Science Citation Index,* and *ISI/BIOMED.*

Contributors

CONSULTING EDITOR

SUJANA S. CHANDRASEKHAR, MD, FACS, FAAOHNS

Consulting Editor, *Otolaryngologic Clinics of North America*, Past President, American Academy of Otolaryngology–Head and Neck Surgery, Secretary-Treasurer, American Otological Society, Partner, ENT & Allergy Associates LLP, Clinical Associate Professor, Department of Otolaryngology–Head and Neck Surgery, Icahn School of Medicine at Mount Sinai, New York, New York; Clinical Professor, Department of Otolaryngology–Head and Neck Surgery, Donald and Barbara Zucker School of Medicine at Hofstra/Northwell, Hempstead, New York

EDITORS

JONI K. DOHERTY, MD, PhD, FACS

Assistant Professor of Clinical Otolaryngology–Head and Neck Surgery, Division of Neurotology, Keck School of Medicine of USC, USC Caruso Department of Otolaryngology–Head and Neck Surgery, Los Angeles, California

MICHAEL SETZEN, MD, FACS, FAAP

Clinical Professor of Otolaryngology, Weill Cornell Medical College, Otolaryngology, PC, Great Neck, New York

AUTHORS

IDO BADASH, MD

Resident Physician, USC Caruso Department of Otolaryngology–Head and Neck Surgery, Los Angeles, California

ALAINA BASSETT, AuD, PhD

Assistant Professor, USC Caruso Department of Otolaryngology–Head and Neck Surgery, Keck School of Medicine of USC, Los Angeles, California

KAEVON BRASFIELD, BS

Keck School of Medicine of USC, University of Southern California, Los Angeles, California

ROBERT G. BRIGGS, MD

Department of Neurological Surgery, Keck School of Medicine of USC, University of Southern California, Los Angeles, California

JOHN PATRICK CAREY, MD

Professor and Chief of Division of Otology, Neurotology, and Skull Base Surgery, Department of Otolaryngology-Head & Neck Surgery, Johns Hopkins School of Medicine, Baltimore, Maryland, USA

WOOSEONG CHOI, BS

Keck School of Medicine of USC, University of Southern California, Los Angeles, California

RAFFAELLO M. CUTRI, BS
Keck School of Medicine of USC, University of Southern California, Los Angeles, California

ROBERT DALLAPIAZZA, MD, PhD
Department of Neurological Surgery, Tulane School of Medicine, Tulane University, New Orleans, Louisiana

JOHN M. DELGAUDIO, MD
Professor, Department of Otolaryngology–Head and Neck Surgery, Emory University School of Medicine, Atlanta, Georgia

JONI K. DOHERTY, MD, PhD, FACS
Assistant Professor of Clinical Otolaryngology–Head and Neck Surgery, Division of Neurotology, Keck School of Medicine of USC, USC Caruso Department of Otolaryngology–Head and Neck Surgery, Los Angeles, California

RYAN E. FLORES, BS
Keck School of Medicine of USC, University of Southern California, Los Angeles, California

ERICK GARCIA, MD
USC Caruso Department of Otolaryngology–Head and Neck Surgery, Keck Medicine of USC, Los Angeles, California

STEVEN L. GIANNOTTA, MD
Department of Neurological Surgery, Keck School of Medicine of USC, University of Southern California, Los Angeles, California

JOHN L. GO, MD
Assistant Professor, Department of Radiology, Keck School of Medicine of USC, Los Angeles, California

HUSEYIN ISILDAK, MD
Department of Otolaryngology–Head and Neck Surgery, Stony Brook University, East Setauket, New York

CHRISTOPHER L. KALMAR, MD, MBA
Department of Plastic Surgery, Vanderbilt University Medical Center, Nashville, Tennessee

PAVAN SURESH KRISHNAN, BA
Clinical Research Coordinator, Department of Otolaryngology–Head and Neck Surgery, Johns Hopkins School of Medicine, Baltimore, Maryland; Medical Student, Virginia Commonwealth University School of Medicine, Richmond, Virginia

MATTHEW R. LARK, DDS
Diplomate American Board of Orofacial Pain; Fellow, American Academy of Orofacial Pain, Master, ICOI, Assistant Professor, University of Toledo Medical Center, Faculty U Michigan School of Dentistry

DARRIN J. LEE, MD, PhD
Department of Neurological Surgery, Neurorestoration Center, Keck School of Medicine of USC, University of Southern California, Los Angeles, California

ALEXANDER LERNER, MD
Assistant Professor, Department of Radiology, Keck School of Medicine of USC, Keck Medical Center of USC, University of Southern California, Los Angeles, California

JEFFREY LIAW, MD
Department of Otolaryngology–Head and Neck Surgery, University of Missouri, Columbia, Missouri

ISABELLE MAGRO, MD, MS
USC Caruso Department of Otolaryngology–Head and Neck Surgery, Keck School of Medicine of USC, Los Angeles, California

AMAR MIGLANI, MD
Department of Otolaryngology–Head and Neck Surgery, Mayo Clinic, Phoenix, Arizona; Department of Otolaryngology–Head and Neck Surgery, Medical University of South Carolina, Charleston, South Carolina

SARAH E. MOWRY, MD, FACS
Associate Professor, Otolaryngology Residency Program Director, Department of Otolaryngology, Case Western Reserve University, University Hospitals, Cleveland Medical Center, Cleveland, Ohio

HENNA D. MURTHY, MD
Resident Surgeon, Department of Otolaryngology, Case Western Reserve University, Cleveland, Ohio

MARGARET NURIMBA, MD
USC Caruso Department of Otolaryngology–Head and Neck Surgery, Keck School of Medicine of USC, Los Angeles, California

DOROTHY W. PAN, MD, PhD
Resident Physician, USC Caruso Department of Otolaryngology–Head and Neck Surgery, Keck School of Medicine of USC, University of Southern California, Los Angeles, Los Angeles, California

VIJAY A. PATEL, MD
Division of Otolaryngology–Head and Neck Surgery, Children's Hospital Los Angeles, Los Angeles, California

MARISA C. PENN, BS
Keck School of Medicine of USC, University of Southern California, Los Angeles, California

SEAN P. POLSTER, MD
Department of Neurological Surgery, University of Pittsburgh Medical Center, Pittsburgh, Pennsylvania

JONATHAN J. RUSSIN, MD
Department of Neurological Surgery, Neurorestoration Center, Keck School of Medicine of USC, University of Southern California, Los Angeles, California

ROBERT A. SAADI, MD
Department of Otolaryngology–Head and Neck Surgery, University of Arkansas, Little Rock, Arkansas

RODNEY J. SCHLOSSER, MD
Department of Otolaryngology–Head and Neck Surgery, Medical University of South Carolina, Department of Surgery, Ralph H. Johnson VA Medical Center, Charleston, South Carolina

DEJAN SHAKYA
Dornsife College of Letters, Arts and Science, University of Southern California, Los Angeles, California

NASIM SHEIKH-BAHAEI, MD, PhD
Assistant Professor, Department of Radiology, Keck School of Medicine of USC, Los Angeles, California

SEIJI B. SHIBATA, MD, PHD
USC Caruso Department of Otolaryngology–Head and Neck Surgery, University of Southern California, Los Angeles, California

ZACHARY SOLER, MD, MSc
Department of Otolaryngology–Head and Neck Surgery, Medical University of South Carolina, Charleston, South Carolina

DONALD R. TANENBAUM, DDS, MPH
Diplomate, American Board of Orofacial Pain; Fellow, American Academy of Orofacial Pain, Clinical Assistant Professor, Hofstra North Shore-LIJ School of Medicine, Clinical Assistant Professor, Department of Oral and Maxillofacial Surgery, School of Dental Medicine at Stony Brook University, Section Head, Facial Pain and Dental Sleep Medicine, Department of Dental Medicine, Long Island Jewish Medical Center

ERIK VANSTRUM, BA
Medical Student, Keck School of Medicine of USC, University of Southern California, Los Angeles, California

NATHALIA VELASQUEZ, MD
Rhinology Fellow, Department of Otolaryngology–Head and Neck Surgery, Emory University School of Medicine, Atlanta, Georgia

KEVIN WU, BS
Keck School of Medicine of USC, University of Southern California, Los Angeles, California

SHENG ZHOU, MD
Resident Physician, USC Caruso Department of Otolaryngology–Head and Neck Surgery, Los Angeles, California

Contents

Headaches are a global health problem and are encountered by a variety of specialties, including otolaryngologists. These patients can present as a challenge, but an understanding of primary and secondary headache disorders and the accompanying broad differential diagnosis is critical. For secondary headache disorders, a differential diagnosis categorized by anatomic location can help organize the evaluation of these patients, which can then be narrowed by the history and examination findings. Additional ancillary tests such as laboratories and imaging can further aid in diagnosis but are not always necessary.

Patients will continue to present to the otolaryngologist's office with "sinus headaches" as their primary complaint. Otolaryngologists should take particular care in establishing a precise diagnosis. A thorough clinical history, comprehensive head and neck examination, well-performed nasal endoscopy, and imaging as necessary are essential components for effective diagnosis and treatment plan implementation. It is fundamental to acknowledge the criteria for diagnosing the various headache disorders that may disguise themselves as sinonasal complaints. Moreover, this patient population accurately diagnosed and treated will be extremely grateful for someone pointing them in a direction to obtain the relief they truly need.

Novel medical devices are emerging as low-risk treatment options for patients suffering from sinus headaches. Early trends for the treatment of sinus headaches using medical devices are following the more established primary headache literature. There are two categories of devices with early data supporting use, which may serve as useful adjuncts to conventional pharmacotherapy in the management of sinus headaches not caused by sinusitis: transcutaneous electrical neurostimulation and acoustic vibration with oscillating expiratory pressure. There is currently a paucity of high-level evidence and further studies are needed. Initial reports suggest these interventions are low risk, but longer follow-up is necessary.

VM is a common yet debilitating migraine variant that has taken many monikers in the past. As a relatively new diagnostic entity, public and provider awareness of this disorder can be improved. Symptoms include vertigo episodes in addition to photophobia, phonophobia, nausea, and headache. Diagnosis is primarily based on clinical history as pathognomonic signs via testing are not reliable. Standardized treatment algorithms have yet to be created and current recommendations have been adopted from migraine guidelines.

Patients often report symptoms of headache and dizziness concomitantly. Symptoms of dizziness can be explored with a comprehensive vestibular assessment, allowing for the investigation of central and peripheral vestibular system contributions to symptoms of dizziness. Patients who report both symptoms of headache and dizziness demonstrate abnormalities of the vestibular system which can be measured quantitatively. Completion of comprehensive vestibular testing can help to guide diagnosis and strategies for intervention.

Imaging plays an important role in identifying the cause of the much less common secondary headaches. Such headaches may be caused by a variety of pathologic conditions which can be categorized as intracranial and extracranial. Idiopathic intracranial hypertension imaging findings include "empty sella," orbital changes, and dural venous sinus narrowing. Intracranial hypotension (ICH) is frequently caused by CSF leaks. Imaging findings include loss of the CSF spaces, downward displacement of the brain, as well as dural thickening and enhancement. Severe cases of ICH may result in subdural hematomas. A variety of intracranial and skull base tumors may cause headaches due to dural involvement. Extracranial tumors and lesions that frequently present with headaches include a variety of sinonasal tumors as well as mucoceles. Neurovascular compression disorders causing headaches include trigeminal and glossopharyngeal neuralgia. Imaging findings include displacement and atrophy of the cranial nerve caused by an adjacent arterial or venous structure.

Idiopathic intracranial hypertension (IIH) is a triad of headaches, visual changes, and papilledema in the absence of a secondary cause for elevated intracranial pressure. There is an association with obesity, and the incidence is rising in parallel with the obesity epidemic. Sometimes these patients present to an otolaryngologist with complaints like tinnitus, dizziness, hearing loss, and otorrhea or rhinorrhea from cerebrospinal fluid leak. IIH diagnosis in conjunction with neurology and ophthalmology, including neuroimaging and lumbar puncture with opening pressure, is key to managing of this condition. Otolaryngologists should recognize IIH as a possible diagnosis and initiate appropriate referrals and treatment.

Though there have been considerable strides in the diagnosis and care of orofacial pain disorders, facial neuralgias, and myofascial pain dysfunction syndrome remain incredibly cumbersome for patients and difficult to manage for providers. Cranial neuralgias, myofascial pain syndromes, temporomandibular dysfunction (TMD), dental pain, tumors, neurovascular pain, and psychiatric diseases can all present with similar symptoms. As a result, a patient's quest for the treatment of their orofacial pain often begins on the wrong foot, with a misdiagnosis or unnecessary procedure, which makes it all the more frustrating for them. Understanding the natural history, clinical presentation, and management of facial neuralgias and myofascial pain dysfunction syndrome can help clinicians better recognize and treat these conditions. In this article, we review updated knowledge on the pathophysiology, incidence, clinical features, diagnostic criteria, and medical management of TN, GPN, GN, and MPDS.

Facial pain is a common medical complaint that is easily misdiagnosed. As a result, this pain often goes mistreated. Despite this, there are a variety of pharmacologic, surgical, and neuromodulatory options for the treatment of facial pain. In this review, the authors detail the forms of facial pain and their treatment options. They discuss the common medications used in the first-line treatment of facial pain and the second-line surgical and neuromodulatory options available to patients when pharmacologic options fail.

Pediatric headache is a common medical complaint managed across multiple subspecialties with a myriad of unique factors (clinical presentation and disease phenotype) that make accurate diagnosis particularly elusive. A thorough understanding of the stepwise approach to headache disorders in children is essential to ensure appropriate evaluation, timely diagnosis, and efficacious treatment. This work aims to review key components of a comprehensive headache assessment as well as discuss primary and secondary headache disorders observed in children, with a particular focus on clinical pearls and "red flag" symptoms necessitating ancillary diagnostic testing.

OTOLARYNGOLOGIC CLINICS
OF NORTH AMERICA

FORTHCOMING ISSUES

August 2022
Gender Affirmation Surgery in Otolaryngology
Regina Rodman and C. Michael Haben, *Editors*

October 2022
Complementary and Integrative Medicine and Nutrition in Otolaryngology
Michael D. Seidman and Marilene B. Wang, *Editors*

December 2022
Updates in Pediatric Otolaryngology
Romaine F. Johnson and Elton M. Lambert, *Editors*

RECENT ISSUES

April 2022
Pituitary Surgery
Jean Anderson Eloy, Christina H. Fang and Vijay Agarwal, *Editors*

February 2022
Business of Otolaryngology: 2022
Stephen P. Cragle and Eileen H. Dauer, *Editors*

December 2021
Childhood Hearing Loss
Nancy M. Young and Anne Marie Tharpe, *Editors*

SERIES OF RELATED INTEREST

Facial Plastic Surgery Clinics
Available at: https://www.facialplastic.theclinics.com/

Erratum

In the article, "Complications in Endoscopic Pituitary Surgery," by Joshua Vignolles-Jeong et. al., published in the April 2022 issue (Volume 55, number 2, pages 161), the additional author to be included is:

Douglas Hardesty, MD

The Ohio State University Wexner Medical Center Department of Neurosurgery, 460 W 10th Ave, Columbus, OH, 43210

And in Table 4 on page 5, the correct rate of hematoma after pituitary is 0.77 percent.

Otolaryngol Clin N Am 55 (2022) xiii
https://doi.org/10.1016/j.otc.2022.05.007
0030-6665/22/
oto.theclinics.com

Foreword

Healing Headaches: The Otolaryngology Perspective

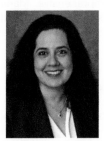

Sujana S. Chandrasekhar, MD, FACS, FAAOHNS
Consulting Editor

The word "headache" may be used by a patient to describe various types and degrees of head, face, and neck discomfort and may be accompanied by various symptoms. Likewise, the patient may present to a number of different types of health care providers, including primary care, internal medicine, neurology, otolaryngology, ophthalmology, dentistry, chiropractic, and more. Even more likely, patients are prone to self-diagnose and treat themselves with over-the-counter medications and treatments, which are often ineffective and can delay appropriate management.

Globally, the World Health Organization (WHO) reports that among adults aged 18 to 65 years, approximately one-third report migraine. Headache on 15 or more days every month affects 1.7% to 4% of the world's adult population. In the Global Burden of Disease Study, updated in 2013, migraine on its own was found to be the sixth highest cause worldwide of years lost due to disability, and headache disorders collectively were third highest.[1]

According to WHO, headache disorders impose a recognizable burden on sufferers, including sometimes substantial personal suffering, impaired quality of life, and financial cost. Repeated headache attacks, and often the constant fear of the next one, damage family life, social life, and employment. The long-term effort of coping with a chronic headache disorder may also predispose the individual to other illnesses. For example, anxiety and depression are significantly more common in people with migraine than in non-migraineur healthy individuals.

What, then, is the Otolaryngologist's role in the evaluation and management of the patient who experiences headache? Drs Michael Setzen and Joni Doherty, Guest Editors of this issue of *Otolaryngologic Clinics of North America* on Headache, have indeed provided a comprehensive and cohesive set of articles as a resource for ENTs as well as all other professionals managing the care of these individuals. This issue covers contributions from the paranasal sinuses, the vestibular system,

Otolaryngol Clin N Am 55 (2022) xv–xvi
https://doi.org/10.1016/j.otc.2022.03.003
0030-6665/22/© 2022 Published by Elsevier Inc.

oto.theclinics.com

temporomandibular joint dysfunction and arthralgia, neuralgia and atypical pain, and idiopathic intracranial hypertension. The judicious application and appropriate role of neuroimaging are discussed. Special populations need special attention. These include children, adolescents, and pregnant women. Hemifacial and circumscribed but intense headaches pose their own challenges.

Each issue of *Otolaryngologic Clinics of North America* seeks to be a current and thorough resource for the evaluation and management of patients with a particular disorder. Drs Setzen's and Dr Doherty's issue, Comprehensive Management of Headache for the Otolaryngologist, meets and exceeds expectations, as it is valuable for all who work to reduce the burden of this disease. I congratulate them and all of the authors featured in this issue.

Sujana S. Chandrasekhar, MD, FACS, FAAOHNS
Consulting Editor
Otolaryngologic Clinics of North America
Past President
American Academy of Otolaryngology–
Head and Neck Surgery

Secretary-Treasurer
American Otological Society

Partner, ENT & Allergy Associates LLP
18 East 48th Street, 2nd Floor
New York, NY 10017, USA

Clinical Professor, Department of Otolaryngology–
Head and Neck Surgery Zucker School of Medicine at Hofstra-Northwell
Hempstead, NY, USA

Clinical Associate Professor
Department of Otolaryngology–
Head and Neck Surgery
Icahn School of Medicine at Mount Sinai
New York, NY, USA

E-mail address:
ssc@nyotology.com
www.ears.nyc

REFERENCE

1. Available at: https://www.who.int/news-room/fact-sheets/detail/headache-disorders. Accessed March 13, 2022.

Preface

Comprehensive Headache Evaluation and Management for the Otolaryngologist

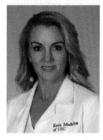 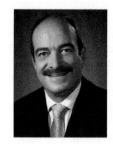

Joni K. Doherty, MD, PhD, FACS   Michael Setzen, MD, FACS, FAAP
Editors

Abbreviations	
HA	Headache
VM	Vestibular migraine
TN	Trigeminal neuralgia
GN	Geniculate neuralgia
MVD	Microvascular decompression

This issue takes us through the most common to rare headache causes and their presentation, essential to more complex evaluation, diagnosis, and management of headaches for comprehensive otolaryngologists, rhinologists, and neurotologists. Primary headaches are the most common headache disorders. The most common forms are tension-type headaches, migraine, and cluster headaches. Knowing the clinical presentation coupled with taking a thorough history and performing a thorough physical examination usually helps arrive at a correct diagnosis. Particular attention should be paid to unusual clinical presentations.

Further diagnostic workup should be performed in the presence of atypical and worrisome signs (eg, sentinel headache). Maintaining a high level of suspicion for virulence and a structured approach to evaluating all patients with headaches is the key to timely diagnosis of secondary headaches. We have contributions from neurotologists, rhinologists, neuroradiologists, neurosurgeons, and even a dental standpoint of temporomandibular joint disorders evaluation and management.

Many patients present to their physicians with a headache or midfacial pain and are certain it is a "sinus headache" and presume an underlying infection. Specialists of all

Otolaryngol Clin N Am 55 (2022) xvii–xviii
https://doi.org/10.1016/j.otc.2022.03.002
0030-6665/22/© 2022 Published by Elsevier Inc.

types, especially otolaryngologists, neurologists, allergists, internists, and emergency physicians, are confronted almost daily with patients saying, "I have a sinus headache, and I need antibiotics." This initiates a series of questions for the physician because several kinds of headaches occur with symptoms in this location. Also, the diagnosis is challenging because there are frequently associated symptoms of nasal congestion that accompany the headache and the common onset of headache with barometric change. These symptom groups can be present in both sinus headaches and migraine. "The role of the otolaryngologist in the evaluation and management of 'sinus headache'" describes headaches ascribed to other causes, in particular, migraine, as well as headaches that are a result of sinusitis. This issue addresses the need for the expertise of an otolaryngologist, who can obtain a history of nasal and sinus disease, evaluate the interior of the nose, and correlate it to a computed tomographic scan, along with the collaboration of neurologists/headache specialists. Because headaches are often a symptom of potentially dangerous conditions that may need emergency workup and referral to the appropriate physician, this issue identifies these emergency conditions for the clinician.

Neuropathic facial pain is caused by vascular compression of the trigeminal nerve in the prepontine cistern. It is characterized by an intermittent prickling or stabbing component or a constant burning, searing pain. Medical treatment consists of anticonvulsant medication. Neurosurgical treatment may require microvascular decompression of the trigeminal nerve.

The approach to the subject of headache in this issue provides information of importance to not only otolaryngologists but also emergency physicians, allergists, internists, pediatricians, pulmonologists, and family practitioners, who frequently see and manage headache and sinus patients. It provides direct clinical information on history, differential diagnosis, laboratory testing and imaging, treatment options, and suggestions for when to refer. It demonstrates the need for a multispecialty team approach in evaluating the headache patient, particularly the patient reporting a "sinus headache" that can be anything but a sinus headache.

Joni K. Doherty, MD, PhD, FACS
Division of Neurotology
Keck School of Medicine of USC
USC Caruso Family Department
of Otolaryngology–
Head and Neck Surgery
1450 San Pablo Street, Suite 5700
Los Angeles, CA 90033, USA

Michael Setzen, MD, FACS, FAAP
Weill Cornell Medical College
Otolaryngology, PC
600 Northern Boulevard, Suite 113
Great Neck, NY 11021, USA

E-mail addresses:
JoniDoherty@gmail.com (J.K. Doherty)
MichaelSetzen@gmail.com (M. Setzen)

The Role of the Otolaryngologist in the Evaluation and Management of Headache

Henna D. Murthy, MD[a], Sarah E. Mowry, MD[a,b],*

KEYWORDS

- Headache • Otolaryngologist • Secondary headaches • History and physical

KEY POINTS

- Headaches are the number one neurologic disorder and have become a global health problem with high economic costs.
- A large differential diagnosis should be kept in mind, including primary and secondary headache disorders. Categorizing based on anatomic location can help organize secondary headache etiologies.
- A comprehensive headache history, focused head and neck, and neurologic physical examination are keys to narrowing the differential diagnosis.

INTRODUCTION

Headaches and migraines are a global health problem and affect the quality of life, workplace loss of productivity, and have high economic costs. Globally, an estimated 47% of adults have an active headache disorder, of which 10% have migraines and 40% have tension-type headaches.[1] According to the Global Burden of Disease 2015 (GBD2015) studies, these conditions have negatively impacted disability-adjusted life years (DALYs) and are ranked in the top 10 causes for years lived with disability (YLDs).[2]

These patients can present as a challenge in diagnosis, workup, management, and definitive treatment. Headaches are associated with a wide variety of etiologies ranging from life-threatening intracranial tumors or intracranial bleeding to benign primary headaches, such as migraines or tension-type headaches. Another challenge arises as presentation and management can be encountered by a variety of physicians, such as

a Department of Otolaryngology, Case Western Reserve University, 10900 Euclid Avenue, Cleveland, OH 44106, USA; b Department of Otolaryngology, University Hospitals, Cleveland Medical Center, 11100 Euclid Avenue, LKS 5405, Cleveland, OH 44106, USA
* Corresponding author: Department of Otolaryngology, University Hospitals, Cleveland Medical Center, 11100 Euclid Avenue, LKS 5405, Cleveland, OH 44106.
E-mail address: Sarah.Mowry@UHhospitals.org

Otolaryngol Clin N Am 55 (2022) 493–499
https://doi.org/10.1016/j.otc.2022.02.001
0030-6665/22/Published by Elsevier Inc.
oto.theclinics.com

primary care, neurology, neurosurgery, cardiology, otolaryngology, ophthalmology, pain management, oral surgery, and dental medicine specialists. The goal of this article is to present common etiologies of headaches and migraines and to focus on pertinent history and diagnostic tests for otolaryngologic causes.

Headaches are the most common neurologic disorder.[1] They are classified as primary or secondary headaches. Primary headaches are idiopathic and have no underlying cause, with the most common being tension-type headaches, migraines, and cluster headaches. Secondary headaches are the result of another condition, such as headaches attributed to trauma, vascular disorders, substances or their withdrawal, and so forth. The International Classification of Headache Disorders (ICHD) establishes criteria based on the characteristics of the headache and describes 14 different categories.[3,4] Headache or facial pain attributed to disorders of the cranium, neck, eyes, ears, nose, sinuses, teeth, mouth, or other facial or cervical structures are a distinct ICHD category. This secondary headache diagnosis is used for a new headache or pre-existing headache that is exacerbated in conjunction with a disorder of the cranium, neck, eyes, ears, nose, sinus, teeth, or mouth. **Box 1** lists causes for secondary headaches organized by anatomic location which could be considered as otolaryngologic headaches.[4–10] This may be a helpful way to organize a differential when assessing patients.

Primary Versus Secondary Headaches

A general understanding of primary headaches will assist in timely diagnosis and treatment. According to the ICHD, there are 4 broad categories of primary headaches including migraine, tension-type, trigeminal-autonomic cephalgia, and other primary headache disorders. There are more than 20 subclassifications within these categories. In general, it is important to differentiate the duration of episodes as less than or greater than 4 hours per day, and the frequency as less than or greater than 15 days per month.[6]

Tension-type headaches are the most prevalent headache globally with a lifetime prevalence of 78%. This type of headache is most prevalent between the ages of 30 to 39 and is slightly higher in women across all demographics.[11] Tension-type headaches are usually described as mild to moderate, bilateral or band-like pressure and tightness. Episodes last from 30 minutes to 7 days, can be waxing and waning, and are not exacerbated by routine physical activity. With more severe cases, patients may also describe throbbing or pulsatile pain and photophobia, which can make it difficult to differentiate from migraines.[4,9]

Migraines are the second most prevalent primary headache, and according to the GBD2015, are the third-highest cause of disability globally in people younger than 50 year old.[4] Episodes can start as early as childhood or teenage years.[12] They are categorized into 2 major types: migraine with or without aura. An aura is described as a focal neurologic symptom that occurs before or at the onset of a migraine and fully resolves spontaneously. These auras can range from visual disturbances, sensory abnormalities, aphasia, hemiplegia, or vertigo. Migraines are usually described as unilateral pulsating pain in the temple but can also be bitemporal or involve the whole head. It has a gradual onset with a crescendo of pain rated moderate to severe. Associated symptoms include nausea, emesis, photophobia, and phonophobia. The episodes last 4 to 72 hours and are worse with activity resulting in patients seeking a dark and quiet room for relief.[4,9,12] These patients can be seen in an otolaryngologist's office as there is a known association between migraines and vestibular symptoms. Episodic vertigo can occur in up to 25% of migraine patients, and these vertiginous episodes can have an abrupt onset, last days, and often occur during headache-free times.[13]

Box 1
Causes of secondary headache catagorized by location in the head and neck

Intracranial
- Mass or lesion (tumor, cyst, abscess)
- Hemorrhage
- Low CSF pressure syndromes
- High CSF pressure syndromes
- Infectious (Lyme, HIV, encephalitis, meningitis, and so forth)
- Chiari malformation
- Trauma related/Whiplash
- Noninfectious, inflammatory intracranial disease

Neurovascular
- Transient ischemic attack or cerebrovascular accident
- Arteriovenous malformation
- Carotid or vertebrobasilar artery dissection
- Dural sinus thrombosis
- Giant cell arteritis
- Trigeminal neuralgia
- Glossopharyngeal neuralgia

Neck
- Cervicogenic
- Craniocervical dystonia
- Retropharyngeal tendonitis

Eyes
- Acute angle-closure glaucoma
- Ocular inflammatory disorders
- Acute refractory disorders
- Trochlear headache

Ears
- Mass or lesion
- Otitis externa or media
- Vestibular migraine
- Motion sickness
- Visual-vestibular mismatch
- Meniere's disease

Nose/paranasal sinuses
- Nasopharyngeal disorders or tumors
- Acute rhinosinusitis
- Chronic or recurring rhinosinusitis
- Mucosal contact points

Teeth/masticatory muscles/TMJ
- Tooth impaction or infection
- Temporomandibular joint disorders
- Myofascial pain

Endocrine
- Hypothyroidism
- Hyperprolactinemia
- Pituitary apoplexy
- Menstrual or hormone related

Other
- Substance use or its withdrawal
- Medication overuse
- Exposure to toxins (carbon monoxide, nitric oxide)
- Hypoxia or hypercapnia
- Arterial hypertension

Cluster headaches are a subcategory of trigeminal-autonomic cephalgia and are separated into episodic and chronic. Although not as prevalent as tension-type or migraine headaches, they are one of the most severe primary headache disorders. Cluster headaches are usually described as quick onset, unilateral, deep, and constant pain near the temple or eye. It reaches maximum intensity within minutes and episodes last 15 minutes to 3 hours. Associated symptoms include ipsilateral lacrimation, ocular erythema, nasal congestion, rhinorrhea, pallor, diaphoresis, or Horner syndrome.[9,12]

Secondary headaches with red flag symptoms should also be considered and high degree of suspicion should be held if they present in the office although these patients are more commonly assessed in an emergency facility. A common mnemonic used is SNOOP4:[14]

- Systemic signs such as fever, chills, weight loss, myalgia, or diaphoresis can point toward infection, malignancy, vasculitis, or inflammatory disease. If a patient has a history of malignancy, then metastasis should always be kept in mind.
- Neurologic signs such as motor, sensory, speech, vision, cognitive, or balance abnormalities should be taken seriously.
- Sudden onset or thunderclap headache can indicate intracerebral hemorrhage, stroke, arterial dissection, venous sinus thrombosis, hypertensive crisis, or pituitary apoplexy.
- Age of onset less than 5 years or greater than 65 years points more toward a secondary headache, as primary headache disorders are not common.
- A change in the pattern of a patient with prior headache, usually with a new symptom should prompt looking for a secondary cause.
- Headaches that are precipitated by Valsalva maneuvers could indicate a Chiari malformation, intracranial mass lesion, hydrocephalus, intracranial hypertension or hypotension, or vascular etiology and may deserve imaging.
- Postural changes aggravating a headache are suspicious for abnormal intracranial pressure whether it is increased or decreased.
- Papilledema should raise concern for an intracranial abnormality or hypertension.

Headache History

As with any new concern, a complete history is a key to narrowing down the differential diagnosis for a patient with headaches. When taking the history, use open-ended questions to inquire about the onset, location/radiation, duration, frequency, character, severity, aggravating factors, and relieving factors. To improve accuracy, the query may be framed as "How many days a month are you completely headache-free?" If a headache is present for more than 15 days per month, it may fall into the category of chronic daily headaches. For the duration, many headaches are divided into short (<4 hours) or long (>4 hours) duration and the use of medication for relief should be specified.[14] Additional associated symptoms with a temporal relationship to the headache onset or fluctuation can further narrow our differential. Incorporate questions such as the history of trauma, muscle tension, neck pain, vision changes, light or sound sensitivity, hearing loss, tinnitus (+/− pulsatile), vertigo, otalgia, aural fullness, otorrhea, nasal congestion or obstruction, nasal discharge, hyposmia, facial pain or pressure, teeth clenching or grinding, dental pain or recent dental work, and nausea or vomiting. Other clues can be obtained from a patient's past medical history, current or new medications, blood thinners, immunosuppression, and recent travel or exposure to sick contacts.[9]

A personal or family history of headaches and migraines are key factors as well. According to the National Headache Foundation, 70% to 80% of migraine sufferers have a family history of migraines, and less than half have received a diagnosis by a medical professional. There is also an association between earlier age of onset, a higher number of medication days, and migraine with aura with a family history of migraine.[15] It is also imperative to keep in mind that a patient with a primary headache disorder, such as migraines, can also suffer from a secondary headache disorder that would exacerbate their "normal" headache symptoms.[16]

Physical Examination

After the headache history is obtained, further information can be gathered during the physical examination. The examination should consist of a complete head and neck examination, neurologic examination including cranial nerve assessment, and possibly nasal endoscopy. Other specialists will be relying on an otolaryngologist to specifically examine and comment on the ears, nose and paranasal sinuses, oral cavity, and neck. The addition of clinical examination findings can aid in the correct diagnosis or referral.

A systematic approach should be used when considering the etiology of a headache. **Fig. 1** is a flow chart that can be used as a guide when encountering these patients, although it is not all-inclusive.

Diagnostic Tests

While headaches can be a symptom of a vast range of diseases, after a thorough history and physical, the differential can usually be narrowed. Although at times, additional diagnostic testing is required to help rule in or rule out diagnoses. Basic laboratory studies such as CBC, coagulation studies, TSH, and inflammatory markers (ie, ESR, CRP) can be helpful in pointing toward an etiology such as infectious, hemorrhagic, hypothyroidism, vasculitis, or other inflammatory conditions. If there is a concern for central nervous system infection or CSF pressure abnormalities contributing to the headache a lumbar puncture can be performed.

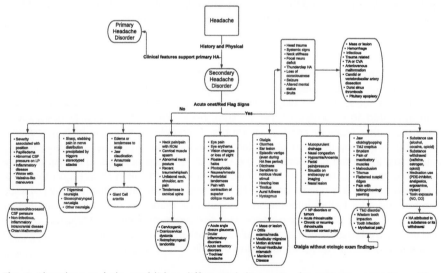

Fig. 1. Flowchart to help establish a differential diagnosis of a patient presenting with a headache complaint. The differential includes primary headache disorders, secondary headaches with red flag symptoms, and secondary headaches without red flap symptoms. Some key history and physical examination findings for each category are listed. It is not exhaustive. CO, carbon monoxide; CSF, cerebrospinal fluid; CVA, cerebrovascular accident; HA, headache; LP, lumbar puncture; NO, nitric oxide; NP, nasopharyngeal; ROM, range of motion; TIA, transient ischemic attach; TMJ, temporomandibular joint.

If further information is needed, then diagnostic imaging studies can be used. Regarding nasal or paranasal sinus symptoms, imaging is not recommended for uncomplicated acute viral or bacterial rhinosinusitis.[17] Complicated acute bacterial rhinosinusitis would include concern for soft tissue, orbital or intracranial spread, severe headache, facial swelling, cranial nerve palsies, malignancy, recent facial trauma or surgery, or an immunocompromised state. Plain film X-rays are not recommended by the American College of Radiology as they are inaccurate and only have moderate sensitivity and specificity. Appropriate imaging modalities for the paranasal sinuses include computed tomography (CT) of the sinuses. Complicated acute bacterial sinusitis should be assessed using CT sinus with contrast or magnetic resonance (MR) with gadolinium to detect extra-sinus involvement.[17] Dr DelGaudio's article will delve into sinus headaches more thoroughly.

Otologic causes often require CT scans of the temporal bone without contrast which provide details of bony structures such as the ossicles, osseous labyrinth, and skull base. An MRI of the internal auditory canal with and without gadolinium provides information about the membranous labyrinth, nerves, cerebellopontine angle, and brain.[18] In addition to imaging, if a vestibular etiology is suspected, a vestibular workup can be considered. Subsequent articles in the issue address these.

For intracranial processes, if an acute hemorrhage or stroke is suspected then a CT head without contrast is usually the first step obtained in an emergency setting. For other less acute intracranial etiologies, an MRI brain with and without gadolinium provides a vast majority of information needed for primary headaches and some secondary headaches.

Overall, laboratories and imaging can aid in the diagnosis of the etiology of headaches, especially if the symptoms are not adding up, but are not always required. The cost versus benefit of each test and the risk of radiation exposure should always be weighed when obtaining these ancillary studies. As always, if imaging is obtained, it is the provider's responsibility to review the scans themselves.

SUMMARY

There are many etiologies of headaches that providers encounter. As an otolaryngologist, our role can include diagnosing primary headaches, such as vestibular migraines or tension-type headaches, to diagnosing and managing secondary headaches or facial pain attributed to disorders of the cranium, neck, eyes, ears, nose, sinuses, teeth, mouth, or other facial or cervical structures. A complete headache history focusing on timing, frequency, duration, characteristics, associated symptoms, and family history is the most important component of the work up of these patients. The next step is a complete head and neck and neurologic physical examination focused on the ears, nose and paranasal sinuses, oral cavity, and neck. Lastly, additional ancillary studies can be ordered if further information is needed for diagnosis or the symptomatology is not adding up. Categorizing secondary headache etiology by anatomic location and using a systematic approach in evaluating patients with headache as demonstrated by the flow chart can assist in narrowing the differential diagnosis.

CLINICS CARE POINTS

- A comprehensive history and physical is crutial to diferentiate a primary from secondary headache disorder.
- A high index of suspicion should be maintained to identify serious underlying pathology as a cause of headache.

- The role of the otolaryngologist is to identify pathology of the head and neck which can contribute to headache and to provide treatment or appropriate referrals.

DISCLOSURE

Dr S.E. Mowry is a paid consultant for Cochlear Americas and Otomed. Educational consultant for Stryker with travel expenses covered.

REFERENCES

1. Jensen R, Stovner LJ. Epidemiology and comorbidity of headache. Lancet Neurol 2008;7(4):354–61.
2. Saylor D, Steiner TJ. The global burden of headache. Semin Neurol 2018;38(2): 182–90.
3. Rizzoli P, Mullally WJ. Headache. Am J Med 2018;131(1):17–24.
4. Olesen J, Steiner TJ, Bendtsen L, et al. The international classification of headache disorders, 3rd edition (ICHD-3) Abbreviated pocket version. 2018 (2988368):28. Available at: https://www.ihs-headache.org/binary_data/3330_ichd-3-pocket-version.pdf%0Ahttps://www.ihs-headache.org/ichd-guidelines. Accessed October 2, 2021.
5. Kim R, Patel ZM. Sinus headache: differential diagnosis and an evidence-based approach. Otolaryngol Clin North Am 2020;53(5):897–904.
6. Bigal ME, Lipton RB. The differential diagnosis of chronic daily headaches: an algorithm-based approach. J Headache Pain 2007;8(5):263–72.
7. Mehle ME, Schreiber CP. What do we know about rhinogenic headache? Otolaryngol Clin North Am 2014;47(2):255–68.
8. Chandrasekhar SS. Vertiginous headache and its management. Otolaryngol Clin North Am 2014;47(2):333–41.
9. Baraness L, BA. Acute headache. In: StatPearls [internet]. StatPearls Publishing. doi:32119397. Available at: https://www.ncbi.nlm.nih.gov/books/NBK554510/. Accessed September 28, 2021.
10. Tran TM, McClelland CM, Lee MS. Diagnosis and management of trochleodynia, trochleitis, and trochlear headache. Front Neurol 2019;10:1–11.
11. Crystal SC, Robbins MS. Epidemiology of tension-type headache. Curr Pain Headache Rep 2010;14(6):449–54.
12. Feoktistov A, Diamond M. Diagnosing and understanding adult headache. Otolaryngol Clin North Am 2014;47(2):175–85.
13. Baloh RW. Neurotology of migraine. Headache 1997;37(10):615–21.
14. Chiang BC, Vanderpluym J. Diagnosing secondary headaches. Practical Neurology 2020;31–5.
15. Pelzer N, Louter MA, van Zwet EW, et al. Linking migraine frequency with family history of migraine. Cephalalgia 2019;39(2):229–36.
16. Friedman BW, Grosberg BM. Diagnosis and management of the primary headache disorders in the emergency department setting. Emerg Med Clin North Am 2009;27(1):71–87.
17. Rosenfeld RM, Piccirillo JF, Chandrasekhar SS, et al. Clinical practice guideline (update): Adult sinusitis. Otolaryngol Head Neck Surg 2015;152:S1–39.
18. Jackler TK, Ear EI. Computed tomography and magnetic resonance imaging of the inner ear. Otolaryngol Head Neck Surg 1988;99(5):494–504.

The Role of the Otolaryngologist in the Evaluation and Management of "Sinus Headache"

Nathalia Velasquez, MD[a], John M. DelGaudio, MD[b],*

KEYWORDS

- Headache • Sinus headache • Tension-type headache
- Medication overuse headache • Cluster headache • Giant cell arteritis • Migraine

KEY POINTS

- Approximately 50% of the adult population worldwide is affected by a headache disorder.
- Headache is a common presenting symptom in the otolaryngology practice and often presents a diagnostic dilemma.
- Complete history and physical, including nasal endoscopy and imaging, when indicated, are paramount to guide to the correct diagnosis.
- Patients will believe pain or pressure over the sinuses is sinonasal in origin until proven otherwise.
- Working knowledge of common headache diagnostic criteria will facilitate the initial evaluation and guide appropriate treatment of the patient who presents with a headache disorder.

INTRODUCTION

Headache is a common pain condition worldwide and one of the most significant contributors to disability. It is estimated that approximately one-half of the adult population is affected by a headache disorder every year.[1] Despite being a common symptom, it is difficult to evaluate, given its wide range of clinical presentations and etiologies. The International Headache Society (IHS) has published a system of classification and operational diagnostic criteria for headaches based on clinical consensus, including primary headaches, secondary headaches, painful lesions of

[a] Department of Otolaryngology/Head and Neck Surgery, Emory University School of Medicine, 550 Peachtree Street Northeast, 11th Floor, Atlanta, GA, USA; [b] Department of Otolaryngology/Head and Neck Surgery, Emory University School of Medicine, 550 Peachtree Street Northeast, Suite 1135, Atlanta, GA 30308, USA
* Corresponding author.
E-mail address: jdelgau@emory.edu

Otolaryngol Clin N Am 55 (2022) 501–518
https://doi.org/10.1016/j.otc.2022.02.009
0030-6665/22/© 2022 Elsevier Inc. All rights reserved.

oto.theclinics.com

the cranial nerves, and other facial pain disorders (**Box 1**).[2] Primary headaches represent idiopathic pain conditions without underlying disorders, whereas secondary headaches disorders occur when a definitive cause or relevant underlying disease is present. The most common types of primary headaches are tension-type headaches (TTHs), migraines, and cluster headaches (CHs), which affect approximately 40%, 10%, and 1% of the adult population, respectively.[3]

Many of these patients often present to the otolaryngologist with "sinus headache," which is a widely used terminology in the medical field. Patients with pain or pressure in or around the maxillary, ethmoid, or frontal regions as well as mandibular or temporal pain, often blame the sinuses for this pain based on the rationale that if a structure is in direct proximity where the pain or pressure is located, it is likely the cause of the problem.[4] Hence, the crucial role of the otolaryngologist in the diagnostic and therapeutic approach to these patients, which in many cases may represent a diagnostic challenge because of the associated systemic complaints and overlapping symptomatology common to many headache etiologies. Therefore, having a working knowledge of common headache diagnostic criteria and a straightforward algorithm for clinical decision-making will facilitate the initial evaluation and guide appropriate treatment of the patient who presents with a headache disorder.

This review discusses the role of the otolaryngologist in the evaluation and treatment of the patient with a headache disorder, as well as the latest evidence-based diagnostic criteria and treatment for the most common diagnoses that can mimic "sinus headache," including TTH, medication overuse headache (MOH), hemicrania continua (HC), CH, giant cell arteritis (GCA), and migraine. Trigeminal neuralgia and temporomandibular disorder (TMD) are being discussed in other sections of this issue.

PATIENT EVALUATION AND CLINICAL APPROACH

The most critical question in evaluating headache history is to establish whether the headache is of primary or secondary type. Primary headaches are recurrent

---

Box 1
International classification of headache disorders, 3rd ed. (ICHD-3)

Primary headaches
- Migraine
- Tension-type
- Trigeminal autonomic cephalalgias (eg, cluster headache)
- Other primary headache disorders (eg, cold-stimulus headache, primary cough headache)

Secondary headaches
- Headache attributed to any of the following: head or neck trauma, cranial or cervical vascular disorder, nonvascular intracranial disorder, substance use or withdrawal, infection, disturbance of homeostasis, psychiatric disorder
- Headache or facial pain attributed to disorder of the cranium, neck, eyes, ears, nose, sinuses, teeth, mouth, or other facial or cranial structures (eg, acute, chronic or recurring rhinosinusitis, temporomandibular disorder

Painful lesions of the cranial nerves and other facial pain
- Pain attributed to a lesion or disease of the trigeminal nerve, glossopharyngeal nerve, nervus intermedius, and central idiopathic pain.

Data from Headache Classification Committee of the International Headache Society (IHS). The International Classification of Headache Disorders, 3rd edition (ICHD-3). Cephalalgia. 2018;38(1):1-211.

headaches. The new-onset headache should undergo assessment for the secondary causes. In recurrent headaches, the next important question is if the current episode is like prior headaches. If this headache is similar to the previous headaches, a primary headache disorder is the most likely diagnosis. If the present headache is different from the previous headache episodes, an evaluation for the secondary causes is necessary.[4]

Headache is defined in terms of frequency, duration, and severity and in terms of quality, size, and accompanying factors such as photophobia, nausea, or vomiting. Asking about the intensity and pain distribution is helpful because higher pain levels and unilaterality are associated with migraines or CHs. Daily and constant pain is unlikely to be of sinonasal origin.[5] Pressing symmetric pain in the face and temples is indicative of tension-type pain, which is rarely severe and may be associated with "trigger points" located in the neck, shoulders, and head muscles. Palpation of the temporomandibular joints for tenderness on jaw opening and percussion of the teeth may be helpful, as is the examination of cranial nerves, particularly the trigeminal nerve.[6]

The key to finding the correct diagnosis in each individual presenting with headache is to perform a stepwise, comprehensive evaluation of the patient, including an extensive history, thorough head and neck examination (including neurologic examination), nasal endoscopy, and imaging, if indicated. The main goal is to diagnose the true cause of the symptoms and rule out any potential otolaryngologic causes.[7] Therefore, a complete history and nasal endoscopy (preferably witnessed by the patient on a monitor) become essential to demonstrate the presence or absence of purulent nasal discharge, loss of sense of smell, and other features diagnostic of acute and chronic rhinosinusitis that will help to differentiate these conditions. It is also important to consider that the combination of different diagnostic modalities can provide more of the information necessary to elucidate each case.[8]

RHINOGENIC AND SINUS HEADACHE

First published in 1997 and then revised in 2007 and 2015, a Rhinosinusitis Task Force (RTF) established by the American Academy of Otolaryngology–Head and Neck Surgery designated cardinal symptoms for the diagnosis of acute and chronic rhinosinusitis (**Box 2**). Other cardinal symptoms must accompany facial pain or pressure to warrant an acute or chronic rhinosinusitis diagnosis.[9] Likewise, the most recent International Classification of Headache Disorders (ICHD-3) by the IHS also considers headache attributed to acute rhinosinusitis in the category of secondary headaches (**Boxes 3** and **4**), with the stipulation that other signs and/or symptoms of acute or chronic rhinosinusitis are present. Therefore, "sinus headaches" should be understood as pain arising from inflammatory sinonasal conditions, such as rhinosinusitis.[2] In some scenarios, it is important to keep in mind that migraines and TTHs can be erroneously diagnosed as headaches secondary to acute or chronic rhinosinusitis, given the similarity in pain location and, in the case of migraine, because of the commonly accompanying nasal autonomic symptoms.[10]

Falco and colleagues found no correlation between pain severity, location, and radiologic findings of disease, measured with Lund-MacKay score, in patients with either CRS with or without nasal polyposis, demonstrating that facial pain in CRS is not predicted by the radiographic extent of disease. The location and severity of facial pain reported by the patient is not a reliable marker of the anatomic location and severity of sinonasal inflammation.[11] Al Hashel and colleagues evaluated 130 patients between 2010 and 2012 with a diagnosis of migraine headache based on IHS criteria.

Box 2
Cardinal symptoms for acute and chronic rhinosinusitis in adults—Rhinosinusitis Task Force (RTF)

Acute rhinosinusitis
Up to 4 weeks of purulent nasal drainage (anterior, posterior, or both) accompanied by nasal obstruction, facial pain-pressure-fullness, or both:
- Purulent nasal discharge is cloudy or colored, in contrast to the clear secretions that typically accompany viral upper respiratory infection and may be reported by the patient or observed on physical examination.
- Nasal obstruction may be reported by the patient as nasal obstruction, congestion, blockage, or stuffiness, or may be diagnosed by physical examination.
- Facial pain-pressure-fullness may involve the anterior face, periorbital region, or manifest with headache that is localized or diffuse.

Chronic rhinosinusitis
Twelve weeks or longer of 2 or more of the following signs and symptoms:
- Mucopurulent drainage (anterior, posterior, or both).
- Nasal obstruction (congestion).
- Facial pain-pressure-fullness.
- Decreased sense of smell.
AND inflammation is documented by one or more of the following findings:
- Purulent (not clear) mucus or edema in the middle meatus or anterior ethmoid region.
- Polyps in nasal cavity or the middle meatus.
- Radiographic imaging showing inflammation of the paranasal sinuses.

Data from Rosenfeld RM, Piccirillo JF, Chandrasekhar SS, et al. Clinical practice guideline (update): adult sinusitis. *Otolaryngol Head Neck Surg.* 2015;152(2 Suppl): S1-S39.

All patients had a previous diagnosis of sinusitis. One hundred and six of these patients (81.5%) were misdiagnosed as sinusitis, 56% by their primary care physician, and 44% by an otolaryngologist. The misdiagnoses were significantly more common in chronic migraine patients ($P < .0001$). The mean time to correct diagnosis was

---

Box 3
Diagnostic criteria for headache attributed to acute rhinosinusitis (ICHD-3)

Description
Headache caused by acute rhinosinusitis and associated with other symptoms and/or clinical signs of this disorder.

Diagnostic criteria
A. Any headache fulfilling criterion C.
B. Clinical, nasal endoscopic, and/or imaging evidence of acute rhinosinusitis.
C. Evidence of causation demonstrated by at least 2 of the following:
   1. Headache has developed in temporal relation to the onset of rhinosinusitis.
   2. Either or both of the following:
      a. headache has significantly worsened in parallel with worsening of the rhinosinusitis.
      b. headache has significantly improved or resolved in parallel with improvement in or resolution of the rhinosinusitis.
   3. Headache is exacerbated by pressure applied over the paranasal sinuses.
   4. In the case of unilateral rhinosinusitis, headache is localized and ipsilateral to it.
D. Not better accounted for by another ICHD-3 diagnosis.

Data from Headache Classification Committee of the International Headache Society (IHS). The International Classification of Headache Disorders, 3rd edition (ICHD-3). *Cephalalgia.* 2018;38(1):1-211.

Box 4
Diagnostic criteria for headache attributed to chronic rhinosinusitis (ICHD-3)

Description
  Headache caused by a chronic infectious or inflammatory disorder of the paranasal sinuses
  and associated with other symptoms and/or clinical signs of the disorder.

Diagnostic criteria
A. Any headache fulfilling criterion C.
B. Clinical, nasal endoscopic, and/or imaging evidence of current or past infection or other
   inflammatory process within the paranasal sinuses.
C. Evidence of causation demonstrated by at least 2 of the following:
   1. Headache has developed in temporal relation to the onset of chronic rhinosinusitis.
   2. Headache waxes and wanes in parallel with the degree of sinus congestion and other
      symptoms of chronic rhinosinusitis.
   3. Headache is exacerbated by pressure applied over the paranasal sinuses.
   4. In the case of unilateral rhinosinusitis, headache is localized and ipsilateral to it.
D. Not better accounted for by another ICHD-3 diagnosis.

Data from Headache Classification Committee of the International Headache Society (IHS). The
International Classification of Headache Disorders, 3rd edition (ICHD-3). Cephalalgia.
2018;38(1):1-211.

7.7 years overall and 11 years for misdiagnosed patients.[12] Similarly, Cady and Schreiber found that over 80% of patients presenting with "sinus headaches" met IHS criteria for migraines and were successfully treated after making the correct diagnosis.[13,14]

Patients presenting with facial pain should only be diagnosed with a sinus-related headache if they have a good correlation between the anatomic location of pain and findings of obstructive inflammatory disease on a computed tomography (CT) scan. In addition, the clinical characteristics of facial pain should be consistent with sinus disease. This includes consistent and not episodic pain. Pain that lasts for only a few hours or less and recurs at weekly or monthly intervals is not likely sinus-related and is much more likely a primary headache condition. It is frequently challenging to convince patients who have self-diagnosed or physician-diagnosed "sinus-headache" that their sinuses are not the problem, as they have been told for months to years that the cause of their headache is their sinuses, and this has been positively reinforced by the use of medications for sinusitis, such as antibiotics and topical and systemic steroids and decongestants. Furthermore, the suspicion for other causes of facial pain should be sought in cases where the pain is out of proportion to the degree of disease; the location does not correlate with the site of the disease, pain is brought on by weather changes, allergy, temperature changes, sleep disturbance, foods or stress, and more importantly when the sinuses are normal on a CT scan.[15]

Recently, contact point headache has been the subject of controversy regarding both its pathogenesis and treatment. It is thought to be secondary to mucosal contact points in the sinonasal cavity, in the absence of inflammatory signs, hyperplastic mucosa, purulent discharge, sinonasal polyps, or masses. It may result from pressure on the nasal mucosa due to anatomic variations, among which the septal deviation, septal spur, and concha bullosa are the most commonly observed.[16] It is unclear if this subset is a significant contributor to the pathogenesis of rhinogenic pain or "sinus headache."

In a retrospective study of approximately 900 patients, Abu-Bakra and Jones evaluated the correlation between headache and nasal mucosal contact points, identifying that the percentage of mucosal contact was the same in patients who experienced a headache and those who did not, suggesting this correlation might be purely coincidental.[17] In a 10-year longitudinal study by Welge-Leussen and colleagues. including patients with refractory cluster or migraine headache and nasal contact points treated surgically, 30% remained pain-free, 35% had significant improvement, and 35% received no benefit from surgery. Also, some patients with initial improvement had recurrent headaches, possibly indicating that the contact point was a trigger for underlying migraine headaches.[18] Moreover, Wang and colleagues investigated the correlation between nasal anatomic abnormalities and mucosal contact points with respect to headache presentation for 2 years. Mucosal contact was observed in 85.9% of patients with refractory headache, but also in 80.4% of patients without a headache. Of all anatomic abnormalities detected, septal deviation was the most frequent (41.1%), followed by middle turbinate pneumatization or concha bullosa (32.4%). Septal deviation with lateral nasal wall contact was the only significant abnormality ($P < .05$) that was more frequent in the headache group (55.1%) than among patients without a headache (40.2%).[19] Thus, mucosal contact may be an aggravating trigger for subsequent migraine or tension headache diagnoses coupled with pain origination.[20] Furthermore, Benin and colleagues described similar findings in a retrospective study including patients with refractory migraine, evidence of contact points on imaging, and positive response to topical anesthetic to the contact area. After surgical correction, mean headache frequency, headache severity, and headache-related disability were reduced significantly, suggesting that for selected patients with refractory headaches, demonstrable contact points, and positive response after topical anesthesia, a surgical approach toward the triggering factor may be useful.[21]

Often in these studies, complications from surgery are not reported and follow-up is lacking. Despite these shortcomings, there seems to be a select patient population who may possibly benefit from directed nasal surgery. They are those who have contact points, have failed medical therapy directed at primary headache diagnoses by a neurologist, have otherwise normal endoscopy and CT scan, and have improvement in headache symptoms after local application of an anesthetic to the contact point.[7] Even in this patient population, an otolaryngologist should hold a lengthy discussion with respect to risks, benefits, and alternatives, with emphasis on the fact that surgery may not alleviate the facial pain and/or headache.

TENSION-TYPE HEADACHE

TTH is the most common form of primary headache.[12] TTH occurs repetitively and can be categorized into episodic TTH (with frequent and infrequent subtypes) and chronic TTH. The differentiating factor for these is the frequency of headache episodes (**Box 5**).[4] The IHS classified chronic TTH as 15 or more headache days per month in the absence of rhinogenic symptoms or signs (**Box 6**).[2] A Danish epidemiologic study revealed that about 78% of the adult population experiences at least one episode of TTH in their lives. TTH is also more common in women in comparison with men (3:1 ratio) with an average age of presentation between 25 and 30 years.[22]

TTH are recurrent headaches, characterized by bilateral "band-like," mild to moderate dull, tightening (nonpulsatile) headache around the frontal or temporal region, which can extend all the way around to include parietal and occipital regions as well. Owing to the overlap in location of the frontal sinuses, it can be mistaken for frontal sinus disease. It can also be confused with TMD when the pain is predominantly located in the temporal region.[7] These patients may also complain of shoulder or neck muscle pain as well as sleep disturbances. In addition, TTH pain is usually not

Box 5
Classification of tension-type headache (ICHD-3)

Tension-type headache
2.1 Infrequent episodic tension-type headache
    2.1.1 Infrequent episodic tension-type headache associated with pericranial tenderness
    2.1.2 Infrequent episodic tension-type headache not associated with pericranial tenderness
2.2 Frequent episodic tension-type headache
    2.2.1 Frequent episodic tension-type headache associated with pericranial tenderness
    2.2.2 Frequent episodic tension-type headache not associated with pericranial tenderness
2.3 Chronic tension-type headache
    2.3.1 Chronic tension-type headache associated with pericranial tenderness
    2.3.2 Chronic tension-type headache not associated with pericranial tenderness
2.4 Probable tension-type headache
    2.4.1 Probable infrequent episodic tension-type headache
    2.4.2 Probable frequent episodic tension-type headache
    2.4.3 Probable chronic tension-type headache

Data from Headache Classification Committee of the International Headache Society (IHS). The International Classification of Headache Disorders, 3rd edition (ICHD-3). Cephalalgia. 2018;38(1):1-211.

aggravated by physical activity such as walking or climbing stairs. Therefore, these patients can perform their routine activities, unlike patients with migraines, who usually feel debilitated and opt to stay in the quiet, dark rooms. Symptoms of nausea, vomiting, photophobia, or phonophobia are typically absent or are very mild. These features, when present, easily differentiate TTH from migraines.[23] Although the physical examination is usually unremarkable in patients affected by TTH, nasal endoscopy and CT scan if necessary to confirm or rule out pathologies in this region can help distinguish TTH from the other causes of headache.

    The treatment of TTH is complex and involves a wide range of medications including nonsteroidal anti-inflammatory drugs (NSAIDs), acetaminophen, muscle relaxants, and antidepressants. During the acute TTH episode, NSAIDs are the mainstay

Box 6
Diagnostic criteria for chronic tension-type headache (ICHD-3)

Diagnostic criteria
A. Headache occurring on greater than 15 d/mo on average for greater than 3 months (>180 d/y), fulfilling criteria B–D.
B. Lasting hours to days, or unremitting
C. At least 2 of the following 4 characteristics:
    1. Bilateral location.
    2. Pressing or tightening (nonpulsating) quality.
    3. Mild or moderate intensity.
    4. Not aggravated by routine physical activity such as walking or climbing stairs.
D. Both of the following:
    1. No more than one of photophobia, phonophobia, or mild nausea.
    2. Neither moderate or severe nausea nor vomiting.
E. Not better accounted for by another ICHD-3 diagnosis.

Data from Headache Classification Committee of the International Headache Society (IHS). The International Classification of Headache Disorders, 3rd edition (ICHD-3). Cephalalgia. 2018;38(1):1-211.

treatment modality. Recent metanalysis studies suggest that ibuprofen, 400 mg, combined with acetaminophen, 1000 mg, are the best pharmacologic agents for acute treatment of TTH, whereas the use of 500 mg dose of aspirin alone was shown to be equivalent to placebo.[22,24,25] Patients should always be warned about the overuse of over-the-counter medications as it may lead to MOH. In patients with chronic TTH, the goal is to reduce the frequency of episodes with the use of preventive medication. Tricyclic antidepressants, more specifically amitriptyline, have been extensively studied and are the most effective treatment modality for chronic TTH. Several studies have tested and compared different doses of amitriptyline against other antidepressants and placebo, and it has been found that doses up to 75 mg are effective in most patients.[24,26,27] Amitriptyline should be started on a low dose (10 mg to 25 mg per day) and titrated by 10 to 25 mg weekly until the therapeutic effect is achieved, or side effects appear. Significant clinical effects are usually seen by the end of 1 week and should be apparent by 3 to 4 weeks of treatment. Evidence for the efficacy of muscle relaxants in TTH is weak, and there is a risk for habituation.[24] Within the non-pharmacologic treatments physical therapy (relaxation, exercise, and posture improvement programs), cognitive-behavioral counseling and biofeedback have also shown improvement in both acute and chronic TTH.[28]

MEDICATION OVERUSE HEADACHE

MOH is a very complex diagnosis. Chronic forms of headache, such as chronic migraine or chronic TTH, often involve a high and daily intake of combination analgesics and acute headache medications, such as NSAIDs and triptans. Paradoxically, the liberal use of analgesics often results in worsening the chronic headache, which itself is indistinguishable from the original headache and frustratingly refractory to analgesia. MOH, also known as rebound headache, is common and affects 1.5% to 3% of the population.[29] The latest International Classification of Headache Disorders (ICHD-3) describes MOH as a headache that is present on 15 or more days per month developing as a consequence of regular overuse of acute or symptomatic headache medication (**Box 7**).[2]

The diagnosis of MOH is extremely important clinically. Again, the key to full understanding is the clinical history. If a physician takes the time to listen to patients and validate their headaches and pain, the reception to a diagnosis of MOH is different than when patients feel they were not heard. Also, it is only a trusting patient who divulges to a doctor the extent of medication overuse.[7] Clinical features depend on the substance of overuse. For example, patients overusing ergot or analgesics suffer from

---

Box 7
Diagnostic criteria for medication overuse headache (ICHD-3)

Diagnostic criteria
A. Headache occurring on greater than 15 d/mo in a patient with a preexisting headache disorder.
B. Regular overuse for greater than 3 months of one or more drugs that can be taken for acute and/or symptomatic treatment of headache (eg, triptans, NSAIDs, opioids, ergotamines, caffeine, or codeine-containing combined analgesics).
C. Not better accounted for by another ICHD-3 diagnosis.

Data from Headache Classification Committee of the International Headache Society (IHS). The International Classification of Headache Disorders, 3rd edition (ICHD-3). Cephalalgia. 2018;38(1):1-211.

a tension-like daily headache, but those patients who overuse triptans complain of migraine-like daily headaches or an increase in the frequency of migraines.[30] When these types of headaches are easily confused with "sinus headache" otolaryngologists are bound to see many patients in their office who are suffering from MOH.

Treatment of MOH has several components. First, patients need education and counseling to reduce the intake of medication for acute headaches. An explanatory brochure is often all that is necessary to prevent or discontinue medication overuse. Second, some patients benefit from drug withdrawal (discontinuation of the overused medication) with the addition of rescue medication. Drug withdrawal is often easier said than done and most patients get worsening headaches before they get better and should therefore be advised of this fact. Withdrawal regimens are determined by what medications are being used. In the case of simple analgesics (acetaminophen, NSAIDs) and triptans, withdrawal should be abrupt. Opioids, however, must be withdrawn slowly and more carefully, and occasionally in an inpatient setting.[29,30] A recent randomized controlled trial showed that complete withdrawal of painkillers for a minimum of 2 months led to a significant reduction in daily headaches and increased quality of life. Partial withdrawal, for example, limiting painkillers to a maximum of 2 days in a given week, was also beneficial but less so than complete withdrawal.[31] In addition, it is well known that the addition of corticosteroids or NSAIDs during the withdrawal process is not helpful and should not be used as a substitute.[32] Finally, preventive drug therapy and nonmedical prevention, including psychological support, might be necessary for patients at the onset of treatment or in patients who do not respond to the first 2 steps.[30]

HEMICRANIA CONTINUA

HC is frequently misdiagnosed as having a rhinogenic source given its symptoms. It presents clinically with a baseline continuous unilateral headache for months that intermittently exacerbates with associated autonomic features characterized by ipsilateral conjunctival injection, tearing, nasal congestion, rhinorrhea, facial sweating, miosis, ptosis, and/or eyelid edema (**Box 8**). HC is included under the classification of trigeminal autonomic cephalalgias (TACs) in ICHD-3 on the basis that the pain is typically unilateral, as are the cranial autonomic symptoms when present.[2] HC is more prevalent in young adults in their third and fourth decades with a mean age of 30 years and a female predominance.[33] The baseline headache in HC is commonly located in the first division of the trigeminal nerve involving the frontal and periorbital regions and occurs on the same side, with a slight preference for the right side. This baseline headache often has superimposed fluctuating headache exacerbations, which may last for a few minutes to days. These exacerbations are also highly variable, with a frequency ranging from more than 20 attacks daily to one attack in 4 months.[34] Migrainous symptoms (nausea, vomiting, photophobia, and phonophobia) are quite common in patients with HC during exacerbations. In Prakash and Patel's study, the mean prevalence of at least one migrainous symptom was 60% with 56% of patients fulfilling the migraine criteria during the exacerbation phase.[35]

A complete response to indomethacin is one of the pathognomonic features of HC, which in addition to being one of the diagnostic criteria, provides excellent relief to the patient. It is proposed that indomethacin is more effective than other NSAIDs, probably due to the highest central nervous system penetration, central serotonergic effects, and inhibition of nitrous oxide-dependent vasodilation.[34,36] In adults, oral indomethacin should be started at a low dose of 25 mg 3 times a day (with meals) with slow titration up to 225 mg daily depending upon response. Patients usually

---

Box 8
Diagnostic criteria for hemicrania continua (ICHD-3)

Description
  Persistent, unilateral headache, associated with ipsilateral conjunctival injection,
  lacrimation, nasal congestion, rhinorrhea, forehead, and facial sweating, miosis, ptosis and/
  or eyelid edema, and/or with restlessness or agitation.

Diagnostic criteria
A. Unilateral headache fulfilling criteria B–D.
B. Present for greater than 3 months, with exacerbations of moderate or greater intensity.
C. Either or both of the following:
    1. At least one of the following symptoms or signs, ipsilateral to the headache:
        a. Conjunctival injection and/or lacrimation.
        b. Nasal congestion and/or rhinorrhea.
        c. Eyelid edema.
        d. Forehead and facial sweating.
        e. Miosis and/or ptosis.
    2. A sense of restlessness or agitation, or aggravation of the pain by movement.
D. Responds absolutely to therapeutic doses of indomethacin.
E. Not better accounted for by another ICHD-3 diagnosis.

Data from Headache Classification Committee of the International Headache Society (IHS). The
International Classification of Headache Disorders, 3rd edition (ICHD-3). Cephalalgia.
2018;38(1):1-211.

---

respond within 24 hours, but some may take up to a week.[33] It is important to keep the patient at a minimum therapeutic dose to avoid any possible adverse effects, which include nausea, vomiting, heartburn, abdominal discomfort, hypertension, renal failure, and liver failure. Most adverse effects to indomethacin are dose-dependent, and maintaining the lowest possible therapeutic dose is recommended.[37] In patients who develop indomethacin-related side effects, other alternative medications should be considered. Various treatments have been found to be effective in case reports and open-label studies, such as COX-2 inhibitors (celecoxib and rofecoxib), topiramate, melatonin, gabapentin, ibuprofen, piroxicam, naproxen, aspirin, verapamil, and steroids.[38] These drugs are not as effective as indomethacin, but they should be tried before interventional options are considered. Other treatment options include off-label use of botulinum toxin-A, occipital nerve stimulation, sphenopalatine ganglion block, and deep brain stimulation with mixed results.[35]

CLUSTER HEADACHE

CH is the most severe primary headache disorder. Its severity has major effects on the patient's quality of life, and in some cases might lead to suicidal ideation. CH is less common than migraine or TTH, with an estimated overall prevalence of 0.2% in the United States. They occur more frequently in men, with a male/female ratio between 3:1 and 6:1. The age of onset varies, with 70% of patients reporting onset before 30 years of age.[39] CHs are classified as one of the subtypes of TACs and are further subdivided into episodic and chronic forms. By definition, CH is characterized by attacks of severe (10/10) unilateral head pain in the orbital, supraorbital, or temporal region lasting between 15 minutes and 3 hours if untreated. The pain is associated with ipsilateral cranial autonomic symptoms such as conjunctival injection, lacrimation, nasal congestion, rhinorrhea, forehead, and facial sweating, ptosis, meiosis, and eyelid edema. Attacks are usually accompanied by restlessness or agitation and unlike patients with migraines, these patients are unable to hold still or lie down (**Box 9**).

Box 9
Diagnostic criteria for cluster headache (ICHD-3)

Description
  Attacks of severe, strictly unilateral pain, which is orbital, supraorbital, temporal, or in any combination of these sites, lasting 15 to 180 minutes and occurring from once every other day to 8 times a day.

Diagnostic criteria
A. At least 5 attacks fulfilling criteria B–D
B. Severe or very severe unilateral orbital, supraorbital, and/or temporal pain lasting 15 to 180 minutes (when untreated)
C. Either or both of the following:
    1. At least one of the following symptoms or signs, ipsilateral to the headache:
        a. Conjunctival injection and/or lacrimation.
        b. Nasal congestion and/or rhinorrhea.
        c. Eyelid edema.
        d. Forehead and facial sweating.
        e. Miosis and/or ptosis.
    2. A sense of restlessness or agitation.
D. Occurring with a frequency between one every other day and 8 per day.
E. Not better accounted for by another ICHD-3 diagnosis.

Data from Headache Classification Committee of the International Headache Society (IHS). The International Classification of Headache Disorders, 3rd edition (ICHD-3). Cephalalgia. 2018;38(1):1-211.

These headaches may occur every other day up to 8 times a day. They usually occur at approximately the same time of day, most often at night. In most patients, the attacks are episodic or occur in "clusters," with daily attacks for weeks to months, followed by a remission for months to years.[2] Triggers include watching TV, alcohol, hot weather, stress, use of nitroglycerin, and sexual activity.[40]

Like all primary headache syndromes, the diagnosis of CH is made clinically based on the patient's history according to the ICHD-3 consensus criteria. It is important for the otolaryngologist to acknowledge these criteria and have a high degree of suspicion, given the potential pathologies that present with similar symptomatology, such as acute sinusitis, GCA, TTH, trigeminal neuralgia, and migraines.[20]

The management strategies in CH are classified into acute and maintenance treatments. For acute treatment, sumatriptan subcutaneous, zolmitriptan nasal spray, and high flow oxygen remain the treatments with a level A recommendation.[41] At least 66% of patients respond to oxygen therapy and it is effective in less than 10 minutes. Other treatment options with some effectiveness in the acute setting include intranasal lidocaine (with reported 33% response), intramuscular octreotide, and intranasal ergotamine.[40,41] It is important to keep in mind that oral medications of any form are not recommended, as the time of onset is often longer than the headache duration.

For maintenance and transitional prophylactic therapy, the only level A recommended therapy by the American Headache Society for the prevention of CHs is suboccipital steroid injections.[41] Adverse events are mild, including transient injection site pain and low-level headache. However, it requires intervention by a headache specialist or anesthesiologist.[42] On the other hand, Verapamil has been historically regarded as the maintenance prophylactic therapy of choice for CH despite only a Level C recommendation and is the most widely prescribed due to its easy access. It is recommended to do regular ECGs to monitor cardiac function when a patient is using this drug. Other pharmacologic options include lithium, oral steroids, valproic acid, melatonin, and intranasal capsaicin.[40]

GIANT CELL ARTERITIS

GCA is the most common primary systemic vasculitis in adults over 50 years of age, affecting women 3 times more often than men. Of all vasculitis and collagen vascular diseases, GCA is the disease most conspicuously associated with headache, which is due to inflammation of cranial arteries, especially branches of the external carotid artery.[43] The variability in the features of headache attributed to GCA is such that any new-onset, unilateral, persisting headache in a patient over 50 years of age should suggest GCA and lead to the appropriate investigations. It may present with a headache as its only symptom, usually with associated scalp hypersensitivity, amaurosis fugax, and/or jaw claudication, which often leads to misdiagnosis as TMD or sinusitis (**Box 10**).[2] The typical described presentation of a swollen, painful temporal artery pulsating on examination may not always be present; however, an elevated erythrocyte sedimentation rate (ESR) > 50 mm/h, C-reactive protein (CRP) > 20 mg/L, or platelets greater than 300×10^9/L have a decent diagnostic utility for GCA and may prompt the physician to perform a temporal artery biopsy.[44] Owing to the variable location of the arteritis within the vessel (skip lesions), false-negative results can be high, but the biopsy likely is more helpful if it is directed by a duplex study to regions that show a halo sign, demonstrating wall thickening.[45]

GCA is considered a medical emergency with devastating outcomes if not treated promptly and correctly. The major risk is blindness due to anterior ischemic optic neuropathy, which can be prevented by immediate medical treatment. The time interval between visual loss in one eye and in the other is usually less than 1 week. Patients with GCA are also at risk of cerebral ischemic events and dementia.[46] These patients should be evaluated by a rheumatologist, and in cases of visual loss by an ophthalmologist ideally on the same day if possible, and in all cases within 3 days. The goal in GCA management is the reduction of ongoing inflammation and prevention of ischemic organ damage. Reduction of serum acute phase reactants such as ESR and CRP can be used as a marker of successful control of inflammation but does

---

Box 10
Diagnostic criteria for giant cell arteritis (ICHD-3)

Description
   Headache caused by and symptomatic of giant cell arteritis (GCA). Headache may be the sole symptom of GCA, a disease most conspicuously associated with headache. The features of the headache are variable.

Diagnostic criteria
A. Any new headache fulfilling criterion C.
B. GCA has been diagnosed.
C. Evidence of causation demonstrated by at least 2 of the following:
   1. Headache has developed in close temporal relation to other symptoms and/or clinical or biological signs of the onset of GCA or has led to the diagnosis of GCA.
   2. Either or both of the following:
      a. Headache has significantly worsened in parallel with worsening of GCA.
      b. Headache has significantly improved or resolved within 3 days of high-dose steroid treatment.
   3. Headache is associated with scalp tenderness and/or jaw claudication.
D. Not better accounted for by another ICHD-3 diagnosis.

Data from Headache Classification Committee of the International Headache Society (IHS). The International Classification of Headache Disorders, 3rd edition (ICHD-3). Cephalalgia. 2018;38(1):1-211.

not always correlate with relapses.[43] Although there is no consensus on the starting or maintenance dose of corticosteroids, it is universally accepted that when GCA is suspected, high doses of systemic corticosteroids should be started while waiting for biopsy results. In cases where there is current or impending vision loss (eg, transient blurred or double vision in the setting of elevated ESR or CRP), pulsed intravenous methylprednisolone, 1000 mg/d, for 3 days is recommended, followed by a maintenance dose of 1 mg/kg of prednisone or equivalent. In less severe but active cases, a starting dose of 40 to 60 mg oral prednisolone or equivalent is recommended with prolonged taper aiming to reach 20 mg prednisolone once the patient has been in remission for at least 4 weeks.[47,48] In addition, in recent prospective, placebo-controlled studies, the IL-6 receptor antibody inhibitor tocilizumab has been shown to reduce cumulative corticosteroid usage and side effects and should be considered as an add-on drug in patients with refractory or relapsing disease, or in whom a risk factor such as diabetes mellitus increases the risk of corticosteroid-associated complications.[48,49]

MIGRAINE

Migraine is the second most common primary headache disorder (TTH being the first) and a common disabling primary headache disorder. Many epidemiologic studies have documented its high prevalence and socioeconomic and personal impacts. In the Global Burden of Disease Study 2015 (GBD2015), it was ranked the third-highest cause of disability worldwide in both men and women under the age of 50 years.[50] According to the headache classification committee of the IHS, migraine can be divided into 2 major subtypes: migraine with and without aura (**Box 11**). They can be further subdivided into episodic and chronic forms (>15 headache days per month for at least 3 months). There are also complications of migraines such as status migrainosus and a persistent aura without infarction.[2]

Migraine classically presents as unilateral pain located in the temple and/or facial region and frequently is accompanied by nasal autonomic symptoms, such as rhinorrhea, nasal congestion, lacrimation, and eye redness, that can be mistaken as a headache secondary to acute or chronic rhinosinusitis.[51] These patients are frequently incorrectly treated with prescription and/or over-the-counter medications for rhinosinusitis, providing inappropriate reinforcement to the patient that their headaches are sinus related. This history subsequently makes it difficult to convince patients that their headaches are not sinus-related, thus providing a challenge for the rhinologist.

Classic migraine patients often start experiencing pain unilaterally and, as pain progresses, it may either migrate to the opposite side or transform into a bilateral global headache. The pain is most often rated by patients as moderate to severe and disabling, and associated with photophobia, phonophobia, nausea, and vomiting. Most patients need to stop or at least significantly reduce their activity during a severe migraine attack and confine themselves to a dark, quiet room. About 20% of all patients with migraine headaches experience migraine aura with a brief presentation of neurologic symptoms preceding the headache.[52] Patients with these classic migraine presentations are easier to diagnose. Unfortunately, many patients who present to the otolaryngologist with "sinus headache" do not have classic migraine. Many do not have an aura, phonophobia, or photophobia. In these patients, correlating the symptoms to the examination and radiologic workup is very important.

Migraine is a primary headache disorder, so the physical examination, including nasal endoscopy, and laboratory findings are usually unremarkable. Advanced imaging such as MRI or CT scan of the head and neck are expected to be negative as well

---

Box 11
Diagnostic criteria for migraine with and without aura (ICHD-3)

Description
  Recurrent headache disorder manifesting in attacks lasting 4 to 72 hours

Diagnostic criteria with aura
A. At least 2 attacks fulfilling criteria B and C.
B. One or more of the following fully reversible aura symptoms:
   1. Visual.
   2. Sensory.
   3. Speech and/or language.
   4. Motor.
   5. Brainstem.
   6. Retinal.
C. At least 3 of the following 6 characteristics:
   1. At least one aura symptom spreads gradually over greater than 5 minutes.
   2. Two or more aura symptoms occur in succession.
   3. Each individual aura symptom lasts 5 to 60 minutes.
   4. At least one aura symptom is unilateral.
   5. At least one aura symptom is positive.
   6. The aura is accompanied, or followed within 60 minutes, by headache.
D. Not better accounted for by another ICHD-3 diagnosis.

Diagnostic criteria without aura
A. At least 5 attacks fulfilling criteria B–D.
B. Headache attacks lasting 4 to 72 hours (when untreated or unsuccessfully treated).
C. Headache has at least 2 of the following 4 characteristics:
   1. Unilateral location.
   2. Pulsating quality.
   3. Moderate or severe pain intensity.
   4. Aggravation by or causing avoidance of routine physical activity (eg, walking or climbing stairs).
D. During headache at least one of the following:
   1. Nausea and/or vomiting.
   2. Photophobia and phonophobia.
E. Not better accounted for by another ICHD-3 diagnosis.

Data from Headache Classification Committee of the International Headache Society (IHS). The International Classification of Headache Disorders, 3rd edition (ICHD-3). Cephalalgia. 2018;38(1):1-211.

---

and these tools should be used not to diagnose migraine headache but to rule out other disorders such as tumors, infections, rhinosinusitis, trauma, and so forth. In most patients, the sinuses will be clear, confirming that the sinuses are not the cause of the headache. In some patients, there may be the coexistence of migraine and rhinosinusitis. In these patients, attributing the headache to the sinus disease should only occur if the site of the sinus disease on the CT scan correlates with the anatomic location of the pain.

Medical management involves the use of medications, categorized as prophylactic, abortive, or rescue based on the onset scenarios: acute or chronic. Rescue or abortive treatments aim to stop the progression of headaches. These include NSAIDs (usually in mild to moderate attacks without nausea or vomiting), triptans (with or without naproxen for moderate to severe attacks), ergots, antiemetics, and dexamethasone (can reduce the recurrence of early headaches).[53,54] Prophylactic treatments, taken regularly, aim to reduce the frequency of the episodes and to improve responsiveness to rescue therapies with impact on the severity and duration of the attack. These include beta-blockers (metoprolol and propranolol), antidepressants (amitriptyline and venlafaxine), anticonvulsants (valproic acid and topiramate), and calcitonin gene-related peptide antagonists (erenumab, remanezumab, and galcanezumab).[55] Moreover, some studies have reported the use of migraine-targeting medications such as sumatriptan and valproate to empirically diagnose migraine in patients presenting with "sinus headache."[56,57] Based on this, it is reasonable to consider a trial of a triptan medication in patients who present to the otolaryngologist complaining of "sinus headache" with a clear nasal endoscopy and CT scan, and in which the symptoms are not consistent with any specific headache syndrome, while the patient is awaiting an appointment with neurology or headache specialist.

SUMMARY

Patients will continue to present to the otolaryngologist's office with "sinus headaches" as their primary complaint. Otolaryngologists should take particular care in establishing a precise diagnosis. A thorough clinical history, comprehensive head and neck examination, well-performed nasal endoscopy, and imaging as necessary are essential components for effective diagnosis and treatment plan implementation. It is fundamental to acknowledge the criteria for diagnosing the various headache disorders that may disguise themselves as sinonasal complaints. Moreover, this patient population accurately diagnosed and treated will be extremely grateful for someone pointing them in a direction to obtain the relief they truly need.

CLINICS CARE POINTS

- Up to 50% of the adult population is affected by a headache disorder, with a very wide range of clinical presentations and etiologies.

- The International Headache Society (IHS) has published a system of classification and operational diagnostic criteria for headaches based on clinical consensus, including primary headaches, secondary headaches, painful lesions of the cranial nerves, and other facial pain disorders.

- The otolaryngologist has a crucial role in the diagnostic and therapeutic approach to the patients who present with headache given the associated systemic complaints and overlapping symptomatology common to many sinonasal and headache etiologies.

- Underlying sinonasal causes of headache are multiple and include acute and chronic rhinosinusitis, mucoceles and intranasal contact points.

- Correct diagnosis is only achieved after a comprehensive evaluation of the patient, including an extensive history, thorough head and neck examination (including neurologic examination), nasal endoscopy, and imaging, if indicated and having the working understanding of the more common headache syndromes and their diagnostic criteria.

DISCLOSURE

N. Velasquez: No financial disclosures. J.M. DelGaudio: Consultant for Medtronic and ProDex.

REFERENCE

1. Hainer BL, Matheson EM. Approach to acute headache in adults. Am Fam Physician 2013;87(10):682–7.
2. Headache classification committee of the international headache society (IHS) The international classification of headache disorders, 3rd edition. Cephalalgia 2018;38(1):1–211.

3. Stovner Lj, Hagen K, Jensen R, et al. The global burden of headache: a documentation of headache prevalence and disability worldwide. Cephalalgia 2007; 27(3):193–210.

4. Shah N, Hameed S. Muscle contraction tension headache. In: StatPearls. Treasure Island (FL): StatPearls Publishing; 2021.

5. Agius AM, Sama A. Rhinogenic and nonrhinogenic headaches. Curr Opin Otolaryngol Head Neck Surg 2015;23(1):15–20.

6. Kamani T, Jones NS. 12 minute consultation: evidence based management of a patient with facial pain. Clin Otolaryngol 2012;37(3):207–12.

7. Patel ZM, Setzen M, Poetker DM, et al. Evaluation and management of "sinus headache" in the otolaryngology practice. Otolaryngol Clin North Am 2014; 47(2):269–87.

8. Cady RK, Dodick DW, Levine HL, et al. Sinus headache: a neurology, otolaryngology, allergy, and primary care consensus on diagnosis and treatment. Mayo Clin Proc 2005;80(7):908–16.

9. Rosenfeld RM, Piccirillo JF, Chandrasekhar SS, et al. Clinical practice guideline (update): adult sinusitis. Otolaryngol Head Neck Surg 2015;152(2 Suppl):S1–39.

10. Eross E, Dodick D, Eross M. The sinus, allergy and migraine study (SAMS). Headache 2007;47(2):213–24.

11. Falco JJ, Thomas AJ, Quin X, et al. Lack of correlation between patient reported location and severity of facial pain and radiographic burden of disease in chronic rhinosinusitis. Int Forum Allergy Rhinol 2016;6(11):1173–81.

12. Al-Hashel JY, Ahmed SF, Alroughani R, et al. Migraine misdiagnosis as a sinusitis, a delay that can last for many years. J Headache Pain 2013;14(1):97.

13. Cady RK, Schreiber CP. Sinus headache or migraine? Considerations in making a differential diagnosis. Neurology 2002;58(9 Suppl 6):S10–4.

14. Schreiber CP, Hutchinson S, Webster CJ, et al. Prevalence of migraine in patients with a history of self-reported or physician-diagnosed "sinus" headache. Arch Intern Med 2004;164(16):1769–72.

15. DelGaudio JM, Wise SK, Wise JC. Association of radiological evidence of frontal sinus disease with the presence of frontal pain. Am J Rhinol 2005;19(2):167–73.

16. Yi HS, Kwak CY, Kim HI, et al. Rhinogenic headache: standardization of terminologies used for headaches arising from problems in the nose and nasal cavity. J Craniofac Surg 2018;29(8):2206–10.

17. Abu-Bakra M, Jones NS. Prevalence of nasal mucosal contact points in patients with facial pain compared with patients without facial pain. J Laryngol Otol 2001; 115(8):629–32.

18. Welge-Luessen A, Hauser R, Schmid N, et al. Endonasal surgery for contact point headaches: a 10-year longitudinal study. Laryngoscope 2003;113(12):2151–6.

19. Wang J, Yin JS, Peng H. Investigation of diagnosis and surgical treatment of mucosal contact point headache. Ear Nose Throat J 2016;95(6):E39–44.

20. Bernichi JV, Rizzo VL, Villa JF, et al. Rhinogenic and sinus headache - Literature review. Am J Otolaryngol 2021;42(6):103113.

21. Behin F, Behin B, Bigal ME, et al. Surgical treatment of patients with refractory migraine headaches and intranasal contact points. Cephalalgia 2005;25(6): 439–43.

22. Stephens G, Derry S, Moore RA. Paracetamol (acetaminophen) for acute treatment of episodic tension-type headache in adults. Cochrane Database Syst Rev 2016;2016(6):CD011889.

23. Derry S, Wiffen PJ, Moore RA, et al. Ibuprofen for acute treatment of episodic tension-type headache in adults. Cochrane Database Syst Rev 2015;2015(7): CD011474.
24. Chowdhury D. Tension type headache. Ann Indian Acad Neurol 2012;15(Suppl 1):S83–8. https://doi.org/10.4103/0972-2327.100023.
25. Moore RA, Wiffen PJ, Derry S, et al. Non-prescription (OTC) oral analgesics for acute pain - an overview of Cochrane reviews. Cochrane Database Syst Rev 2015;2015(11):CD010794.
26. Pfaffenrath V, Diener HC, Isler H, et al. Efficacy and tolerability of amitriptylinoxide in the treatment of chronic tension-type headache: a multi-centre controlled study. Cephalalgia 1994;14(2):149–55.
27. Bendtsen L, Jensen R, Olesen J. A non-selective (amitriptyline), but not a selective (citalopram), serotonin reuptake inhibitor is effective in the prophylactic treatment of chronic tension-type headache. J Neurol Neurosurg Psychiatry 1996; 61(3):285–90.
28. Steger B, Rylander E. HelpDesk Answers: What treatments best prevent chronic tension headaches? J Fam Pract 2015;64(8):493–501.
29. Wakerley BR. Medication-overuse headache: painkillers are not always the answer. Br J Gen Pract 2020;70(691):58–9.
30. Diener HC, Dodick D, Evers S, et al. Pathophysiology, prevention, and treatment of medication overuse headache. Lancet Neurol 2019;18(9):891–902.
31. Nielsen M, Carlsen LN, Munksgaard SB, et al. Complete withdrawal is the most effective approach to reduce disability in patients with medication-overuse headache: a randomized controlled open-label trial. Cephalalgia 2019;39(7):863–72.
32. de Goffau MJ, Klaver ARE, Willemsen MG, et al. The effectiveness of treatments for patients with medication overuse headache: a systematic review and meta-analysis. J Pain 2017;18(6):615–27.
33. Charlson RW, Robbins MS. Hemicrania continua. Curr Neurol Neurosci Rep 2014; 14(3):436.
34. Prakash S, Adroja B. Hemicrania continua. Ann Indian Acad Neurol 2018; 21(Suppl 1):S23–30.
35. Prakash S, Patel P. Hemicrania continua: clinical review, diagnosis, and management. J Pain Res 2017;10:1493–509.
36. Summ O, Andreou AP, Akerman S, et al. A potential nitrergic mechanism of action for indomethacin, but not of other COX inhibitors: relevance to indomethacin-sensitive headaches. J Headache Pain 2010;11(6):477–83.
37. Prakash S, Husain M, Sureka DS, et al. Is there need to search for alternatives to indomethacin for hemicrania continua? Case reports and a review. J Neurol Sci 2009;277(1–2):187–90.
38. VanderPluym J. Indomethacin-responsive headaches. Curr Neurol Neurosci Rep 2015;15(2):516.
39. Rozen TD, Fishman RS. Cluster headache in the United States of America: demographics, clinical characteristics, triggers, suicidality, and personal burden. Headache 2012;52(1):99–113.
40. Hoffmann J, May A. Diagnosis, pathophysiology, and management of cluster headache. Lancet Neurol 2018;17(1):75–83.
41. Robbins MS, Starling AJ, Pringsheim TM, et al. Treatment of cluster headache: the American headache society evidence-based guidelines. Headache 2016; 56(7):1093–106.
42. Blumenfeld A, Ashkenazi A, Grosberg B, et al. Patterns of use of peripheral nerve blocks and trigger point injections among headache practitioners in the USA:

Results of the American Headache Society Interventional Procedure Survey (AHS-IPS). Headache 2010;50(6):937–42.

43. Dinkin M, Johnson E. One giant step for giant cell arteritis: updates in diagnosis and treatment. Curr Treat Options Neurol 2021;23(2):6.

44. Chan FLY, Lester S, Whittle SL, et al. The utility of ESR, CRP and platelets in the diagnosis of GCA. BMC Rheumatol 2019;3:14.

45. Chrysidis S, Duftner C, Dejaco C, et al. Definitions and reliability assessment of elementary ultrasound lesions in giant cell arteritis: a study from the OMERACT Large Vessel Vasculitis Ultrasound Working Group. RMD Open 2018;4(1): e000598.

46. Garvey TD, Koster MJ, Warrington KJ. My treatment approach to giant cell arteritis. Mayo Clin Proc 2021;96(6):1530–45.

47. Mackie SL, Dejaco C, Appenzeller S, et al. British Society for Rheumatology guideline on diagnosis and treatment of giant cell arteritis. Rheumatology (Oxford) 2020;59(3):e1–23.

48. Hellmich B, Agueda A, Monti S, et al. 2018 Update of the EULAR recommendations for the management of large vessel vasculitis. Ann Rheum Dis 2020;79(1): 19–30.

49. Stone JH, Tuckwell K, Dimonaco S, et al. Trial of tocilizumab in giant-cell arteritis. N Engl J Med 2017;377(4):317–28.

50. Steiner TJ, Stovner LJ, Vos T. GBD 2015: migraine is the third cause of disability in under 50s. J Headache Pain 2016;17(1):104.

51. Feoktistov A, Diamond M. Diagnosing and understanding adult headache. Otolaryngol Clin North Am 2014;47(2):175–85.

52. Becker WJ. Acute MIGRAINE TREATMENT IN Adults. Headache 2015;55(6): 778–93.

53. Hsu YC, Lin KC. Taiwan headache society TGSOTHS. Medical treatment guidelines for acute migraine attacks. Acta Neurol Taiwan 2017;26(2):78–96.

54. Tfelt-Hansen PC. Evidence-based guideline update: pharmacologic treatment for episodic migraine prevention in adults: report of the Quality Standards subcommittee of the American Academy of Neurology and the American Headache Society. Neurology 2013;80(9):869–70.

55. Kari E, DelGaudio JM. Treatment of sinus headache as migraine: the diagnostic utility of triptans. Laryngoscope 2008;118(12):2235–9.

56. Ishkanian G, Blumenthal H, Webster CJ, et al. Efficacy of sumatriptan tablets in migraineurs self-described or physician-diagnosed as having sinus headache: a randomized, double-blind, placebo-controlled study. Clin Ther 2007;29(1): 99–109.

57. Maurya A, Qureshi S, Jadia S, et al. Sinus Headache": Diagnosis and Dilemma?? An Analytical and Prospective Study. Indian J Otolaryngol Head Neck Surg 2019; 71(3):367–70.

Novel Devices for Sinus Headache

Amar Miglani, MD[a,b],*, Zachary Soler, MD, MSc[b], Rodney J. Schlosser, MD[b,c]

KEYWORDS

- Sinus headaches • Medical devices • Treatment of sinus headaches
- Acoustic vibration with oscillating expiratory pressure
- Transcutaneous microcurrent electrical neurostimulation

KEY POINTS

- Comprehensive evaluation of sinus headache should include a thorough head and neck examination, including neurologic examination, nasal endoscopy, CT scan, and application of International Headache Society criteria.
- Early studies suggest that microcurrent electrical nerve stimulation and acoustic vibrations with oscillating expiratory pressure are low-risk interventions that may serve as useful adjuncts to conventional pharmacotherapy in the management of sinus headaches that are not caused by sinusitis.
- There is a need for further high-level studies supporting the use of low-risk medical devices for the treatment of sinus headache.

INTRODUCTION
Defining Sinus Headache

Sinus headache is a frequently misused but common presenting chief complaint in otolaryngology practices. It frequently refers to facial pain, pressure, or headache in the sinonasal or facial region and often represents a primary headache disorder.[1,2] Most patients presenting with sinus headaches in the absence of objective sinonasal inflammation fulfill the International Headache Society (IHS) criteria of migraine headache.[3] Other causes of a sinus headache include cluster headaches, hemicrania continua, and tension headaches, but only a minority present with true sinusitis.

[a] Department of Otolaryngology–Head & Neck Surgery, Mayo Clinic Arizona, Phoenix, AZ, USA; [b] Department of Otolaryngology–Head & Neck Surgery, Medical University of South Carolina, Rutledge Tower,135 Rutledge Avenue, MSC 550, Charleston, SC 29425, USA; [c] Department of Surgery, Ralph H. Johnson VA Medical Center, 109 Bee Street, Charleston, SC 29401, USA
* Corresponding author. Department of Otolaryngology–Head and Neck Surgery, Mayo Clinic Arizona, 5777 East Mayo Boulevard, Phoenix, AZ 85054.
E-mail address: Miglani.amar@mayo.edu

Otolaryngol Clin N Am 55 (2022) 519–529
https://doi.org/10.1016/j.otc.2022.02.002
0030-6665/22/Published by Elsevier Inc.

oto.theclinics.com

Diagnostic Challenges

Numerous factors contribute to the diagnostic challenges of sinus headache patients. The first difficulty is the location of pain, because many patients with sinusitis and sinus headaches localize pain/pressure to similar locations overlying the frontal, periorbital, and maxillary region. Patients naturally assume pain in these locations is from sinusitis. Additionally, several studies have demonstrated an overlap in symptomatology between sinonasal inflammatory disorders and primary headache disorders, and this is further supported by improved recent understanding of migraine pathophysiology. Acute migraines result from primary neuronal dysfunction in which a cortical-spreading depression, self-propagating depolarizing wave spreads across the cerebral cortex and ultimately activates afferent fibers of the trigeminal nerve. Trigeminal nerve activation results in the release of proinflammatory mediators, such as calcitonin-gene-related peptide and substance P, leading to mucosal inflammation and pain amplification. This pathophysiology explains the concurrence of migraine with rhinogenic symptoms including nasal congestion and rhinorrhea.[4] A 2002 study performed by Barbanti and colleagues[5] examining 177 consecutive patients with migraine found that 46% of patients experienced autonomic symptoms including lacrimation, conjunctival injection, eyelid edema, and nasal congestion. Lastly, primary headache disorders and inflammatory nasal pathologies, such as allergic rhinitis and chronic rhinosinusitis, are all widely prevalent conditions affecting 10% to 40% of the general population; therefore, many patients suffer from multiple diagnoses that confound the clinical presentation.[6] Mehle and Kremer[7] looked at 35 patients with a self-diagnosed sinus headache, assessed with IHS criteria for migraine followed by sinus computed tomography (CT) scan. Although 74% of patients met IHS migraine criteria, 20% of these patients meeting migraine criteria also had significant objective evidence of sinonasal inflammation on CT imaging.

Diagnostic Recommendation

In light of the previously mentioned diagnostic challenges, in 2013 Patel and colleagues[8] published an evidence-based guide to diagnosis and treatment of sinus headache. A key takeaway from this guide was the importance of performing a comprehensive evaluation of the patient presenting with a sinus headache. Evaluation should include a thorough head and neck examination including neurologic examination, nasal endoscopy, CT scan, and application of IHS criteria, all while maintaining a high clinical suspicion of a migraine diagnosis.[8]

Burden of Disease and Challenges with Management

Headache disorders are an almost universal human experience. Migraine is the third most prevalent disorder and the seventh-highest cause of disability worldwide. The direct and indirect socioeconomic costs of headaches are estimated at $14 billion per year. Lifelong headache prevalence is 96% with a female predominance. The global active prevalence of tension-type headache is approximately 40% and migraine is 10% to 20%.[9] Many patients with headache are misdiagnosed with sinusitis leading to chronification of the headache. Al-Hashel and coworkers[10] recruited 130 patients with migraine and discovered that the mean delay to diagnosis was 7.8 years with many patients inappropriately managed for sinusitis medically and surgically. Established barriers to headache therapy include failure to consult the appropriate subspecialty professional, failure to arrive at a specific diagnosis, and lack of appropriate acute and preventative therapy.[11] There are frequently long wait times for patients to see neurologists. Many otolaryngologists are unfamiliar with prescribing neuroactive medications. From a patient's perspective, there is a stigma associated with a diagnosis of headache disorders making it difficult sometimes for patients to accept this reality.[12]

Treatment of Sinus Headache

Embedded in the sinus headache patient population is a large group of patients with primary headache disorders. Therefore, much of the therapeutic investigation aimed at the treatment of sinus headaches has mirrored the more established primary headache literature. Several studies evaluating empiric treatment of patients with sinus headache have demonstrated that most patients improve with triptan therapy.[13,14] Perhaps the best study, published in 2007, is a multicenter (26 centers in the United States) randomized, double-blinded, placebo-controlled investigation of sumatriptan for treatment of sinus headaches.[15] Patients with sinus headache fulfilled IHS criteria for migraine, were without active or recent evidence of sinusitis, and had no prior treatment with migraine medications. A statistically significant benefit over placebo was noted with a single 50-mg dose of sumatriptan. Sixty-nine percent and 76% of patients treated with sumatriptan had a positive headache response compared with a placebo response of 43% and 49% at 2 and 4 hours, respectively.

Medical Devices for Headache and Sinus Headache

Just as efficacy for triptans was first demonstrated and popularized in the primary headache literature before use in sinus headache studies, medical devices are following a similar trend. There are currently four Food and Drug Administration–approved minimally invasive and low-risk neuromodulation/neurostimulation devices on the market for primary headache disorders.[16] These devices have distinct targets: two devices target the brain, one targets the vagus nerve, and one targets the supraorbital nerve. Invasive neurostimulation techniques also exist including occipital nerve stimulation, sphenopalatine ganglion stimulation, and ventral tegmental area deep brain stimulation, but these techniques are reserved for patients with refractory primary headache conditions because of risks associated with the procedure. A recent systematic review with meta-analysis investigating neuromodulation techniques for acute abortive and preventive migraine treatment revealed that limited evidence exists and further high-level studies are needed; however, based on available data, supraorbital transcutaneous electrical nerve stimulation, percutaneous electrical nerve stimulation, and high-frequency repetitive transcranial magnetic stimulation over the primary motor cortex were effective at reducing headache, with small to medium magnitude of effect.[17] Vagus nerve stimulation, left prefrontal cortex, and cathodal transcranial direct current stimulation over the motor cortex had no significant effect on headache and heterogeneity was high. Similar devices have recently been developed for patients with sinus headache.

DISCUSSION

There are currently two medical devices under investigation with potential promise for the treatment of patients with sinus headache: transcutaneous electrical nerve stimulation and acoustic vibrations with oscillating expiratory pressure.[18,19] Furthermore, balloon sinuplasty has been studied in this patient population, although the benefit is questionable based on available evidence.[20] **Table 1** highlights the available evidence supporting use of these medical devices.

Table 1
Medical devices for treatment of sinus headache

Study	Year	Study Design	Level of Evidence	Number of Subjects	Study Groups	Protocol	Pain End Points	Conclusion
Microcurrent stimulation								
Maul et al[22]	2019	Randomized, double-blinded, placebo-controlled trial	2	71	Microcurrent therapy Placebo	Device was repetitively applied by each patient to the bilateral periorbital areas for 5 min	Improvement in VAS (0–10) pain scale	Treatment of rhinologic facial pain using this noninvasive microcurrent device is safe and effective in providing rapid relief of nasal/sinus pain
Goldsobel et al[23]	2019	Single-arm, prospective interventional study	3	30	Microcurrent therapy arm	Self-administered therapy to bilateral periorbital regions for 5 min, 1–4 times daily PRN, for 4 wk	Improvement in VAS (0–10) pain scale	Self-administered periorbital microcurrent treatment given at home is efficacious in reducing sinus pain for up to 6 h and reducing moderate pain and congestion over 4 wk with daily use
Acoustic vibration and oscillating expiratory pressure								
Miglani et al (unpublished)	2021	Single-arm, prospective interventional study	3	30	Acoustic vibration and oscillating expiratory pressure arm	Twice daily, 3-min treatments, for 4 wk	Improvement in VAS (0–10) pain scale, Brief Pain Inventory, and McGill Pain Questionnaire	Significant improvement in pain scores at 2 and 4 wk following treatment

Study	Year	Study type		N	Device/arm	Treatment	Outcome measure	Results
Khanwalker et al	2021	Prospective, nonrandomized, interventional cohort	3	50	Acoustic vibration arm	2 sequential 10-min treatment cycles	Improvement in VAS (0–10) pain scale	Patients with some baseline pain and headache experienced a significant improvement after second treatment
Balloon sinuplasty								
Laury et al[20] 2018	2018	Randomized controlled trial	2	35	Balloon sinus dilation Nasal cavity balloon dilation	Office-based procedure where sinus corresponding to location of pain was dilated (ie, maxillary pain then maxillary sinus dilation performed)	Improvement in SNOT-22, HIT-6, and medication usage were assessed	Both groups experienced statistically significant improvements in SNOT-22 and HIT-6, and reported decreased medication usage No significant difference between groups was observed

Abbreviations: HIT-6, Headache Impact Test-6; SNOT-22, Sinonasal Outcome Test-22; VAS, Visual Analog Scale.

Neuromodulation Using Microcurrent Technology for Relief of Sinus Pain

A. Mechanism of action: Neuromodulation modifies the pain system by manipulating central or peripheral pain pathways using electrical or magnetic impulses to reduce pain levels. Initially, neuromodulation was founded in neurosurgery and focused on more destructive procedures before transitioning to minimally invasive procedures. Several targets for neuromodulation exist and include the hypothalamus/ventral tegmental area, sphenopalatine ganglion, occipital nerve, vagus nerve, supraorbital nerve, and cortex.[16] It has been demonstrated that the application of electrical or magnetic stimulation can modify central neurotransmitters involved in pain pathways.[21]

B. Device use: The recently studied microcurrent device (**Fig. 1**A) for management of sinus headaches administers vibrations and microcurrents to the facial skin in a confided, repetitive "H" pattern above and below the bilateral orbits for 5 minutes. This pattern spans between the bilateral supraorbital and infraorbital nerve regions and across the nasal dorsum (**Fig. 1**B).

C. Efficacy: In 2019, a randomized, placebo-controlled, double-blinded trial of microcurrent technology for the relief of sinus pain was performed. Seventy-one patients with facial pain attributed to self-reported nasal/sinus disease were recruited and received 5-minutes of office-based treatment using an active or placebo microcurrent emitter. Active microcurrent treatment had a statistically significant reduction in mean pain score of 1.66 (on Visual Analog Scale 0–10 scale; 29.6%) compared with sham device score reduction of 0.91 (15.9%).[22] In a follow-up single-arm, prospective interventional study, 30 subjects with moderate facial pain (numeric rating scale >5) were given a microcurrent treatment device and instructions for self-administration to the bilateral periorbital regions for 5 minutes.[23] Subjects were instructed to treat themselves once daily and up to four times daily as needed for 4 weeks. Pain was measured acutely and weekly. Microcurrent therapy rapidly reduced the posttreatment numeric rating scale by 1.2 at 10 minutes, 1.6 at

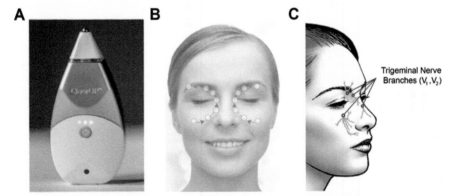

Fig. 1. ClearUP device, which uses microcurrent stimulation with vibration of bilateral supraorbital nerves. (*A*) Image of device. (*B*) Treatment path that subject administers the device. (*C*) Trigeminal nerve fibers that are targeted. (From Goldsobel AB, Prabhakar N, Gurfein BT. Prospective trial examining safety and efficacy of microcurrent stimulation for the treatment of sinus pain and congestion. *Bioelectron Med.* 2019;5(1). https://doi.org/10.1186/s42234-019-0035-x" license under the terms of the Creative Commons Attribution 4.0 International License (http://creativecommons.org/licenses/by/4.0/).)

1 hour, 1.9 at 2 hours, 2.1 at 4 hours, and 2.1 at 6 hours. With daily treatment, a numeric rating scale for pain was reduced by 2.9 (43.3%) after 4 weeks.

D. Risks: Examining the risks and complications of device use, the initial randomized, controlled trial comparing the active device with a sham device found no major complications and one minor complication (transient reddening of the skin stimulated by the device). This minor complication dissipated 15 minutes after use and caused no discomfort or short- or long-term sequelae. In the follow-up prospective, a single-arm study involving 30 subjects, two patients reported transient erythema, one reported headache, and one reported eyelid twitch. All complications were considered minor side effects that resolved without intervention.

E. Satisfaction: In a review of satisfaction ratings, more than 80% of the active treatment arm deemed the device appropriate for treatment and preferred the device over their current treatment regimen. A statistically similar portion of the sham treatment group noted similar satisfaction ratings.

F. Knowledge gaps: To date, a single randomized, placebo-controlled trial exists examining single in-clinic use of the microcurrent device for sinus pain. Additionally, a prospective single-arm study exists researching the daily use of this device. Further high-level randomized controlled trials with longer follow-up are needed.

Acoustic Vibrations with Oscillating Expiratory Pressure

A. Mechanism of action: Much of the mechanism of action of this technology on pain modulation is still unknown. A previous study of acoustic vibrations with oscillating expiratory pressure found significant improvements in objective and subjective metrics of nasal congestion/obstruction suggesting that physiologic changes may occur within the nasal cavity in response to device use. The mechanism by which these changes modulate pain transmission/interpretation in the trigeminal system is still unknown. Prior studies of acoustic energy applied to the nasal cavity have demonstrated increases in nasal nitric oxide levels, which has been shown to possess anti-inflammatory effects.[24] It is also possible that mechanical stimulation of the trigeminal nerve within the sinonasal mucosa downregulates pain while performing nasal breathing against resistance and in the presence of acoustic energy. Ultimately, further research in this space is needed.

B. Device use: There have been two studies investigating the use of acoustic vibrations on nasal congestion and patients noted improvement in secondary symptoms of facial pain and pressure. In a proof-of-concept, single-arm prospective study looking at the use of SinuSonic (SinuSonic, Columbia, SC) technology, which uses acoustic vibrations with oscillating expiratory pressure, subjects used the SinuSonic device for 3 minutes twice daily (unpublished data) **(Fig. 2)**.

C. Efficacy: Twenty-nine patients completed a single-arm 4-week study. Facial pain Visual Analog Scale, brief pain inventory, and McGill Pain Questionnaire demonstrated statistically significant improvements in all pain scores at 4 weeks with approximately 70% of patients achieving a minimal clinically important difference across all metrics.

D. Risks: There were no major complications and only one patient that noted an episode of mild nasal bleeding, which resolved without intervention.

E. Satisfaction: At 4 weeks 86% of subjects stated they would use the device again and recommend the device to others.

F. Knowledge gaps: Further studies are needed. At the present time, data on the use of SinuSonic demonstrate improvement in a single-arm prospective fashion. Further high-level randomized, placebo-controlled clinical trials are needed.

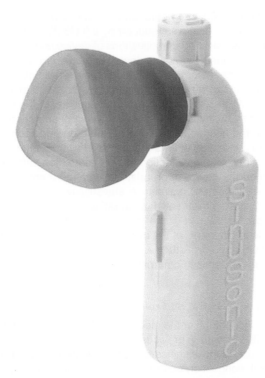

Fig. 2. SinuSonic device, which uses acoustic vibrations with oscillating expiratory pressure. (From Soler ZM, Nguyen SA, Salvador C, et al. A novel device combining acoustic vibration with oscillating expiratory pressure for the treatment of nasal congestion. *Int Forum Allergy Rhinol*. Published online 2020.)

Balloon Sinuplasty

A. Mechanism of action: It is theorized that weather and barometric pressure can trigger sinus headaches. Temperature, pressure, moon phase, pollutants, allergens, and humidity have been implicated in the pathogenesis of sinus headaches but no definitive evidence exists. Given the narrow diameter of sinus ostia, it is hypothesized that even small amounts of inflammation can obstruct the ostia preventing pressure equalization. The proposed mechanism of balloon sinus ostial dilation is widening the narrow sinus ostia to facilitate equalization of pressures across the ostia thus treating sinus headaches.

B. Device use: Balloon sinuplasty is used to dilate the sphenoid sinus ostia, maxillary sinus ostia, and the frontal sinus outflow tract. This is performed under local anesthesia in the clinic or under general anesthesia in an operating room setting.

C. Efficacy: A single prospective, single-blinded randomized, controlled trial at a tertiary care medical center was performed where subjects reported sinus pressure headaches without evidence of mucosal thickening on CT.[25] Subjects were blinded and randomized to undergo balloon dilation of the affected sinus or balloon dilation in the nasal cavity (placebo). Preprocedure and postprocedure Sinonasal Outcome Test-22 scores, Headache Impact Test-6 scores, and medication use was determined at baseline and until 6 months follow-up. The study demonstrated that both arms experienced statistically and clinically significant decreases in

Sinonasal Outcome Test-22 and Headache Impact Test-6 scores from preprocedure to 6 months postprocedure. There were no statistically significant differences between treatment arms. It is unclear why both groups demonstrated a significant improvement. It is possible that medialization of the middle turbinate, which occurred in both groups, could alter airflow patterns resulting in the perceived benefit. Another possibility is a placebo effect in both treatment arms. Lastly, it is possible that simply stimulating the trigeminal nerve system with the use of a balloon intranasally is adequate to modulate the pain pathway regardless of whether the nasal cavity or sinus ostia are stimulated. Further investigation into the use of balloon dilation is warranted.

D. Risks: Risks of balloon sinuplasty are reported to be lower than conventional sinus surgery, but major complications, such as orbital injury, intracranial injury, and skull base injury with cerebrospinal fluid rhinorrhea, have been reported.

E. Satisfaction: Not reported.

F. Knowledge gaps: There is limited evidence supporting the use of balloon sinuplasty for sinus headaches. The currently available study suggests that balloon ostial dilation provides comparable significant improvements when compared with nasal cavity balloon dilation. Further mechanistic studies and studies looking at outcomes are needed.

SUMMARY

Data on the use of medical devices for the treatment of sinus headaches are emerging. Early trends for the treatment of sinus headaches using medical devices are following the more established primary headache literature. Preliminary reports suggest that microcurrent neurostimulation of the supraorbital nerve and acoustic vibration with oscillating expiratory pressure delivered to the nasal cavity may be useful adjuncts for the treatment of sinus headaches, but further high-level studies are needed. Initial reports suggest these interventions are low risk, but longer follow-up is necessary.

CLINICS CARE POINTS

- Sinus headache should be suspected in patients who report facial pain or pressure over the sinonasal region, lack objective evidence of sinonasal inflammation, and fulfill IHS criteria for a migraine headache disorder.

- A comprehensive evaluation should include a thorough head and neck examination, including a neurologic examination, nasal endoscopy, CT scan, and application of IHS criteria.

- Microcurrent neurostimulation of the supraorbital nerve and acoustic vibration with oscillating expiratory pressure seem to be low-risk interventions, but further efficacy data for the treatment of sinus headaches are needed.

- Management of sinus headache should include neurology evaluation, use of appropriate pharmacotherapy (ie, triptans), and optimization of comorbid conditions (ie, allergic rhinitis and chronic sinusitis) if present.

- Microcurrent neurostimulation of the supraorbital nerve or acoustic vibration with oscillating expiratory pressure may be considered as an adjunct for sinus headache treatment.

DISCLOSURE

R.J. Schlosser and Z.M. Soler are consultants for Healthy Humming.

REFERENCES

1. Levine HL, Setzen M, Cady RK, et al. An otolaryngology, neurology, allergy, and primary care consensus on diagnosis and treatment of sinus headache. Otolaryngol - Head Neck Surg 2006. https://doi.org/10.1016/j.otohns.2005.11.024.
2. Cady RK, Dodick DW, Levine HL, et al. Sinus headache: a neurology, otolaryngology, allergy, and primary care consensus on diagnosis and treatment. Mayo Clin Proc 2005;80(7):908–16.
3. Patel ZM, Setzen M, Poetker DM, et al. Evaluation and management of "sinus headache" in the otolaryngology practice. Otolaryngol Clin North Am 2014; 47(2):269–87.
4. Jayawardena ADL, Chandra R. Headaches and facial pain in rhinology. Am J Rhinol Allergy 2018. https://doi.org/10.2500/ajra.2018.32.4501.
5. Barbanti P, Fabbrini G, Pesare M, Vanacore N, Cerbo & R. Unilateral cranial autonomic symptoms in migraine.
6. Lal D, Rounds A, Dodick DW. Comprehensive management of patients presenting to the otolaryngologist for sinus pressure, pain, or headache. Laryngoscope 2015. https://doi.org/10.1002/lary.24926.
7. Mehle ME, Kremer PS. Research submissions sinus CT scan findings in "sinus headache". Migraineurs 2007. https://doi.org/10.1111/j.1526-4610.2007.00811.
8. Patel ZM, Kennedy DW, Setzen M, et al. Sinus headache": rhinogenic headache or migraine? An evidence-based guide to diagnosis and treatment. Int Forum Allergy Rhinol 2013. https://doi.org/10.1002/alr.21095.
9. Rizzoli P, Mullally WJ. Headache. Am J Med 2018;131(1):17–24.
10. Al-Hashel JY, Ahmed SF, Alroughani R, et al. Migraine misdiagnosis as a sinusitis, a delay that can last for many years. 2013. http://www.thejournalofheadacheandpain.com/content/14/1/97.
11. Dodick DW, Loder EW, Manack Adams A, et al. Assessing barriers to chronic migraine consultation, diagnosis, and treatment: results from the Chronic Migraine Epidemiology and Outcomes (CaMEO) study. Headache 2016;56(5): 821–34.
12. Young WB, Park JE, Tian IX, et al. The stigma of migraine. PLoS One 2013;8(1). https://doi.org/10.1371/journal.pone.0054074.
13. Kari E, Delgaudio JM. Treatment of sinus headache as migraine: the diagnostic utility of triptans. Laryngoscope 2008. https://doi.org/10.1097/MLG.0b013e318182f81d.
14. Cady RK, Schreiber CP. Sinus headache or migraine? Neurology 2002;58(9 suppl 6):S10–4.
15. Ishkanian G, Blumenthal H, Webster CJ, et al. Efficacy of sumatriptan tablets in migraineurs self-described or physician-diagnosed as having sinus headache: a randomized, double-blind, placebo-controlled study. Clin Ther 2007;29(1): 99–109.
16. Miller S, Sinclair AJ, Davies B, et al. Neurostimulation in the treatment of primary headaches. Pract Neurol 2016;16(5):362–75.
17. Moisset X, Pereira B, Ciampi de Andrade D, et al. Neuromodulation techniques for acute and preventive migraine treatment: a systematic review and meta-analysis of randomized controlled trials. J Headache Pain 2020;21(1). https://doi.org/10.1186/s10194-020-01204-4.
18. Khanwalkar A, Johnson J, Zhu W, et al. Resonant vibration of the sinonasal cavities for the treatment of nasal congestion. Int Forum Allergy Rhinol 2021;1–4. https://doi.org/10.1002/alr.22877.

19. Soler ZM, Nguyen SA, Salvador C, et al. A novel device combining acoustic vibration with oscillating expiratory pressure for the treatment of nasal congestion. Int Forum Allergy Rhinol 2020. https://doi.org/10.1002/alr.22537.
20. Laury AM, Chen PG, McMains KC. Randomized controlled trial examining the effects of balloon catheter dilation on "sinus pressure"/barometric headaches. Otolaryngol - Head Neck Surg (United States 2018. https://doi.org/10.1177/0194599818772818.
21. Oshinsky ML, Murphy AL, Jr HH, et al. NIH public access. 2015;155(5):1037-1042. doi:.Non-Invasive
22. Maul XA, Borchard NA, Hwang PH, et al. Microcurrent technology for rapid relief of sinus pain: a randomized, placebo-controlled, double-blinded clinical trial. Int Forum Allergy Rhinol 2019;9(4):352–6.
23. Goldsobel AB, Prabhakar N, Gurfein BT. Prospective trial examining safety and efficacy of microcurrent stimulation for the treatment of sinus pain and congestion. Bioelectron Med 2019;5(1). https://doi.org/10.1186/s42234-019-0035-x.
24. Weitzberg E, Lundberg JON. Humming greatly increases nasal nitric oxide. Am J Respir Crit Care Med 2002. https://doi.org/10.1164/rccm.200202-138BC.
25. Alobid I, Benitez P, Pujols L, et al. Severe nasal polyposis and its impact on quality of life. The effect of a short course of oral steroids followed by long-term intranasal steroid treatment. Rhinology 2006.

Vestibular Migraine
Clinical Aspects and Pathophysiology

Pavan Suresh Krishnan, BA[a,b], John Patrick Carey, MD[a,*]

KEYWORDS

- Vestibular migraine • Migraine • Dizziness • Vertigo • Imbalance • Vestibular
- Headache

KEY POINTS

- Vestibular migraine (VM) is the most common cause of episodic vertigo in the US.
- The full mechanism of pathophysiology is thought to mirror that of migraine; however, it has yet to be fully elucidated.
- Symptoms experienced include episodic vertigo along with typical migraine symptoms such as headache, photophobia, phonophobia, sensitivity to motion, and other stimuli.
- Diagnostic criteria rely on patient history as there have not been any clinically useful biomarkers found, to date.
- Treatment success is achievable using a multipronged approach of behavioral change, trigger avoidance, vestibular rehabilitation (VR), and multiple pharmacologic options.

INTRODUCTION

Vestibular migraine (VM), first recognized as a distinct diagnostic entity in 2001 by Neuhauser and colleagues, is a migraine variant characterized by both vestibular and migraine symptoms.[1] Numerous case series established a co-occurrence of vertigo and migraine and described clinical features of patients at this intersection,[1–5] indicating possible similarities in pathophysiology between these phenomena. VM is the most common cause of episodic vertigo, affecting nearly a fourth of patients suffering from dizziness; this number may be an underestimate as only 50% of patients experiencing vertigo are seen in specialty clinics, increasing time to diagnosis and risk of misdiagnosis.[6–8]

It is imperative that otolaryngologists understand the implications of VM as numerous studies have found that vertigo and dizziness are among the strongest

[a] Department of Otolaryngology-Head & Neck Surgery, Johns Hopkins School of Medicine, 601 North Caroline Street, Baltimore, MD 21287, USA; [b] Virginia Commonwealth University School of Medicine, 1201 East Marshall Street, Richmond, VA 23298, USA
* Corresponding author: 601 N Caroline St 6th Floor, Baltimore, MD 21287
E-mail address: jcarey@jhmi.edu
Twitter: @pkrishhh (P.S.K.)

Otolaryngol Clin N Am 55 (2022) 531–547
https://doi.org/10.1016/j.otc.2022.02.003
0030-6665/22/© 2022 Elsevier Inc. All rights reserved.

contributors to disability, decreased work productivity, increased superfluous health care spending, and lower quality of life.[9] What makes VM a difficult diagnosis for most practitioners is the presence of vestibular symptoms in only 50% of headache episodes,[1] symptom-overlap with other vestibular disorders, lack of objective signs and testing, and varied temporal associations of symptoms. It is up to otolaryngologists, as often the primary physicians caring for dizzy patients, to recognize symptoms, explore causes, and adequately manage these, often treatable, symptoms.

BACKGROUND
History

The earliest descriptions of migraine as a syndrome can be dated back to 3000 BC in Mesopotamian poems.[10] However, the link between vertigo and migraine was first fully contemplated in 1873 by English physician Edward Liveing. He contended that individuals with migraine suffered from an unstable nervous system secondary to medullary lesions that irregularly accumulate tension, eventually discharging into a "nerve-storm."[11] The same year, Latham advanced a competing theory focusing on cerebral vessels' constriction dilatation inducing aura and pain, respectively.[12] In 1888, Gowers united rival camps of thought postulating that migraine must primarily be a neurologic abnormality that is secondary to variations in cranial vessel caliber.[13]

About 50 years later, Wolff's experimentation (often on himself) showed that migraine and aura are associated with vasoconstriction and vasodilatation, respectively.[14] In 1941, Lashley published the evolution of his own scintillating scotomas during migraine episodes, proposing that the pathophysiology of migraine is localized to the frontal cortex, initiated by a "wave of strong excitation" followed by inhibition.[15] These inferences were supported by laboratory experiments by Leão (**Fig. 1**), eliciting and recording waves of depression of electrical activity in the cerebral cortex of various animal models.[16] An association between neuronal abnormalities and

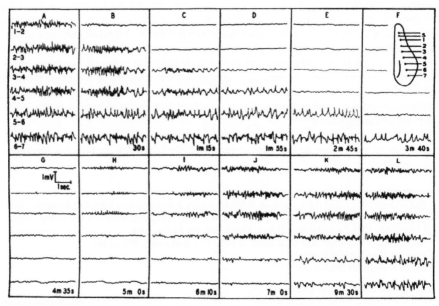

Fig. 1. Leao's spreading depression. (*From* Ref.[16])

corresponding vasomotor changes in cerebral vessels was later corroborated by blood flow imaging studies, positron emission tomography (PET), magnetoencephalography, and functional magnetic resonance imaging.[17]

Through ensuing systematic epidemiologic studies, vestibulocochlear disturbances gained credibility as part of the migraine prodrome and possible migraine equivalent, despite the acknowledged difficulties proving a causal relationship between migraine and its transitory symptoms.[2,3,5] Due to the lack of uniform diagnostic criteria, VM went by many monikers: migraine-associated dizziness, migraine-related dizziness, migraine-related vestibulopathy, migrainous vertigo, and benign recurrent vertigo. Thus, major research advancements and clinical identification of symptoms have been hampered.

In response to a lack of accepted definitions, the Bárány Society, representing the international community of basic scientists, neurologists, and otolaryngologists committed to vestibular research, initiated efforts to classify and define neurotological disorders. In 2009, the Committee for Classification of Vestibular Disorders (ICVD) of the Bárány Society published a consensus definition of VM.[18] The Bárány Society's ICVD subsequently worked in conjunction with the Migraine Classification Subcommittee of the Classification Committee of the IHS, resulting in categories of *Vestibular Migraine* and *Probable Vestibular Migraine*. The final consensus criteria for *Vestibular Migraine* and *Probable Vestibular Migraine* were published in 2012[19] as a joint effort. Only *Vestibular Migraine* criteria were added to the appendix of the International Classification of Headache Disorders (ICHD-3) in 2014,[20,21] citing the need for further validating research.

Definitions

VM was operationally defined in 2001 before becoming established as its own nosologic classification.[1] The current classification includes head-motion induced dizziness with nausea, excluding nonvestibular symptoms such as orthostatic dizziness or panic symptoms. Future classification versions may redefine the criteria to include the many patients experiencing other forms of dizziness.

Due to the lack of pathognomonic physical examination signs and laboratory assessments, the diagnosis of VM relies on the clinical history and the exclusion of another vestibular diagnosis to better account for the presentation. Patients under suspicion for VM must undergo vestibular and neurologic testing to rule out other differential diagnoses[19,20] (**Table 1**).

Epidemiology

Prevalence estimates have ranged from 7% to 16%; however, these were calculated from samples of patients presenting to specialty clinics, not a true sampling of the population.[1,6–8,22] Neuhauser and colleagues found a lifetime prevalence of 0.98% among the adult German population.[8] The most recent population-based cross-sectional study of US adults reported VM as the most common cause of episodic dizziness with a 1-year prevalence of 2.7% (**Fig. 2**). It is important to note that this is most likely an underestimate given lack of proper awareness of this migraine variant at the time, 4 years before consensus criteria were defined. Formeister and colleagues also estimated that about 50% of patients with VM are not being seen in specialty dizzy clinics that would be familiar with this diagnosis.[23] This allows for improper diagnoses and increased time to diagnosis, an issue that is prevalent in the vestibular disorder community.[24–26]

VM has a female preponderance ranging from 75% to 94% of individuals with VM.[8,23] On average, individuals develop symptoms of vertigo 8.4 years after the first

Table 1
Neuhauser vs. Consensus criteria

Neuhauser et al Operational criteria (2001)		Lampert et al Consensus criteria (2012)	
Definite Migrainous Vertigo	**Probable Migrainous Vertigo**	**Vestibular Migraine**	**Probable Vestibular Migraine**
Episodic vestibular symptoms of at least moderate severity (rotational vertigo, other illusory self or object motion, positional vertigo, ie, sensation of imbalance or illusory self or object motion that is provoked by head motion)	Episodic vestibular symptoms of at least moderate severity (rotational vertigo, other illusory self or object motion, positional vertigo, head motion intolerance)	At least 5 episodes with vestibular symptoms of moderate or severe intensity, lasting 5 min to 72 h	At least 5 episodes with vestibular symptoms of moderate or severe intensity, lasting 5 min to 72 h
Migraine according to the IHS criteria	At least one of the following: migraine according to the criteria of the IHS; migrainous symptoms during vertigo; migraine-specific precipitants of vertigo, for example, specific foods, sleep irregularities, hormonal changes; response to antimigraine drugs	Current or previous history of migraine with or without aura according to the International Classification of Headache Disorders (ICHD)	Only one of the criteria B and C for vestibular migraine is fulfilled (migraine history or migraine features during the episode)
At least one of the following migrainous symptoms during at least 2 vertiginous attacks: migrainous headache, photophobia, phonophobia, visual or other auras	Other causes ruled out by appropriate investigations	One or more migraine features with at least 50% of the vestibular episodes: headache with at least 2 of the following characteristics: one-sided location, pulsating quality, moderate or severe pain intensity, aggravation by routine physical activity; photophobia and phonophobia; visual aura	Not better accounted for by another vestibular or ICHD diagnosis
Other causes ruled out by appropriate investigations		Not better accounted for by another vestibular or ICHD diagnosis	

(From:Refs[1,19]).

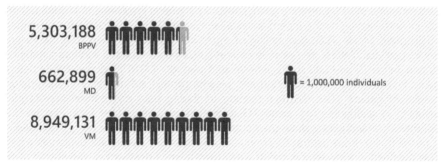

Fig. 2. Number of Cases in 2020 According to 1-year Prevalence Data per US Census Bureau (*Data from* Refs.[23,25,26,53])

onset of migraine[27] and age of onset typically ranges from 37 to 53.2 years.[23] Migraine headaches typically start earlier in life than VM[1,5,6] but then decrease in frequency with age.[28] Often the otolaryngologist will see a patient with VM who considers themselves to no longer have migraine because headaches are either absent or less frequent or severe.

VM can also present in the pediatric population, manifesting as benign paroxysmal vertigo of children. Symptoms of vertigo or disequilibrium coupled with anxiety, nystagmus, and vomiting recur for months to years and eventually give way to migraine in many such individuals.[29]

THEORIES OF PATHOGENESIS

The pathophysiology of VM is not fully known; however, the growing body of knowledge regarding migraine in general points to possible central as well as peripheral mechanisms. In the cerebral cortex, evidence suggests that visual auras are due to cortical spreading depression (CSD), a transient, reversible wave of depolarization triggered by the activation of cortical pyramidal cells.[3,5] Ion channels in the neuronal membranes may have inherent properties that confer not only susceptibility to CSD but also sensory hypersensitivity at baseline. The sensory hypersensitivity and lack of habituation to repetitive stimuli may explain, for example, the sensitivity to visual motion often seen in VM. If CSD arises or spreads to the vestibular cortex or vestibular nuclei, acute vestibular symptoms may arise. However, the vestibular symptoms that would arise from this do not fit the characteristics of aura in terms of duration, nystagmus patterns, and lack of other cerebellar symptoms.[30,31]

Electrophysiologic and neuroimaging studies have determined that multisensory integration occurs at the vestibular thalamus, specifically the ventral posterolateral (VPL) and ventral posteromedial (VPM) nuclei, and the vestibular cortex, specifically the insular, parietal operculum, temporoparietal junction, posterior parietal, cingulate, somatosensory, and frontal cortices. Sensitization at the level of the thalamus in addition to the convergence of sensory modalities at the level of the cortex causes perceptual hypersensitivity common in patients with VM.[30] These areas integrate multiple senses, and their dysfunction may explain the sensitivity to combinations of visual and vestibular stimulation. Thus, VM can be described as central hypersensitization and aberrant sensory integration in terms of vestibulo-thalamic-cortical processing.

The "vascular theory" of migraine held that ischemia was caused by vasospasm, but the duration of symptoms, oculomotor findings, as well as central dysfunction during episodes of VM made vestibulo-cochlear ischemia an unlikely explanation for most presentations of VM. Current evidence favors peripheral involvement through a more complex mediation by the trigeminovascular system (TVS): CSD activates meningeal nociceptors of the TVS, comprising of trigeminal nuclei, ganglion (TG), nerve and meningeal vasculature. The release of vasoactive neuropeptides such as neurokinin A, substance P, and calcitonin gene-related peptide (CGRP) induces sterile neurogenic inflammation: vasodilatation and plasma protein extravasation. Inflammatory mediators induce TG excitation causing throbbing pain and central sensitization resulting in allodynia. The same TG excitation may reach the inner ear via the ophthalmic branch, as well as the cochlear nucleus and superior olivary complex— a possible link from central to peripheral cochlear and vestibular dysfunction.[30,31] This connection was demonstrated when long-latency nystagmus was shown to be induced through trigeminal electrical stimulation in patients with migraine.[32]

Genetic variants predispose individuals to VM by creating functional impairments in ion channels and receptors at various levels of vestibular processing. However, as in other vestibular disorders, genetic contributions to VM are not fully elucidated. Family studies report autosomal dominant inheritance with high penetrance in women. Candidate genes that have been shown to be mutated in other disorders of episodic vertigo such as familial hemiplegic migraine type 1, spinocerebellar ataxia type 6, and episodic ataxia type 2 do not seem to be susceptible loci in VM.[30,31] Other loci have been implicated in VM such as 1p36, 5q35, 11q22 to 23, and 22q12. Family aggregation studies showed a sibling recurrence risk ratio of 4 to 10, suggesting that there is higher familial prevalence of VM than that of the general population. Other genetic association studies have found allelic variants in *HTR6*, *PRG*, and *TRP*.[22] These findings plus clinical heterogeneity indicate that VM is a complex polygenic disease.

SYMPTOMATOLOGY

Patients with VM are typically migraineurs who also experience episodes of true vertigo lasting minutes to days[5] that can be spontaneous, positional, or visual in nature. Positional vertigo, experienced by 40% to 70% of patients with VM, is often experienced if head position is maintained (unlike BPPV).[33] Such patients present with head-motion intolerance, like motion sickness, and even visual-motion intolerance. Vertigo episodes vary in severity, duration, and frequency not only between patients but also in individual patients over time. VM is one of the only vestibular syndromes that can have attacks ranging from a few minutes to days or weeks. Other features which vary include episode recovery time and temporality of association between vertigo and migraine headaches.[1,5,7,33]

In some cases, headache is not reported, and patients may instead suffer from other migraine symptoms such as photophobia or phonophobia[1,4]; in fact, headache-free intervals before vertigo begins can last several years.[33,34] Migraine and dizziness diaries may help patients record precipitants (menstruation, sleep abnormalities, stress, specific foods, and stimuli) and episode features for accurate diagnosis.

Hearing loss and tinnitus have both been reported in patients with VM and may be transient and nonprogressive. However, severe fluctuating HL may indicate concomitant Meniere's disease (MD).[3,35,36]

Patients with VM also experience decreased quality of life,[6] more anxiety, agoraphobia, and distress[37,38] which may contribute to aggravated VM symptoms, creating a positive feedback cycle. The intersection of migraine, vertigo, and anxiety has been explored in several epidemiologic studies and has been termed "Migraine-Anxiety Related Dizziness (MARD)" by Furman and colleagues,[39] who proposed common pathophysiology related to monoaminergic pathways.

VM diagnostic criteria were made rigorous for research purposes; however, in clinical practice, VM should be suspected in any patient with migraine features experiencing vertigo or in any patient experiencing symptom resolution after starting antimigraine medications. Clinical heterogeneity remains a diagnostic challenge when approaching patients with VM; therefore, it is imperative that any connections between vertiginous and migraine symptoms must be interrogated.

EVALUATION

Patients being evaluated for possible VM should have neurologic and neurotologic evaluations to rule out other vestibular syndromes according to the ICVD criteria. Most patients with VM will have normal results on audiometric, caloric, and vestibular evoked myogenic potential testing (VEMP).[40]

During attacks of vertigo in VM, nystagmus has been observed with both central and peripheral features, including sponataneous as well as positional nystagmus. However, in one case series, low velocity, sustained central positional nystagmus occurred in all 26 patients of the VM cohort.[40–42] Severe vertical positional nystagmus has also been reported in patients.[5] When patients were allowed to record their nystagmus occurring at home, spontaneous vertical nystagmus was found to be highly specific for VM, while direction-changing horizontal nystagmus characterized attacks of MD.[41]

There are few testing abnormalities in interictal periods that are specific to VM, which is why diagnostic criteria are based on clinical history. It is important to note that testing discrepancies may be attributed to patients' recency of latest episodes

Table 2 Behavioral modifications for VM	
• Reduce stressors	
• Adhere to a regular sleep schedule	
• Stay hydrated	
• Maintain an active lifestyle and manage weight	
• Avoid sudden changes in barometric pressure	
• Avoid regular analgesic use	
• Avoid fasting	
• Adhere to a migraine diet and avoid:	• Chocolate
	• Alcohol (especially red wine)
	• Aged cheese
	• Monosodium glutamate (found in fast food, soy sauce, yeast, meat tenderizers)
	• Foods high in sodium (ie, processed foods, cured meats)
	• Citrus
	• Caffeine (ie, soda, coffee, energy drinks)

Data from:Refs[54,55].

Table 3
Oral supplements for VM

Agent	Mechanism of Action	Therapeutic Indication	Dose/day; length of time	Adverse Effects	Comments
Magnesium (chelated)	Inhibits NMDA glutamate receptors thereby reducing neuronal hyperexcitability	Prophylaxis; aura and menstrual migraine	400–600 mg; 3–4 mo	Diarrhea, flushing	Reduced headache duration and intensity; Category D in pregnancy
Riboflavin (Vitamin B2)	Rescue mitochondrial energy production	Prophylaxis	400 mg; at least 3 mo	Diarrhea, polyuria	Reduced headache frequency; not recommended for children
Coenzyme Q10 (CoQ10)	Rescue mitochondrial energy production	Prophylaxis	100 mg three times a day; at least 3 mo	Anorexia, dyspepsia, nausea, diarrhea, rash	Reduced headache frequency and nausea

Data from:Refs[55,56].

Table 4
Vestibular suppressants

Agent	Dosage	Sedation	Time to Onset (Mode)	Length of Relief (Mode)	Adverse Effects
Meclizine	12.5–100 mg every 4–6 h	High risk	1 h (oral)	24 h	Blurred vision, sedation, urinary retention, dry mouth
Dimenhydrinate	50 mg every 4–6 h	Low risk	Immediate (IV) 20–30 m (IM) 15–30 m (oral)	3–6 h	See above
Clonazepam	0.25–0.5 mg twice/day	Mild risk	20–60 m (oral)	6–12 h	Respiratory depression, bradycardia, confusion, drug dependency, acute withdrawal syndrome
Diazepam	2–10 mg twice/day	High risk	1–5m (IV) 30 m (oral)	15–60 m (IV) 3–8h (oral)	See above
Lorazepam	0.5 mg twice/day	Mild risk	1–3 m (IV) 15–30 m (IM) 20–30 m (oral)	6–8h (IV/IM) 12–24 h (oral)	See above
Scopolamine	0.5 mg patch every 3 d	Low risk	4h (transdermal)	72 h	Topical allergy, tachyarrhythmia, prostatic enlargement

*Data from:*Refs[55,57].

Table 5
Antiemetics

Agent	Dosage (Mode)	Time to Onset (Mode)	Length of relief (Mode)	Adverse Effects
Diphenhydramine	25–50 mg (oral) every 6–8 h 10–50 mg (IM/IV)	15–30 m (oral) Immediate (IV)	4–8 h (oral) 6–8 h (IM/IV)	Blurred vision, urinary retention, sedation
Dimenhydrinate	50–100 mg every 4–6 h (oral/IM/IV)	15–30 m (oral) 20–30 m (IM) Immediate (IV)	3–6 h	Blurred vision, sedation, urinary retention, dry mouth
Metoclopramide	10 mg (oral) three times/d 10 mg (IM)	30–60 m (oral) 10–15 m (IM) 1–3 m (IV	1–2 h	Extrapyramidal effects, hypotension, QT prolongation, sedation
Ondansetron	4–8 mg (oral) 8 mg (sublingual) 4–16 mg (IV)	30 m (oral)	2 h (oral)	Headache, diarrhea, fever
Prochlorperazine	5–10 mg (oral) every 6–8 h 5–10 mg (IM)	30–40 m (oral) 10–20 m (IM)	3–12 h (oral) 3–4 h (IM)	Sedation, extrapyramidal effects
Promethazine	25 mg (oral) every 6–8 h 12.5 mg (IM) every 6–8 h 25 mg (rectal) every 12 h	20 m (oral) 5 m (IV)	4–12 h (oral)	Sedation, extrapyramidal effects

Data from: Refs[55,57]

Table 6
Migraine prophylaxis

Agent	Dosage	Benefit	Possible Adverse Effects	Comments	Reference
Propranolol	40–240 mg/d	Reduced frequency and severity of vertigo episodes	Fatigue, hypotension, impotence, depression	For patients with hypertension, palpitations, tachycardia, or anxiety symptoms	Salviz, M., Yuce, T., Acar, H., Karatas, A. & Acikalin, R. M. Propranolol and venlafaxine for vestibular migraine prophylaxis: A randomized controlled trial. The Laryngoscope 126, 169–174 (2016).
Verapamil	80–480 mg/d	Reduced frequency and severity of vertigo and headache episodes	Constipation, weight loss, sedation	For patients with seasonal migraine, hypertension, or comorbid MD	Kaya, I. et al. Can verapamil be effective in controlling vertigo and headache attacks in vestibular migraine accompanied with Meniere's disease? A preliminary study. J Neurol 266, 62–64 (2019).
Amitriptyline	25–75 mg/d	Reduced frequency of vertigo episodes	Weight gain, dry mouth, constipation, sedation	For patients with depressive and sleep disturbance symptoms	Görür, K., Gür, H., Ismi, O., Özcan, C. & Vayisoğlu, Y. The effectiveness of propranolol, flunarizine, amitriptyline, and botulinum toxin in vestibular migraine complaints and prophylaxis: a nonrandomized controlled study. Braz J Otorhinolaryngol S1808-8694(21)00,026–4 (2021).

(continued on next page)

Table 6
(continued)

Agent	Dosage	Benefit	Possible Adverse Effects	Comments	Reference
Topiramate	50–100 mg/d	Reduced frequency and severity of vertigo episodes	Paresthesias, fatigue, memory issues	50 and 100 mg dose regimens are similar in efficacy	Gode, S. et al. Clinical assessment of topiramate therapy in patients with migrainous vertigo. Headache 50, 77–84 (2010)..
Lamotrigine	100 mg/d	Reduced frequency of vertigo and headache episodes	Blurred vision, skin rash, ataxia, headache, weight gain	Effective against aura	Bisdorff, A. R. Treatment of migraine-related vertigo with lamotrigine an observational study. Bull Soc Sci Med Grand Duche Luxemb 103–108 (2004).
Acetazolamide	250–500 mg/d	Reduced frequency and severity of vertigo and headache episodes	Paresthesias	High risk for adverse effects	Çelebisoy, N. et al. Acetazolamide in vestibular migraine prophylaxis: a retrospective study. Eur Arch Otorhinolaryngol 273, 2947–2951 (2016).
Venlafaxine	37.5–150 mg/d	Reduced frequency and severity of vertigo episodes	Nausea, insomnia	For patients with comorbid severe depression	Salviz, M., Yuce, T., Acar, H., Karatas, A. & Acikalin, R. M. Propranolol and venlafaxine for vestibular migraine prophylaxis: A randomized controlled trial. Laryngoscope 126, 169–174 (2016).

Drug	Dose	Benefit	Adverse effects	Indication	Reference
Sertraline	25–150 mg/d	Improved dizziness and psychiatric symptoms	Fatigue, sexual adverse effects, dulled mentation	For patients with comorbid psychiatric symptoms	Staab, J. P., Ruckenstein, M. J., Solomon, D. & Shepard, N. T. Serotonin reuptake inhibitors for dizziness with psychiatric symptoms. Arch Otolaryngol Head Neck Surg 128, 554–560 (2002).
Botulinum toxin (Botox)	155 units total	Reduced frequency of vertigo episodes and severity of headache	Minor pain, muscular weakness, skin reaction	For severe headache symptoms	Görür, K., Gür, H., İsmi, O., Özcan, C. & Vayisoğlu, Y. The effectiveness of propranolol, flunarizine, amitriptyline, and botulinum toxin in vestibular migraine complaints and prophylaxis: a nonrandomized controlled study. Braz J Otorhinolaryngol S1808-8694(21)00,026–4 (2021)

and variability in definitions of VM. Additionally, abnormal testing caused by disturbed physiology may dissipate between episodes.

TREATMENT

Given the heterogeneity of presenting symptoms in VM, treatment approaches range from dietary and behavioral modification (**Table 2**), supplements (**Table 3**), acute abortifacients, prophylactic medications, vestibular rehabilitation (VR), and alternative approaches. There are currently no approved, standardized treatment protocols for VM that have been studied systematically. Most treatments are based on the extrapolation of data from trials using antimigraine medications to reduce the frequency and/or severity of migraine headaches.

For the treatment of acute VM episodes that disrupt lifestyle, vestibular suppressants (**Table 4**) and antiemetics (**Tables 5** and **6**) should be considered. Special considerations of comorbidities and potential adverse effects must be made by the physician and patient. Triptans can also be used if the patient commonly suffers from migraine headaches with or without vertigo spells; however, no placebo-controlled trials are conclusive. Case reports in India have shown acute episodes of VM lasting greater than 1 day aborted by intravenous methylprednisolone (1000 mg/d) within 6 hours after oral drugs proved ineffective.[43] Noninvasive vagus nerve stimulation (nVNS) is a novel option for acute treatment. This therapy is thought to induce electrophysiologic change in the trigemino-vestibulo-vagalconnections of the nucleus tractus solitarius (NTS) and dorsal motor vagus nucleus (DMX).[44] Recently, placebo-controlled trial of galcanezumab and ubrogepant, CGRP antagonists were shown to reduce headache days and relieve headache pain in migraine patients within 2 hours, respectively.[45,46] Galcanezumab is currently undergoing the first placebo-controlled trial for the acute treatment of VM.[47]

Prophylactic treatment of VM essentially follows migraine headache prophylaxis guidelines (**Table 6**). Prophylaxis should be considered in patients experiencing attacks significantly affecting activities of daily living despite acute treatment, at least 3 debilitating episodes per month, and contraindication to or failure of acute treatment modalities.[48] The specific agent should be chosen based on comorbid conditions and side effect profile. If episode frequency fails to reduce by 50% after 2 months, then consider replacing agents.[49]

Other nonpharmacologic treatments such as VR are critical adjuncts to management, aiding vestibular compensation through neuroplasticity and anxiety reduction.[50] Regimented yoga routines have shown to improve postural control and enhance cervical VEMP responses, which may be attributed to plastic changes in the sacculocollic pathways of the vestibular system and increased muscular strength.[51] The first randomized controlled trial (RCT) investigating the efficacy of acupuncture in VM prophylaxis compares acupuncture to venlafaxine, a serotonin-norepinephrine reuptake inhibitor for VM prophylaxis, and should be completed in 2023.[52,]

SUMMARY

Though VM is the most common cause of episodic vertigo, consensus diagnostic criteria were only established in 2012, which has helped accelerate research efforts to better understand its pathophysiologic mechanisms and develop treatment strategies. No reliable patterns in imaging or objective testing have been found, so the diagnosis relies on collecting a thorough clinical history. VM pathogenesis has not yet been fully elucidated. However, theories involving CSD, trigeminovascular inflammation, central hypersensitivity via sensory dysregulation, and genetic predisposition have been put forth. Treatment strategies should be based on patient symptoms and migraine guidelines, with novel modalities currently undergoing clinical trials.

CLINICS CARE POINTS

- Recognize that VM is common. Diagnosis is largely based on history.
- Headaches do not have to be present with all spells and may only have been in the past.
- Successful treatment of VM depends on a multimodal approach involving acute and prophylactic pharmacologic agents, dietary trigger avoidance, selective nutrient supplementation, and physical therapy.
- Lifestyle changes including sleep regulation should be initiated.
- Behavioral change should be the first therapeutic measure and requires strict adherence.
- Use acute vestibular suppressants and antiemetics to control symptoms according to patient comorbidities and tolerance.
- Start prophylactic treatment if episodes are not sufficiently controlled.
- Titrate dose until effective; if efficacy is not shown after 2 months, consider a different agent.

DISCLOSURE

This was supported in-part by funding from the American Otological Society (Fellowship Grant, PSK). The authors disclose no conflicts of interest or sponsorships.

REFERENCES

1. Neuhauser H, Leopold M, von Brevern M, et al. The interrelations of migraine, vertigo, and migrainous vertigo. Neurology 2001;56:436–41.
2. Kayan A, Hood JD. Neuro-otological manifestations of migraine. Brain 1984;107:1123–42.
3. Cutrer FM, Baloh RW. Migraine-associated dizziness. Headache 1992;32:300–4.
4. Johnson GD. Medical management of migraine-related dizziness and vertigo. Laryngoscope 1998;108:1–28.
5. Dieterich M, Brandt T. Episodic vertigo related to migraine (90 cases): vestibular migraine? J Neurol 1999;246:883–92.
6. Neuhauser HK, Radtke A, von Brevern M, et al. Migrainous vertigo: prevalence and impact on quality of life. Neurology 2006;67:1028–33.
7. Van Ombergen A, Van Rompaey V, Van de Heyning P, et al. Vestibular migraine in an otolaryngology clinic: prevalence, associated symptoms, and prophylactic medication effectiveness. Otol Neurotol 2015;36:133–8.
8. Neuhauser HK, Radtke A, von Brevern M, et al. Burden of dizziness and vertigo in the community. Arch Intern Med 2008;168:2118.
9. Kovacs E, Wang X, Grill E. Economic burden of vertigo: a systematic review. Health Econ Rev 2019;9:37.
10. Pearce JM. Historical aspects of migraine. J Neurol Neurosurg Psychiatr 1986;49:1097–103.
11. Liveing Edward. On megrim, sick headache, and some allied disorders: a contribution to the pathology of nerve-storms. London: J. & A. Churchill; 1873.
12. Latham P W On. Sick-Headache. Br Med J 1873;1:7–8.

13. Gowers SWR. A manual of diseases of the nervous system. P. Blakiston, Son & Company; 1898.
14. Wolff HG. Headache and other head pain. Headache and other head pain 1948;648.
15. Lashley KS. Patterns of cerebral integration indicated by the scotomas of migraine. Arch Neurpsych 1941;46:331.
16. Leão AAP. Spreading depression of activity in the cerebral cortex. J Neurophysiol 1944;7:359–90.
17. Hadjikhani N, Sanchez del Rio M, Wu O, et al. Mechanisms of migraine aura revealed by functional MRI in human visual cortex. Proc Natl Acad Sci U S A 2001; 98:4687–92.
18. Bisdorff A, Von Brevern M, Lempert T, et al. Classification of vestibular symptoms: Towards an international classification of vestibular disorders. J Vestib Res 2009; 19:1–13.
19. Lempert T, Olesen J, Furman J, et al. Vestibular migraine: diagnostic criteria. J Vestib Res 2012;22:167–72.
20. Headache Classification Committee of the International Headache Society (IHS). The international classification of headache disorders, 3rd edition. Available at: https://www.ichd-3.org/. Accessed September 25, 2021.
21. Lempert T, Neuhauser H. Epidemiology of vertigo, migraine and vestibular migraine. J Neurol 2009;256:333–8.
22. Paz-Tamayo A, Perez-Carpena P, Lopez-Escamez JA. Systematic review of prevalence studies and familial aggregation in vestibular migraine. Front Genet 2020; 11:954.
23. Formeister EJ, Rizk HG, Kohn MA, et al. The epidemiology of vestibular migraine: a population-based survey study. Otol Neurotol 2018;39:1037–44.
24. To-Alemanji J, Ryan C, Schubert MC. Experiences engaging healthcare when dizzy. Otol Neurotol 2016;37:1122–7.
25. von Brevern M, Radtke A, Lezius F, et al. Epidemiology of benign paroxysmal positional vertigo: a population based study. J Neurol Neurosurg Psychiatr 2007;78: 710–5.
26. Alexander TH, Harris JP. Current epidemiology of meniere's syndrome. Otolaryngol Clin North Am 2010;43:965–70.
27. Thakar A, Anjaneyulu C, Deka RC. Vertigo syndromes and mechanisms in migraine. J Laryngol Otol 2001;115:782–7.
28. de Rijk P, Resseguier N, Donnet A. Headache characteristics and clinical features of elderly migraine patients. Headache 2018;58:525–33.
29. van de Berg R, Widdershoven J, Bisdorff A, et al. Vestibular migraine and recurrent vertigo of childhood: diagnostic criteria consensus document of the classification committee of vestibular disorders of the bárány society and the international headache society. VES 2021;31:1–9.
30. von Brevern M, Lempert T. Vestibular migraine. Handb Clin Neurol 2016;137:301–16.
31. Huang T-C, Wang S-J, Kheradmand A. Vestibular migraine: an update on current understanding and future directions. Cephalalgia 2020;40:107–21.
32. Marano E, Marcelli V, Di Stasio E, et al. Trigeminal stimulation elicits a peripheral vestibular imbalance in migraine patients. Headache 2005;45:325–31.
33. Furman JM, Marcus DA, Balaban CD. Migrainous vertigo: development of a pathogenetic model and structured diagnostic interview. Curr Opin Neurol 2003; 16:5–13.
34. Park JH, Viirre E. Vestibular migraine may be an important cause of dizziness/vertigo in perimenopausal period. Med Hypotheses 2010;75:409–14.

35. Johnson GD. Medical management of migraine-related dizziness and vertigo. Laryngoscope 1998;108:1–28.
36. Radtke A, von Brevern M, Neuhauser H, et al. Vestibular migraine: long-term follow-up of clinical symptoms and vestibulo-cochlear findings. Neurology 2012;79:1607–14.
37. Kutay Ö, Akdal G, Keskinoğlu P, et al. Vestibular migraine patients are more anxious than migraine patients without vestibular symptoms. J Neurol 2017;264:37–41.
38. Clark MR, Heinberg LJ, Haythornthwaite JA, et al. Psychiatric symptoms and distress differ between patients with postherpetic neuralgia and peripheral vestibular disease. J Psychosom Res 2000;48:51–7.
39. Furman JM, Balaban CD, Jacob RG, et al. Migraine-anxiety related dizziness (MARD): a new disorder? J Neurol Neurosurg Psychiatr 2005;76:1–8.
40. Young AS, Nham B, Bradshaw AP, et al. Clinical, oculographic, and vestibular test characteristics of vestibular migraine. Cephalalgia 2021;41:1039–52.
41. Young AS, Lechner C, Bradshaw AP, et al. Capturing acute vertigo: a vestibular event monitor. Neurology 2019;92:e2743–53.
42. Polensek SH, Tusa RJ. Nystagmus during attacks of vestibular migraine: an aid in diagnosis. Audiol Neurootol 2010;15:241–6.
43. Prakash S, Shah ND. Migrainous vertigo responsive to intravenous methylprednisolone: case reports. Headache: The J Head Face Pain 2009;49:1235–9.
44. Beh SC, Friedman DI. Acute vestibular migraine treatment with noninvasive vagus nerve stimulation. Neurology 2019;93:e1715–9.
45. Dodick DW, Lipton RB, Ailani J, et al. Ubrogepant for the treatment of migraine. N Engl J Med 2019;381:2230–41.
46. Stauffer VL, Dodick DW, Zhang Q, et al. Evaluation of galcanezumab for the prevention of episodic migraine: The EVOLVE-1 randomized clinical trial. JAMA Neurol 2018;75:1080–8.
47. University of California, San Francisco. A pilot trial of galcanezumab for vestibular migraine 2020. Available at. https://clinicaltrials.gov/ct2/show/NCT04417361.
48. Ailani J, Burch RC, Robbins MS, et al. the B. of D. of the A. H. the american headache society consensus statement: update on integrating new migraine treatments into clinical practice. Headache: The J Head Face Pain 2021;61:1021–39.
49. von Brevern M, Lempert T. Vestibular migraine: treatment and prognosis. Semin Neurol 2020;40:83–6.
50. Alghadir AH, Anwer S. Effects of vestibular rehabilitation in the management of a vestibular migraine: a review. Front Neurol 2018;9:440.
51. Shambhu T, Kumar SD, Prabhu P. Effect of practicing yoga on cervical vestibular evoked myogenic potential. Eur Arch Otorhinolaryngol 2017;274:3811–5.
52. Hu T. The efficacy and safety of acupuncture for prophylaxis of vestibular migraine 2020. Available at. https://clinicaltrials.gov/ct2/show/NCT04664088.
53. Bureau, U. C. U.S. Census bureau today delivers state population totals for congressional apportionment. Census.gov. Available at. https://www.census.gov/library/stories/2021/04/2020-census-data-release.html.
54. American Headache Society. Diet and migraine [online image]. Retrieved October 10, 2021 2019. Available at. https://americanheadachesociety.org/wp-content/uploads/2018/05/DietMigraine.pdf.
55. Shen Y, Qi X, Wan T. The treatment of vestibular migraine: a narrative review. Ann Indian Acad Neurol 2020;23:602–7.
56. Tepper SJ. Nutraceutical and other modalities for the treatment of headache. CONTINUUM: Minneap Minn 2015;21:1018.
57. Hain TC, Yacovino D. Pharmacologic treatment of persons with dizziness. Neurol Clin 2005;23:831–53.

Exploring Vestibular Assessment in Patients with Headache and Dizziness

Alaina Bassett, AuD, PhD[a],*, Erik Vanstrum, BA[b]

KEYWORDS

• Vestibular migraine • Dizziness • Vertigo • Migraine • Posttraumatic headache

KEY POINTS

- Due to the prevalence of headache and dizziness as chief complaints, the coincidence of these symptoms is common.
- Most literature evaluating vestibular function in headache patients involves those experiencing persistent dizziness following traumatic brain injury (TBI) and vestibular migraine (VM).
- The pathophysiology underlying both VM and migraine remains poorly understood but is thought to involve central hyperexcitability, sensory dysmodulation, and parallel activation of nociceptive pathways.
- Patients with VM and TBI demonstrate abnormalities in oculomotor assessment, which includes saccades, gaze, smooth pursuit, and optokinetic testing.
- Vestibular evoked myogenic potential studies may play a role in distinguishing VM from other vestibular disorders, including Meniere's disease (MD).

INTRODUCTION

The chief complaints of dizziness and headache each, respectively, generate a broad range of potential diagnoses. The vague nature of these symptoms is such that even when they present coincidently, identifying the underlying diagnosis remains challenging. Quantitative measurements of vestibular function in these patients can provide diagnostic insight.

Dizziness and vertigo are commonly reported features of migraine headaches.[1] The presentation of vestibular symptoms in addition to migraine headache can stem from numerous peripheral and central vestibular disorders. In cases of traumatic brain injury (TBI) and issues of vestibular migraine (VM), persistent dizziness and headache are

[a] Caruso Department of Otolaryngology – Head and Neck Surgery, Keck School of Medicine of the University of Southern California, 1640 Marengo Street, Suite 100, Los Angeles, CA 90033, USA; [b] Keck School of Medicine of the University of Southern California, 1975 Zonal Avenue, Los Angeles, CA 90033, USA
* Corresponding author.
E-mail address: alaina.bassett@med.usc.edu

Otolaryngol Clin N Am 55 (2022) 549–558
https://doi.org/10.1016/j.otc.2022.02.004
0030-6665/22/© 2022 Elsevier Inc. All rights reserved.

oto.theclinics.com

often reported.[2] Vestibular testing provides the medical team with an opportunity to systematically explore the function of the peripheral and central vestibular system with controlled stimuli. While other diagnoses also present with coincident headache and vertigo, including idiopathic intracranial hypertension, vascular accidents, and Meniere's disease (MD), much of the literature on vestibular testing has focused on TBI and VM. The purpose of this article is to offer a review of this literature on TBI and VM that is of particular interest to the vestibular audiologist and otolaryngologist.

Nomenclature and Definition

Vestibular assessment refers to evaluating the peripheral and central vestibular systems through bedside or outpatient testing of quantitative measures. For this article, the peripheral vestibular system is defined as the disorders of cranial nerve VIII and all distal structures.[3] The central vestibular system will refer to the cerebral vestibular pathways (eg, the vestibular nuclei).[3] Vestibular testing includes but is not limited to the completion of videonystagmography (VNG), video head impulse testing (vHIT), and vestibular evoked myogenic potential testing (VEMP). VNG encompasses oculomotor testing, positioning, positional testing, and caloric irrigation (water or air).

The spectrum of TBI can range from sports-related concussions to mild-through severe- TBI. The level of severity regarding the head injury can be quantified using a variety of standardized scales.[4] Following a TBI event, patients most frequently report posttraumatic headaches and dizziness.[5] The identification of an event resulting in TBI guides the suspected posttraumatic headache diagnosis. This differs from VM, which is characterized by transient vestibular symptoms and migraine headaches. Clinical identification of VM is complicated by a significant overlap of symptoms with other vestibular disorders. For this reason, the historical nomenclature and diagnostic criteria for VM can be convoluted. Terms such as migraine-associated dizziness/vertigo and migrainous vertigo have previously been used in the literature.[6] Adoption of the name VM incorporates the primary symptomatology. It is consistent with validated consensus diagnostic criteria put forth by the International Headache Society and the committee for the International Classification of Vestibular Disorders of the Bárány Society.[7] Since its creation in 2012, this diagnostic definition has been used throughout the literature to reduce VM's clinical heterogeneity.

Epidemiology

In a review of 20.6 million adult visits in the ambulatory care setting, the prevalence of dizziness visits was 8.8 per 1000.[8] Dizziness is a leading reported chief complaint seen by primary care physicians.[8,9] Of reported medical visits for dizziness, three-quarters of encounters are linked to unspecified causes.[8] When presenting to primary care, a fraction of patients (16%) receive a diagnosis on the first presentation.[10] The multifactorial expression of dizziness often leads to visits with additional specialists including neurologists, and otolaryngologists.[8]

A recent systematic review estimated the prevalence of VM to be 1% to 3% with notable variation by race/ethnicity in the US: 3.13% in African, 2.64% in European, and 1.07% in Asian descendant populations.[11] Due to the overlap in symptomatology, among other conditions presenting with vertigo or dizziness, there can be a considerable challenge in making a diagnosis.[12] Population analysis suggests that only 10% of those meeting VM diagnostic criteria are told that migraine is the cause of their dizziness.[13] Differential diagnoses that can share symptom presentation with VM include an ischemic event, MD, vestibular neuritis (VN), and Benign Paroxysmal Positional Vertigo (BPPV).[7] Missed diagnosis and misdiagnosis are common occurrences, and estimations of VM as a cause for vestibular disturbance may be severely underappreciated.

It is estimated that 69 million individuals worldwide will sustain a TBI each year.[14] TBI is the leading cause of dizziness in adults under the age of 40.[15] TBI can result in devastating physical and functional injuries, and outcomes can range from complete recovery to death.[5] Centers for Disease Control records indicate that adults over the age of 75 demonstrate the highest rate of TBI-related hospitalization.[16] Unfortunately, trends in TBI-related deaths over the past 18 years suggest that TBI-related suicide deaths surpassed motor vehicle accidents nationwide.[17]

Demographic Risk Factors

While all individuals are at risk for sustaining TBI, certain groups are more likely to develop long-term health problems from their acquired injuries.[18] Racial and ethnic minorities demonstrate an increased risk for sustaining a TBI and poorer health outcomes following the event.[18] Lack of insurance is identified as a contributing factor to the decreased in-patient and out-patient health care utilization.[18]

There are higher rates of VM in female patients with an estimated female: male ratio of 1.5 to 5:1.[6,11,19] Female patients can note worsening symptoms during menopause.[20] Despite the female preponderance, there is no clear relationship between VM and hormonal profile. VM can first arise at any age, though generally between 8 and 50 years with median ages mid-30s to 40s.[21,22]

Migraine commonly presents before the development of vestibular symptoms. In a cohort of 279 patients, migraine preceded vestibular symptoms by ~15 years.[21] Synchronous onset of migraine and vestibular symptoms can also occur, notably earlier in life with more severe symptoms.[20] In a systematic review of VM prevalence, Paz-Tamayo *et al.* show the onset for synchronous migraine and vertigo was 23 ± 10 years, while the onset in patients with an asynchronous presentation was 24 ± 9 years for migraine and 35 ± 12 years for vertigo.[11]

PATHOPHYSIOLOGY

The pathophysiology underlying both VM and migraine continues to be explored.

Central hyperexcitability is a commonly cited mechanism underlying general migraine. Those with VM may require a lower threshold for the activation of vestibular pathways. For instance, perceived thresholds for a coplanar canal and otolith signaling (ie, roll tilt about an earth-horizontal axis) are lower among patients with VM than migraineurs and healthy controls.[23]

Sensory dysmodulation, the principle by which exposure to one stimulus can extend to other sensory stimuli, has also been postulated.[22] Migraine patients develop nystagmus on painful trigeminal stimulation, whereas healthy controls do not.[24] Patients with VM have altered visuospatial processing, both when positionally challenged and in a head-upright position.[22]

To explain both vestibular and migraine symptoms, investigators have proposed parallel activation of vestibular and nociceptive pathways. Basic science experiments demonstrated shared neurotransmitter signaling mechanisms between trigeminal and vestibular ganglia.[25,26] Imaging studies revealed the convergence of these neural pathways on the brainstem and in higher cerebral processing centers, including the thalamus.[27] Functional MRI revealed increased thalamic activation in patients with VM as compared with migraineurs and healthy controls.[28] Further, the degree of thalamic hyperactivity correlates with the frequency of VM attacks. These same brain structures are also noted to be involved in the processing of anxiety, suggesting a possible explanation for the high levels of mental health comorbidities seen in patients with VM.[29]

Dysfunction of the peripheral vestibular system may be implicated in migraine attacks as well. Pain in migraine is attributed to the trigeminovascular-mediated vasodilation of blood vessels, brain and blood components release, and subsequent inflammation of the meninges.[30] The trigeminovascular system also supplies the inner ear, and mouse models suggest that similar extravasation may cause local inflammation and disruption of electrolyte homeostasis of inner ear structures, including the eighth cranial nerve.[25]

These multiple lines of evidence suggest VM is multi-factorial in origin and could include both labyrinthine and neurologic dysfunction.[23] Findings consistent with both origins are demonstrated in obtained audiovestibular assessments.

CLINICAL PRESENTATION

In complex presentations such as VM and TBI, the patient's case history and reported symptoms are pivotal in guiding care. Classification of VM is dependent on the clinical features reported by the patient.[7] Integration of clinical features and comprehensive clinical assessments of the inner ear provide value in guiding treatment decisions. **Box 1** uses the international classification of vestibular disorders consensus document to define vertigo, dizziness, vestibulo-visual, and postural symptoms.[31]

Often patients with central and peripheral system involvement will demonstrate a combination of vestibular symptoms (eg, vertigo and postural symptoms). The diversity of vestibular symptoms reported by patients with VM can lead to confusion in obtaining a diagnosis.[32] Comprehensive case history questions provide an improved classification of vestibular symptoms by determining the type of symptoms (ie, vertigo, dizziness, vestibulo-visual, and postural), triggering events, duration, headache symptoms, and relieving activities.[31,32] Auditory and vestibular symptoms may differ during the ictal and interictal periods of VM and patients in acute stages of TBI.[32,33] Patients may require comparison of multiple vestibular assessments to monitor for changes in case presentation or newly reported vestibular symptoms unrelated to the suspected diagnosis.

Oculomotor Assessment

Examining eye movements by completing an oculomotor test battery allows evaluating the integrity of central and peripheral vestibular systems. Ocular motor assessments include completing saccades testing, gaze testing, smooth pursuit, and optokinetic testing.[28] The presence of eye movements can vary based on the patient's ictal or interictal status. Oculomotor abnormalities have been observed in patients with VM and TBI, yet these symptoms can also be demonstrated in patients who have migraine without dizziness.[2,21,34]

Box 1
Defining characteristics of reported vestibular and balance symptoms[30]

Vertigo
  The sensation of self-motion when no self-motion is occurring or the distortion of self-motion with head movement.

Dizziness
  Sensation of impaired spatial orientation without a false send of motion

Vestibulo-Visual Symptoms
  Visual symptoms resulting from vestibular system involvement or the connection between the visual and vestibular systems

Postural Symptoms
  Balance symptoms related to maintenance of postural stability, occurring only while upright

Positioning and Static Positional Testing

The manipulation of the head's orientation relative to gravity modulates the "neural tone" of the vestibular system.[35] The term "positioning" refers to the orientation that the head must be positioned to elicit symptoms, such as those completed during the diagnostic maneuvers to identify BPPV.[28] BPPV is a common and treatable disorder of the peripheral vestibular system.[36] Reported BPPV rates related to TBI range from 4.3% to 45%.[37–40] In VM, nystagmus characteristics can cause confusion when determining if symptoms are related to mechanical BPPV. Patients will report brief, discrete episodes of vertigo triggered by changes in head position.[41] In VM, nystagmus is often observed but not in relation to a specific canal, and symptoms may be poorly lateralized.[36]

Static positional testing will typically include a sitting, supine, lateral right, and left lateral position with fixation removed.[28,33] Spontaneous nystagmus (eg, patient sitting upright with fixation removed) is reported during both ictal and interictal phases of VM.[33,42] The characteristics of ictal spontaneous nystagmus vary with reported horizontal, vertical, and torsional components.[33] During the interictal phase, the prevalence of spontaneous nystagmus is lower and demonstrates a significantly reduced slow component velocity compared with the ictal presentation.[33,43]

Caloric Irrigation

Completion of caloric irrigation explores the low-frequency response of the VOR. Caloric irrigation with either warm (excitatory) or cool (inhibitory) air or water generates a temperature gradient, which changes the density of the endolymph in the horizontal canal of the irrigated ear. Completing all 4 irrigations allows for the calculation of unilateral weakness (UW%), the difference in caloric response between the right and left ears. Completion of caloric irrigation for patients with VM or TBI demonstrates variable results.[2] Reported caloric weaknesses range from 21% to 63% in patients with sports-related concussions and TBI.[44,45] In cases of VM, 19%-36% of patients demonstrate abnormal caloric responses.[46] Unfortunately, caloric irrigation can be a noxious experience for some patients. Previously reported work by Vitkovic and colleagues indicates that patients with definite migrainous vertigo were four times more likely to experience an emetic response to calorics than any other migraine category.[47]

Video Head Impulse Testing

High frequency vestibular ocular reflex responses (VOR) of all 6 semicircular canals can be evaluated using vHIT testing. Results generate a gain value, which calculates the relationship between eye movement and head movement during the head impulse. Reduced gain, the relationship between eye movement and head movement, and the presentation of saccadic intrusions for high-frequency semicircular canal function can indicate peripheral vestibular system involvement. Abnormal vHIT results have been reported between 11% and 67% in patients with VM.[46,48] For patients with VM, results may be influenced by ictal or interictal symptom presentation.[33] The relationship between horizontal canal vHIT gain and caloric irrigation should be evaluated in cases whereby MD is suspected. Patients with MD may demonstrate vHIT gain values within normal limits and reduced caloric responses for the involved ear.[49]

Vestibular Evoked Myogenic Potential

VEMP testing uses sound to stimulate the peripheral vestibular system, specifically the otolithic organs. Two types of VEMP tests can be completed, cervical and ocular.

Cervical VEMP (cVEMP) explores the sacculo-collic response of ipsilateral sternoclei-domastoid in response to the activation of the saccule. Ocular VEMP (oVEMP) demonstrates the activation of the utricle, and recorded responses can be observed from the ipsilateral or contralateral extraocular muscles. Characteristics explored when evaluating VEMP testing include presence/absence, amplitude, and latency.[50,51] Administrative parameters such as stimuli and adequate muscle contraction can influence the presence of VEMP responses. Age-related changes have also been identified for both oVEMP and cVEMP.[52–54]

VEMP results have recently been discussed to distinguish VM from other otologic conditions, such as MD.[50,51,55] In the initial episodes of MD, diagnosis may be challenging as patients may present with only vestibular symptoms.[7] It is important to note that clinical cases have been documented whereby patients experience trauma and develop posttraumatic MD.[56] Abnormalities of oVEMP and cVEMP responses can present in both MD and VM. Evidence of reduced amplitude and absence of responses is reported unilaterally and bilaterally in patients with MD and VM.[50,51] However, the obtained patterns of reduced or absent response can suggest VM over MD. Saccular dysfunction (cVEMP) is more common in patients with MD than patients with VM.[51,55] Rizk and colleagues report that a present cVEMP in either ear or a present oVEMP in the suspected ear has a 93% chance of ruling out MD.[51] Patients with VM are more likely to demonstrate abnormal oVEMP responses and normal cVEMP responses.[50] Longitudinal evaluation of VEMP thresholds reveals that patients with MD develop a permanent otolithic loss compared with fluctuant loss observed in patients with VM.[55] Completion of longitudinal assessment in addition to monitory VEMP patterns might assist in differentiating between VM and MD.[55]

TREATMENT AND MANAGEMENT

Treatment strategies for VM have been adopted from those of classic migraine.[22] Symptoms are managed with a combination of lifestyle and dietary modification, vestibular rehabilitation (VR), and activities that promote spatial awareness (eg, dancing) and medication.

VR and physical therapy can promote recovery in patients with VM, especially those experiencing dizziness or imbalance between acute episodes.[57] A detailed audiovestibular assessment will assist physical therapists in developing rehabilitative strategies. A recent review of 5 studies investigating the effectiveness of VR shows consistent positive benefits to patients with VM in scores of dizziness/vertigo, activity confidence levels, headache, and measures of anxiety/depression.[58] In one report, VR potentiated benefits in those receiving pharmacologic intervention.[59] Further, a recent meta-analysis of 2 studies (cumulative cohort of n = 48 patients) showed patients experienced decreased frequency of vertigo attacks.[60] However, most experiments do not include control groups and variably include participants with multiple causes of dizziness; thus, the interpretation of these results is mixed, and a more robust evaluation is required to support evidence-based recommendations.[58] It should be noted that no downsides to VR were reported.

SUMMARY

Vestibular laboratory testing allows for the exploration of both the peripheral and central vestibular systems. While such testing is valuable in evaluating patients experiencing headache and concomitant vestibular dysfunction, further research is required to solidify its role in providing reliable diagnoses. The underlying mechanisms underlying vestibular symptoms in those experiencing headaches remain poorly understood; advances in delineating these mechanisms may improve the vestibular audiologist's ability for testing and interpretation.

CONFLICTS OF INTEREST

A. Bassett serves on the Specialty Representative Advisory Committee board for the Association of the Migraine Disorders. No Financial interest.

REFERENCES

1. Calhoun AH, Ford S, Pruitt AP, et al. The Point Prevalence of Dizziness or Vertigo in Migraine – and Factors That Influence Presentation. Headache. J Head Face Pain 2011;51(9):1388–92.
2. Chan TLH, Hale TD, Steenerson KK. Vestibular Lab Testing: Interpreting the Results in the Headache Patient with Dizziness. Curr Neurol Neurosci Rep 2020; 20(6):16.
3. Thompson TL, Amedee R. Vertigo: a review of common peripheral and central vestibular disorders. Ochsner J 2009;9(1):20–6.
4. Malec JF, Brown AW, Leibson CL, et al. The mayo classification system for traumatic brain injury severity. J Neurotrauma 2007;24(9):1417–24.
5. Defrin R. Chronic post-traumatic headache: clinical findings and possible mechanisms. J Man Manipulative Ther 2014;22(1):36–43.
6. Neuhauser H, Leopold M, Brevern M von, et al. The interrelations of migraine, vertigo, and migrainous vertigo. Neurology 2001;56(4):436–41.
7. Lempert T, Olesen J, Furman J, et al. Vestibular migraine: Diagnostic criteria. J Vestib Res 2012;22(4):167–72.
8. Dunlap PM, Khoja SS, Whitney SL, et al. Assessment of Health Care Utilization for Dizziness in Ambulatory Care Settings in the United States. Otol Neurotol 2019; 40(9):e918–24.
9. Sloane PD. Dizziness in primary care. Results from the National Ambulatory Medical Care Survey. J Fam Pract 1989;29(1):33–8.
10. Adams ME, Marmor S. Dizziness Diagnostic Pathways: Factors Impacting Setting, Provider, and Diagnosis at Presentation. Otolaryngol Head Neck Surg 2021. https://doi.org/10.1177/01945998211004245. 01945998211004245.
11. Paz-Tamayo A, Perez-Carpena P, Lopez-Escamez JA. Systematic Review of Prevalence Studies and Familial Aggregation in Vestibular Migraine. Front Genet 2020;11:954.
12. Stevens SM, Rizk HG, Golnik K, et al. Idiopathic intracranial hypertension: Contemporary review and implications for the otolaryngologist. The Laryngoscope 2018;128(1):248–56.
13. Formeister EJ, Rizk HG, Kohn MA, et al. The Epidemiology of Vestibular Migraine: A Population-based Survey Study. Otology & Neurotology 2018;39(8):1037–44.
14. Dewan MC, Rattani A, Gupta S, et al. Estimating the global incidence of traumatic brain injury. J Neurosurg 2019;130(4):1080–97.
15. Chamelian L, Feinstein A. Outcome after mild to moderate traumatic brain injury: The role of dizziness. Arch Phys Med Rehabil 2004;85(10):1662–6.
16. Centers for Disease Control and Prevention. Surveillance Report of Traumatic Brain Injury-related Hospitalizations and Deaths by Age Group, Sex, and Mechanism of Injury—United States, 2016 and 2017. Centers for Disease Control and Prevention, U.S. Department of Health and Human Services. 2021.

17. Daugherty J, Waltzman D, Sarmiento K, et al. Traumatic Brain Injury–Related Deaths by Race/Ethnicity, Sex, Intent, and Mechanism of Injury — United States, 2000–2017. MMWR Morb Mortal Wkly Rep 2019;68(46):1050–6.

18. Gao S, Kumar RG, Wisniewski SR, et al. Disparities in Health Care Utilization of Adults With Traumatic Brain Injuries Are Related to Insurance, Race, and Ethnicity: A Systematic Review. J Head Trauma Rehabil 2018;33(3):E40–50.

19. Feigin VL, Nichols E, Alam T, et al. Global, regional, and national burden of neurological disorders, 1990–2016: a systematic analysis for the Global Burden of Disease Study 2016. The Lancet Neurol 2019;18(5):459–80.

20. Yan M, Guo X, Liu W, et al. Temporal Patterns of Vertigo and Migraine in Vestibular Migraine. Front Neurosci 2020;14:341.

21. Teggi R, Colombo B, Albera R, et al. Clinical Features, Familial History, and Migraine Precursors in Patients With Definite Vestibular Migraine: The VM-Phenotypes Projects. Headache: The J Head Face Pain 2018;58(4):534–44.

22. Huang T-C, Wang S-J, Kheradmand A. Vestibular migraine: An update on current understanding and future directions. Cephalalgia 2020;40(1):107–21.

23. King S, Wang J, Priesol AJ, et al. Central Integration of Canal and Otolith Signals is Abnormal in Vestibular Migraine. Front Neurol 2014;5. https://doi.org/10.3389/fneur.2014.00233.

24. Marano E, Marcelli V, Stasio ED, et al. Trigeminal Stimulation Elicits a Peripheral Vestibular Imbalance in Migraine Patients. Headache: The J Head Face Pain 2005;45(4):325–31.

25. Koo J-W, Balaban C. Serotonin-Induced Plasma Extravasation in the Murine Inner Ear: Possible Mechanism of Migraine-Associated Inner ear Dysfunction. Cephalalgia 2006;26(11):1310–9.

26. Balaban CD. Migraine, vertigo and migrainous vertigo: Links between vestibular and pain mechanisms. J Vestib Res 2011;21(6):315–21.

27. Tedeschi G, Russo A, Conte F, et al. Vestibular migraine pathophysiology: insights from structural and functional neuroimaging. Neurol Sci 2015;36(S1):37–40.

28. Dieterich M, Obermann M, Celebisoy N. Vestibular migraine: the most frequent entity of episodic vertigo. J Neurol 2016;263(S1):82–9.

29. Moskowitz MA. Pathophysiology of Headache—Past and Present. Headache. J Head Face Pain 2007;47(s1):S58–63.

30. Bisdorff A, Von Brevern M, Lempert T, et al. Classification of vestibular symptoms: Towards an international classification of vestibular disorders. J Vestib Res 2009;19(1,2):1–13.

31. Beh SC, Masrour S, Smith SV, et al. The Spectrum of Vestibular Migraine: Clinical Features, Triggers, and Examination Findings. Headache: The J Head Face Pain 2019;59(5):727–40.

32. Young AS, Nham B, Bradshaw AP, et al. Clinical, oculographic, and vestibular test characteristics of vestibular migraine. Cephalalgia 2021;41(10):1039–52.

33. McCaslin DL. Electronystagmography/videonystagmography. Plural Pub; 2013.

34. Radtke A, von Brevern M, Neuhauser H, et al. Vestibular migraine: Long-term follow-up of clinical symptoms and vestibulo-cochlear findings. Neurology 2012;79(15):1607–14.

35. Coats AC. Computer-quantified positional nystagmus in normals. Am J Otol 1993;14(5):314–26.

36. Argaet EC, Bradshaw AP, Welgampola MS. Benign positional vertigo, its diagnosis, treatment and mimics. Clin Neurophysiol Pract 2019;4:97–111.

37. Marcus HJ, Paine H, Sargeant M, et al. Vestibular dysfunction in acute traumatic brain injury. J Neurol 2019;266(10):2430–3.
38. Davies RA, Luxon LM. Dizziness following head injury: a neuro-otological study. J Neurol 1995;242(4):222–30.
39. Alsalaheen BA, Mucha A, Morris LO, et al. Vestibular rehabilitation for dizziness and balance disorders after concussion. J Neurol Phys Ther 2010;34(2):87–93.
40. Calzolari E, Chepisheva M, Smith RM, et al. Vestibular agnosia in traumatic brain injury and its link to imbalance. Brain 2021;144(1):128–43.
41. von Brevern M, Radtke A, Lezius F, et al. Epidemiology of benign paroxysmal positional vertigo: a population based study. J Neurol Neurosurg Psychiatr 2007; 78(7):710–5.
42. Calic Z, Nham B, Taylor RL, et al. Vestibular migraine presenting with acute peripheral vestibulopathy: Clinical, oculographic and vestibular test profiles. Cephalalgia Rep 2020;3. https://doi.org/10.1177/2515816320958175. 251581632095817.
43. ElSherif M, Reda MI, Saadallah H, et al. Video head impulse test (vHIT) in migraine dizziness. J Otology 2018;13(2):65–7.
44. JU Toglia, Rosenberg PE, Ronis ML. Posttraumatic Dizziness: Vestibular, Audiologic, and Medicolegal Aspects. Arch Otolaryngol - Head Neck Surg 1970; 92(5):485–92.
45. Zhou G, Brodsky JR. Objective Vestibular Testing of Children with Dizziness and Balance Complaints Following Sports-Related Concussions. Otolaryngol Head Neck Surg 2015;152(6):1133–9.
46. Liu YF, Dornhoffer JR, Donaldson L, et al. Impact of caloric test asymmetry on response to treatment in vestibular migraine. J Laryngol Otol 2021;135(4):320–6.
47. Vitkovic J, Paine M, Rance G. Neuro-Otological Findings in Patients with Migraine- and Nonmigraine-Related Dizziness. Audiol Neurotol 2008;13(2):113–22.
48. Kang WS, Lee SH, Yang CJ, et al. Vestibular Function Tests for Vestibular Migraine: Clinical Implication of Video Head Impulse and Caloric Tests. Front Neurol 2016;7:166.
49. McCaslin DL, Rivas A, Jacobson GP, et al. The Dissociation of Video Head Impulse Test (vHIT) and Bithermal Caloric Test Results Provide Topological Localization of Vestibular System Impairment in Patients With "Definite" Ménière's Disease. Am J Audiol 2015;24(1):1–10.
50. Makowiec KF, Piker EG, Jacobson GP, et al. Ocular and Cervical Vestibular Evoked Myogenic Potentials in Patients With Vestibular Migraine. Otology & Neurotology 2018;39(7):e561–7.
51. Rizk HG, Liu YF, Strange CC, et al. Predictive Value of Vestibular Evoked Myogenic Potentials in the Diagnosis of Ménière's Disease and Vestibular Migraine. Otology & Neurotology 2020;41(6):828–35.
52. Akin FW, Murnane OD, Tampas JW, et al. The Effect of Age on the Vestibular Evoked Myogenic Potential and Sternocleidomastoid Muscle Tonic Electromyogram Level. Ear & Hearing 2011;32(5):617–22.
53. Su H-C, Huang T-W, Young Y-H, et al. Aging Effect on Vestibular Evoked Myogenic Potential. Otology & Neurotology 2004;25(6):977–80.
54. Piker EG, Jacobson GP, Burkard RF, et al. Effects of age on the tuning of the cVEMP and oVEMP. Ear Hear 2013;34(6):e65–73.
55. Dlugaiczyk J, Lempert T, Lopez-Escamez JA, et al. Recurrent Vestibular Symptoms Not Otherwise Specified: Clinical Characteristics Compared With Vestibular Migraine and Ménière's Disease. Front Neurol 2021;12:674092.

56. Bächinger D, Goosmann MM, Schuknecht B, et al. Clinical Imaging Findings of Vestibular Aqueduct Trauma in a Patient With Posttraumatic Meniere's Syndrome. Front Neurol 2019;10:431.

57. von Brevern M, Lempert T. Vestibular Migraine: Treatment and Prognosis. Semin Neurol 2020;40(01):083–6.

58. Alghadir AH, Anwer S. Effects of Vestibular Rehabilitation in the Management of a Vestibular Migraine: A Review. Front Neurol 2018;9:440.

59. Whitney SL, Wrisley DM, Brown KE, et al. Physical Therapy for Migraine-Related Vestibulopathy and Vestibular Dysfunction With History of Migraine. Laryngoscope 2000;110(9):1528–34.

60. Byun YJ, Levy DA, Nguyen SA, et al. Treatment of Vestibular Migraine: A Systematic Review and Meta-analysis. Laryngoscope 2021;131(1):186–94.

Utility of Neuroimaging in the Management of Chronic and Acute Headache

Alexander Lerner, MD*, Nasim Sheikh-Bahaei, MD, PhD, John L. Go, MD

KEYWORDS

- Headache • Idiopathic intracranial hypertension • Intracranial hypotension
- CSF leak • Sinonasal tumor • Glossopharyngeal neuralgia • Trigeminal neuralgia
- MRI

KEY POINTS

- Imaging is critical in evaluation of atypical headaches where it plays an important role in identifying the cause of the much less common secondary headaches.
- Idiopathic intracranial hypertension (IIH) imaging findings include "empty sella," orbital changes, and dural venous sinus narrowing. Orbital changes in IIH include flattening of the posterior globe, optic nerve head hyperintensity and enhancement, and optic nerve tortuosity.
- Intracranial hypotension (ICH) is frequently caused by CSF leaks. Imaging findings include loss of the CSF spaces, downward displacement of the brain, as well as dural thickening and enhancement.
- Extracranial tumors and lesions that frequently present with headaches include a variety of sinonasal tumors as well as mucoceles.
- Neurovascular compression disorders causing headaches include trigeminal and glossopharyngeal neuralgia. Imaging findings include displacement and atrophy of the cranial nerve caused by an adjacent arterial or venous structure.

Primary headaches such as migraine, cluster headache, and tension headache represent most headache cases where imaging is usually unremarkable. However, imaging is critical in the evaluation of atypical headaches where it plays an important role in identifying the cause of the much less common secondary headaches. Such headaches may be caused by a variety of pathologic conditions which can be categorized as intracranial and extracranial. The MR imaging protocol should be carefully selected to evaluate for the clinically suspected diagnosis.

Keck Medical Center of USCD, Department of Radiology, 1500 San Pablo Street, 2nd Floor, Imaging, Los Angeles, CA 90033, USA
* Corresponding author.
E-mail address: lernera@med.usc.edu

Otolaryngol Clin N Am 55 (2022) 559–577
https://doi.org/10.1016/j.otc.2022.02.010
0030-6665/22/© 2022 Elsevier Inc. All rights reserved.
oto.theclinics.com

Abbreviations	
CSF	Cerebrospinal Fluid
MR	Magnetic Resonance
CT	Computed Tomography
MRI	Magnetic Resonance Imaging
TMJ	Temporomandibular Joint
CTA	Computed Tomography Angiography
IAC	Internal Auditory Canal
MRA	Magnetic Resonance Angiography
FLAIR	Fluid Attenuated Inversion Recovery
STIR	Short Tau Inversion Recovery
DTPA	Diethylenetriaminepentaacetic Acid
HRCT	High Resolution CT
FIESTA	Fast Imaging Employing Steady-state Acquisition
CISS	Constructive Interference in Steady-State
FRFSE	Fast Relaxation Fast Spin Echo
ADC	Apparent Diffusion Coefficient
TOF	Time Of Flight
CNV	Cranial Nerve V

IIH imaging findings include "empty sella," orbital changes, and dural venous sinus narrowing. Care should be taken to distinguish primary empty sella from secondary empty sella and normal variation, which are not associated with IIH. Orbital changes in IIH include flattening of the posterior globe, optic nerve head hyperintensity and enhancement, and optic nerve tortuosity. Unilateral or bilateral stenosis of transverse sinuses has been reported in most patients with IIH, which is best assessed on MR or CT venogram.

Intracranial hypotension is frequently caused by CSF leaks. Imaging findings include loss of the CSF spaces, downward displacement of the brain, as well as dural thickening and enhancement. Severe cases of ICH may result in subdural hematomas.

A variety of intracranial and skull base tumors may cause headaches due to dural involvement. Extracranial tumors and lesions that frequently present with headaches include a variety of sinonasal tumors as well as mucoceles.

Neurovascular compression disorders causing headaches include trigeminal and glossopharyngeal neuralgia. Dedicated high-resolution MR cisternography and MR angiography imaging are necessary to demonstrate vascular compression of cranial nerve V and cranial nerve IX in these disorders. Imaging findings include displacement and atrophy of the cranial nerve caused by an adjacent arterial or venous structure.

INTRODUCTION

Most patients with headache referred for imaging suffer from primary headaches such as migraines, cluster headaches, and tension headaches. CT and MRI imaging of the brain in these patients usually reveals no significant abnormality. Focal T2 hyperintensities in supratentorial white matter may be noted in some patients with migraine.[1,2]

However, imaging of atypical headaches is important to identify the cause of the much less common secondary headaches. Such headaches may be caused by a variety of pathologic conditions, which can be categorized as intracranial and extracranial. Intracranial causes include masses and infections of the cerebrum, meninges, and skull. They also include intracranial hemorrhage, dural venous sinus thrombosis, vascular malformations, aneurysms, neurovascular compression, and

CSF flow disorders.[3,4] Extracranial causes include temporal bone pathologic condition, paranasal sinus disease, TMJ disease, and nasopharyngeal carcinoma, as well as many other disorders.[2,5,6] Although some of these disorders may cause acute headaches, we have focused on 4 important categories of chronic secondary headaches: idiopathic intracranial hypertension (IIH), intracranial hypotension (ICH), CSF leak, intracranial and extracranial tumors and lesions, and neurovascular compression disorders.[3]

Noncontrast CT of the head is often used for the initial evaluation of severe atypical acute headaches and is effective at detecting intracranial hemorrhages, hydrocephalus, and large masses. Contrast CT is useful if soft tissue abscess or extracranial mass are suspected. When vascular pathologic condition is suspected, CTA or MRA may be needed for diagnosis. MRI with contrast may be needed to identify and characterize intracranial lesions. The MR imaging protocol should be carefully selected to evaluate for the clinically suspected diagnosis as routine MRI brain will not be effective at diagnosing many disorders such as neurovascular compression, subtle IAC pathologic condition, or smaller sellar and juxtasellar lesions. Optimal imaging protocols are described below for each group of disorders discussed.

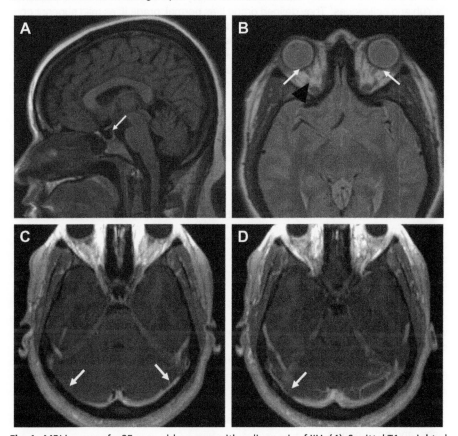

Fig. 1. MRI images of a 25-year-old woman with a diagnosis of IIH. (*A*): Sagittal T1-weighted images demonstrate the empty sella (*white arrow*), (*B*): T2 axial images of the orbits show flattening of the posterior globes (*white arrows*) with tortuosity of the optic nerves and smear sign (*black arrowhead*), and (*C, D*): MRV images demonstrate narrowing and tapering of the distal transverse sinuses (*white arrows*).

IDIOPATHIC INTRACRANIAL HYPERTENSION (BENIGN INTRACRANIAL HYPERTENSION OR PSEUDOTUMOR CEREBRI)

Neuroimaging of Idiopathic Intracranial Hypertension

Techniques: Sagittal T1-weighted images to evaluate the sella turcica and pituitary gland; axial T2 and FLAIR to evaluate the shape of the globe, optical discs, and optic nerves; coronal STIR/T2-weighted images to evaluate the optic nerve diameter, and postcontrast T1-weighted images and diffusion-weighted images for assessment of the optic disc, and CT venogram (CTV) or MR venogram (MRV) to evaluate dural venous sinuses, particularly transverse sinuses.

Sella and pituitary gland: One of the most common radiological findings of IIH is "empty sella" (**Fig. 1**A). By definition, empty sella means partial or complete filling of the sella turcica with CSF with the lack of visible pituitary gland. Although it is present in many patients with IIH and can facilitate the diagnosis in the correct clinical setting, it is a nonspecific finding, commonly seen in the general population or in other causes of IIH including venous sinus thrombosis or intracranial space-occupying lesion.[7,8]

The best method to assess the sella changes in on midsagittal T1-weighted images. There is a five-point grading classification for empty sella based on an article published by Yuh and colleagues[7] They defined grade I: as normal, grade II: as mild superior concavity (sless than one-third height of sella turcica), grade III: moderate concavity (between one-third and two-third height of the sella turcica), grade IV: severe concavity (more than two-third height of the sella turcica), and grade V: no pituitary tissue visible. Partial empty sella is defined as grades III and IV and empty sella as grade V.

It is important to differentiate primary empty sella from secondary in which the actual size of the pituitary gland is reduced. In IIH or other causes of raised intracranial pressure, the changes in the appearance of sella are secondary to increased CSF pressure and intrasellar herniating of the arachnoid matter resulting in deformity but not atrophy of the pituitary gland.[9–11] The same explanation can be applied to healthy controls with defects in the diaphragm sellae, which is a common variation among the normal population.[12,13]

However, based on many morphologic studies, in IIH there is an enlargement of sella turcica and remodeling of the bony structures with a minor contribution from changes in the actual pituitary gland, which can be used to differentiate IIH from secondary empty sella or normal variation.[14] Many studies have evaluated the sella changes over the course of treatment[10,15,16] and showed mild improvement in the appearance of empty sella mainly from the slight increase in the height of the pituitary gland after CSF pressure reduction without any interval change in the appearance of the sella turcica itself.[11]

Empty sella might be present at the subclinical stages of IIH,[7] although some studies have claimed that it reflects the chronicity of raised intracranial pressure with gradual remodeling over time and a 1 mm increase in the width of sella per decade on average.[17,18]

The sensitivity and specificity of empty sella for diagnosis of IIH range from 65% to 80% and 70% to 100% respectively, depending on the definition used,[19] however, using the grading system introduced by Yuh and colleagues,[7] the sensitivity and specificity can improve.[20,21]

Orbital changes: In IIH, there are a constellation of changes involving globe, optic discs, and optic nerves.

Flattening of the posterior globe: Flattening of the normal convexity of the posterior globe is commonly seen in IIH cases (**Fig. 1**B). The normal curve of the posterior sclera is considered as a sign of equilibrium between intracranial and intraocular

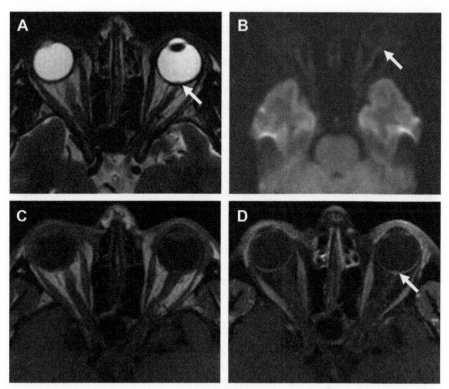

Fig. 2. Orbit images of a case with IIH and papilledema. (*A*): Axial T2-weighted images show minimal protrusion of the optic disc into the globe (*white arrow*), (*B*): Diffusion-weighted images show hyperintensity in the optic disc (*white arrow on B*). (*C, D*) Axial T1-weighted images precontrast and postcontrast demonstrate enhancement of the optic disc (*white arrow on D*).

pressure.[19,22] In severe cases, there is also evidence of protrusion of the optic nerve head into the posterior sclera[21] (**Fig. 2**A). The correlation between MRI and fundoscopy examination has shown that flattening of the globe might precede papilledema, emphasizing the importance of this MRI finding.[23]

The sensitivity and specificity of flattening of the posterior globe is quite variable between different studies, which might be partly due to subjective radiological interpretations, suboptimal reading agreement, and different imaging techniques.[19] Based on prior studies, globe flattening is highly specific for IIH with pooled specificity of 98% but less sensitive at 66% (ranges from 43% to 85%).[17,24]

In a study by Agid and colleagues[21], they claimed that flattening of the sclera is the only radiological sign that conclusively identifies IIH. However, it is important to keep in mind that other causes of raised intracranial pressure or ocular hypotony can display similar appearances on MRI.[25] The globe changes and posterior flattening is reversible and can improve after treatment.[11]

The best MRI sequence for evaluation of the posterior globe flattening or protrusion of the optic disc is axial T2 or FLAIR images.

Optic nerve head hyperintensity and enhancement: There are reports of reduced diffusion and hyperintensity in the head of the optic nerve in cases with papilledema[26,27] (**Fig. 2**B). Some reports have also shown enhancement of the optic disc[28]

(**Fig. 2**C, D), although these findings are not very common. The lack of restricted diffusion or enhancement does not exclude papilledema, but the presence of optic disc enhancement is highly specific (close to 100%) for optic disc edema due to any underlying pathologic conditions because it is rarely reported in normal controls.[21] Hyperintensity on diffusion-weighted images might be dependent on the degree of papilledema because studies with lower grades of papilledema did not find restricted diffusion.[11,27] Based on pathophysiological studies, ischemic changes in ciliary circulation in higher grades of papilledema are responsible for these changes.[26]

The best plane and sequence to evaluate optic disc hyperintensity is on axial diffusion-weighted images and for enhancement is axial postcontrast T1-weighted images with fat suppression.

The thickness of the optic nerve sheath: Many studies have reported distension of the CSF spaces around the optic nerve as a result of increased intracranial pressure. However, there are significant variations across different studies with a wide range of sensitivity from 45% to 89%.[17,21,29] For more accurate definition and diagnosis, certain cutoffs have been defined in large cohort studies using volumetric MRI data. In recent studies on children, we found that a cutoff of 6 mm is highly specific for raised intracranial pressure.[30] The width of the perioptic CSF ring more than 2 mm has also been used in many studies with a pooled sensitivity of 58% and specificity of 89%.[19] The thickness of the nerve sheath usually reduces after treatment; however, it still remains larger than normal controls.[11]

The best plan and sequence to evaluate optic nerve sheath is on coronal STIR or T2-weighted images.

Optic nerve tortuosity: Both horizontal and vertical tortuosities of the optic nerve have been reported in IIH. The kinking of the optic nerve is believed to be secondary to distension of the nerve sheath between 2 fixed points at the 2 ends of the intraorbital segment of the optic nerve.[17,31] On sagittal view the kinked optic nerve with vertical tortuosity seems as "S shape" and on axial view the optic nerve cannot be entirely visualized on one slice, partly obscured by intraorbital fat which is called "smear sign"[17] (see **Fig. 1**B). The tortuosity of the optic nerve in either direction is not a very sensitive finding with a pooled sensitivity of 43%,[19] but the specificity of horizontal tortuosity has been reported to be more than vertical.[22,32] The pooled specificity of optic nerve tortuosity is around 90%.[19]

The best plane and sequence to evaluate horizontal and vertical tortuosity of the optic nerve is axial and sagittal T1-weighted or T2-weighted images.

Cerebral venous sinus imaging: Unilateral or bilateral stenosis of transverse sinuses have been reported in most IIH cases[33,34] (**Fig. 1**C, D). Some studies have even claimed that bilateral stenosis is a pathognomonic finding for this disease[35] and others showed that based on the definition of transverse sinus stenosis 100% of IIH patients have bilateral stenosis on MRV.[36]

Independent of the sensitivity or specificity of this finding, the primary role the venous sinus imaging in cases with raised intracranial pressure is to differentiate the primary (IIH) versus secondary causes of IIH, which can be due to venous sinus thrombosis or rarely dural fistulas.

The changes in the transverse sinus caliber are usually found at the distal two-third of the transverse sinuses at the transition point to the sigmoid sinus.[37] Most of the cases show tapering and smooth narrowing of the lumen (extraluminal, 80%); however, there are also reports of filling defects and abrupt cut off the transverse sinuses (intraluminal, 20%).[19]

There are a few challenges in the evaluation of dural venous stenosis in IIH including significant anatomic variation between cases, lack of standard definition of sinus stenosis, and the use of various imaging techniques across different centers and studies from flow sensitive MRV, contrast-enhanced MRV, and CTV.[19,38] Based on contrast-enhanced MRV, the pooled sensitivity of bilateral transverse sinus stenosis for diagnosis of IIH is estimated to be around 97%.[19]

Another caveat to consider is the lack of knowledge about the role of sinus stenosis on IIH. It is still not clear whether the venous sinus stenosis has a causative role in raised intracranial pressure or is the consequence of it. There are 3 different hypotheses: the sinuses are congenitally narrowed in cases with raised pressure, they are compressed secondary to raised intracranial pressure, and there is an acquired stenosis.[38] Despite all these uncertainties, several studies have shown that intravascular intervention with stenting of the transverse sinuses results in significant improvement in the clinical symptoms and CSF opening pressure in IIH cases.[38,39]

The best sequences to assess the dural venous sinuses are MRV or CTV with 3D reformatting in all 3 planes.

Less common radiological findings: Enlargement of the optic canal has been reported in some patients with IIH, which might be primary changes contributing to worsening of the papilledema or secondary to raised CSF pressure over the time.[19]

Cerebral tonsillar herniation has been seen in some patients with IIH. The association between Chiari malformation I and IIH is complex and not clearly understood because many studies have shown cases with Chiari may have imaging findings compatible with raised IIH; however, tonsillar displacement is seen in some of the patients with IIH.[40]

Slitlike ventricles have also been reported in older imaging studies with prominent ventricle horns.[19]

Spontaneous CSF leak, meningoceles, and meningoencephaloceles have also been reported in IIH cases, particularly through basal skull foramina. Widening foramen oval or Meckel cave has also been seen in some studies.[19]

INTRACRANIAL HYPOTENSION AND CSF LEAK

A common presentation of ICH is a headache. Due to the leakage of CSF from the subarachnoid space, a decrease in the volume of CSF intracranially results in a compensatory increase in either arterial input or decreased venous output based on the Monro-Kellie doctrine to maintain intracranial pressure.[41–43] The venous distension in the dura results in headaches. Patients with ICH present with orthostatic headaches that begin 20 to 30 minutes after rising in the morning from sleep and persist throughout the day.[44,45] Diagnosis of ICH is made by lumbar puncture with opening pressure less than 6 cm of H_2O.

The neuroimaging of ICH is best made with an initial MRI of the brain with contrast. Relevant imaging findings include loss of the CSF space due to the decreased presence of CSF. This is best seen as effacement of the prepontine and basilar cisterns and downward displacement of the brain on sagittal images, loss of the pontomedullary angle on sagittal images, tonsillar ectopia below the foramen magnum, dural thickening, and enhancement that seems as pachymeningeal thickening and can be mistaken for subdural hematomas on noncontrast studies. Severe cases of ICH may result in rupture of the subdural veins and true subdural hematomas. Due to the decreased amount of CSF, venous engorgement may be seen with an increased size of the venous sinuses. Due to the downward displacement of the brainstem and traction on the lower cranial nerves (CN), lower cranial neuropathy may result. CT imaging may also demonstrate effacement of the basilar cisterns and downward

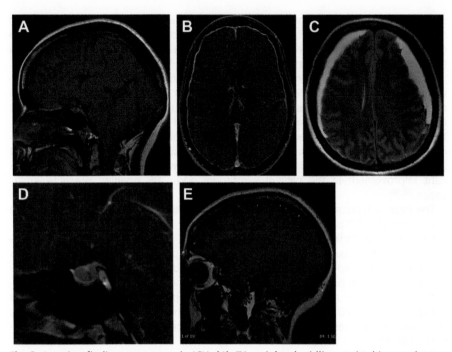

Fig. 3. Imaging findings were seen in ICH. (*A*): T1-weighted midline sagittal image demonstrating loss of the CSF space anterior to the brainstem, loss of the pontomedullary junction, and tonsillar ectopia. (*B*): Postcontrast T1-weighted axial image demonstrating diffuse pachymeningeal enhancement. (*C*): T2-weighted axial image demonstrating bilateral subdural hematomas. Note the presence of fluid levels in the dependent portion of the collections. (*D*): Postcontrast T1-weighted midline sagittal image demonstrating pituitary enlargement. (*E*): Right parasagittal T1-weighted image demonstrating distension of the signal flow void of the right transverse sinus.

displacement of the brain on sagittal reconstructions. Bilateral subdural effusions may also be seen[46–49] (**Fig. 3**).

Although the most common cause of ICH is due to a spinal cause, such as rupture of a perineural cyst or a CSF-venous fistula, defects of the anterior, central skull base, or temporal bone may be the root cause. The patient's clinical presentation will direct what type of neuroimaging is required. CSF rhinorrhea is commonly the result of a defect of the anterior skull base, commonly the cribriform plate. Due to the rise of obesity, unusual causes of defects have been described, in particular, associated with the paranasal sinuses, especially along the lateral wall of the sphenoid sinuses. CSF otorrhea may be the result of a defect of the tegmen tympani or tegmen mastoideum. The cause of these defects in the skull base is felt to be due to the presence of arachnoid granulations adjacent to areas of markedly thin bone resulting in erosion and resultant CSF leak.

The imaging modalities used to diagnose CSF leak from the skull base include nuclear medicine (NM) cisternography, noncontrast high-resolution CT, CT cisternography, and MR cisternography. NM cisternography entails the injection of Indium-DTPA by lumbar puncture, and subsequent imaging of the face after the placement of pledgets within the nasal cavity for the detection of a CSF leak has a high specificity

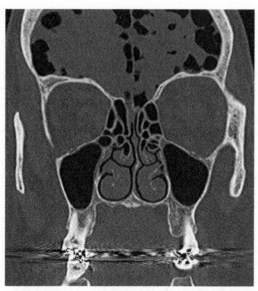

Fig. 4. High-resolution noncontrast coronal CT of the face demonstrates defect of the right cribriform plate and extensive pneumocephalus.

ranging from 76% to 100%, with sensitivity of 100% and accuracy of 90% (10) but does not show the site of the leak. With some of the other imaging modalities, NM cisternography has fallen out of favor.

High-resolution CT of the area of interest is the mainstay in diagnosing a candidate for a source of CSF leak. The current generation of CT scanners allows for sub-millimeter (mm) imaging. CT of the face in the setting of CSF rhinorrhea or CT of the temporal bone for CSF otorrhea should be the principal imaging modality used. Images should be acquired in all 3 orthogonal planes with sub-mm imaging using a bone algorithm.[50] In the setting of CSF leak localization, these studies reported a

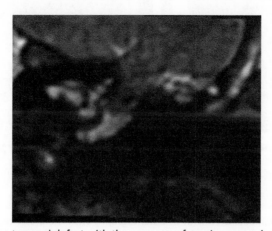

Fig. 5. Left tegmen tympani defect with the presence of meningoencephalocele in the middle ear cavity. Fluid-sensitive thin-section coronal T2-weighted image demonstrates herniation of the temporal lobe into the superior aspect of the middle ear cavity, which is also filled with fluid.

sensitivity and specificity for HRCT of 44% to 100% and 45% to 100%, respectively, with most studies being on the upper end of this scale. Reported positive predictive values and negative predictive values were 100% and 50% to 70%, respectively, with an accuracy of 87% to 93%[50–54] (**Fig. 4**).

MR cisternography, using thin section heavily T2-weighted coronal images, has a reported sensitivity of detecting the site of 56% to 94%, a specificity of 57% to 100%,[44,46,55,56] a positive predictive value of 64% to 92%,[52,55] a negative predictive value of 71%,[55] and an overall accuracy of 78% to 96%.[52,55–57]

MR cisternography may demonstrate a cleft between the subarachnoid space and the superior recess of the nasal cavity, fluid within the nasal cavity, and within the paranasal sinuses. In the setting of a defect of the tegmen tympani, a fluid-filled sac or the brain parenchyma may be seen in the setting of meningocele and meningoencephalocele (**Fig. 5**).

CT cisternography may aid in the diagnosis of active CSF leak but may not demonstrate intermittent leaks. To perform CT cisternography, a noncontrast CT of the area of interest is initially performed using a bone algorithm and reconstructed in the 3 orthogonal planes. Contrast is then injected into the subarachnoid space (10 cc, Isovue 200M contrast, Bracco Diagnostics, 10 cc) by lumbar puncture. With the patient prone, the contrast column is then followed up the thecal sac by placing the patient prone in Trendelenburg position with the head flexed to allow the contrast to go intracranially. The head is positioned so that the area of interest is placed in the dependent position to allow the contrast, which is denser than CSF, to flow to the area of interest. Once contrast is at the area of interest, anterior skull base, central skull base, or temporal bone, another CT study is performed at the area of interest with exact specifications as the precontrast study. The timing of the second contrast is performed without delay (**Fig. 6**).

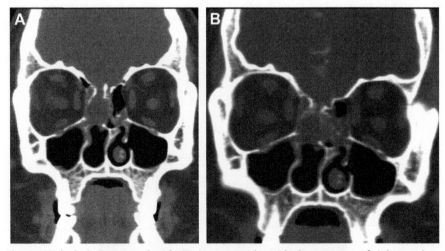

Fig. 6. CSF leak demonstrated with CT cisternography with the presence of right nasal encephalocele. (*A*): Precontrast CT of the face, coronal plane demonstrating a mass in the right nasal cavity with defect of the right cribriform plate. (*B*): Postcisternogram CT of the face, coronal plane demonstrating extension of contrast around the mass in the right nasal cavity below the cribriform plate.

The presence of contrast in the sinonasal cavity due to a defect in the anterior or central skull base, or contrast within the mastoids or middle ear cavity, is positive for a leak.

Another imaging modality used to determine the site of leak is fluorescein imaging. Patients with small leaks of the anterior skull base at the level of the cribriform plate may be difficult to see endoscopically. On injection of fluorescein by lumbar puncture intraoperatively, due to CSF circulation, fluorescein circulates throughout the CSF space quickly. With a Wood's lamp, the site of the CSF leak may be visualized endoscopically during the transnasal approach. Keerl and colleagues[58] assessed 420 applications of IF ranging from 0.5 to 2 mL of 0.5% to 5% fluorescein, which is equivalent to 2.5 to 100 mg. Serious adverse events have been reported, including lower extremity weakness, seizures, cranial nerve deficits, and even death with doses as high as 500 to 1250 mg.

INTRACRANIAL AND EXTRACRANIAL TUMORS AND LESIONS

Headache is the most common presenting symptom of an extra-axial tumor due to dural involvement. Tumors of the skull base may also present with headache and may be a sign of intracranial extension also due to dural involvement. CT and MRI play complementary roles in the evaluation of these tumors. The role of CT is to determine the degree and extent of bony erosion and destruction. MRI is used to characterize the lesion with regard to signal characteristics, the pattern of enhancement, involvement of adjacent structures, and infiltration of the marrow adjacent to the areas of bone destruction. In evaluating a mass, high-resolution MRI with contrast of the area of interest provides excellent detail of the primary tumor and adjacent structures. A noncontrast CT of the area with a bone algorithm demonstrates the site and size of bony involvement to help plan reconstruction. Although a contrast-enhanced CT also provides some information regarding the tumor itself, MRI is superior to CT in

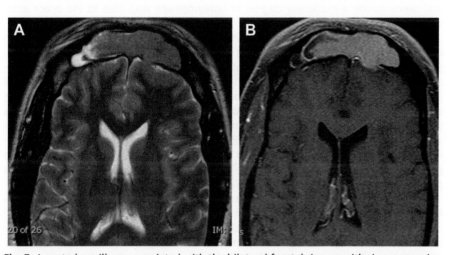

Fig. 7. Inverted papilloma associated with the bilateral frontal sinuses with sinus expansion representing mucocele formation. (*A*): T2-weighted axial image demonstrating a mass filling the left frontal sinus and extending into the right frontal sinus. Note erosion of the posterior table of a portion of the left frontal sinus as well as mucocele formation. The mass is mildly hyperintense in signal intensity relative to gray matter. (*B*): Postcontrast T1-weighted axial image demonstrates homogeneously avid enhancement of the mass.

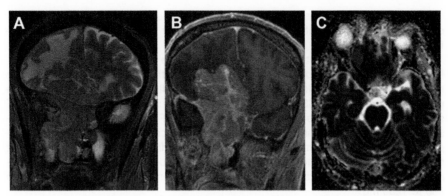

Fig. 8. Esthesioneuroblastoma. (*A*): T1-weighted coronal image demonstrates a large mass associated with the bilateral nasal cavity with superior extension above the anterior skull base with mass effect on the bilateral frontal lobes, right greater than left. The mass is intermediate in signal intensity to gray matter. Also, note the edema associated with the right frontal lobe, which is hyperintense in signal intensity. (*B*): Postcontrast T1-weighted images demonstrate heterogeneous moderate to avid enhancement of the mass. (*C*): ADC map ion the axial plane demonstrates marked decreased signal intensity of the mass, representing a marked reduction in the diffusion coefficient of this lesion.

depicting the internal architecture of the lesion and its effect on the adjacent brain parenchyma.

In the sinonasal cavity, the most common benign tumor is papilloma. These lesions usually occur along the lateral wall of the nasal cavity or middle meatus. On T2-weighted images, these tumors are hyperintense on T2-weighted images with linear stria, which are lower in signal intensity, giving the tumor a cerebriform appearance and demonstrate a moderate degree of enhancement and, due to the linear stria, also have a cerebriform appearance[59,60] (**Fig. 7**).

The most common tumor of the sinonasal cavity is squamous cell cancer, which demonstrates mildly hyperintense signal intensity on T2-weighted images and heterogeneous moderate to avid enhancement.[61] Neuroendocrine tumors, including esthesioneuroblastoma, sinonasal neuroendocrine carcinoma, and sinonasal neuroendocrine undifferentiated carcinoma, are a spectrum of tumors based on the degree of differentiation of the cellular population. This group of tumors demonstrates similar imaging characteristics with intermediate to hypointense signal intensity on T2-weighted images and diffusion restriction on diffusion-weighted images. Esthesioneuroblastomas that extend superior to the anterior skull base may demonstrate the presence of nonenhancing cysts at the tumor brain interface and is believed to be pathognomonic for these tumors[61–63] (**Fig. 8**).

Sinonasal salivary gland malignancies account for up to 3% of head and neck malignancies.[61,64] Aggressive sinonasal tumors may also extend intracranially. The most common minor salivary gland malignancies are adenoid cystic carcinoma, adenocarcinoma, and mucoepidermoid carcinoma. The MR imaging characteristics are fairly nonspecific, although a general rule is that the lower the signal intensity of a mass on T2-weighted images, the more likely it is a malignant tumor.[61,65,66]

Mucoceles of the frontal sinus and frontoethmoidal mucoceles may also present with headache due to sinus expansion and involvement of the adjacent dura[67] (see **Fig. 7**). On CT imaging, mucoceles demonstrate marked thinning or apparent absence

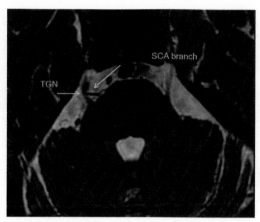

Fig. 9. Axial MR cisternography: Vascular loop of the right SCA (*arrow*) compressing and distorting the midcisternal segment of CN V (*arrow*) in a patient with TN.

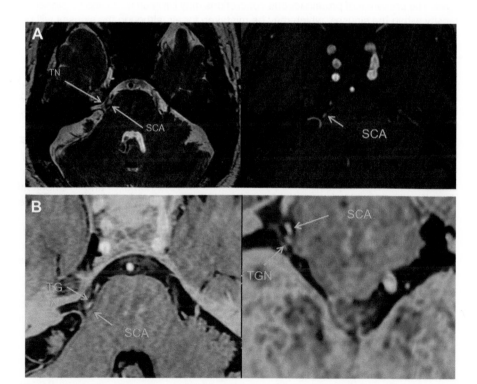

Fig. 10. Axial MR cisternography (*A*): Vascular loop of the right SCA (*arrow*) compressing and distorting the root entry zone of CN V (*arrow*) in a patient with TN. Axial TOF MRA (*B*) confirms the position of the right SCA. Axial and Coronal color-coded MRI and MRA fusion images demonstrate the relationship between the right CNV and the right SCA.

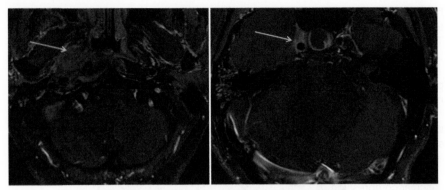

Fig. 11. Axial T1WI postcontrast images in a patient presenting with TN. Images show nasopharyngeal carcinoma (*arrows*) invading the skull base, right Meckel cave, and right cavernous sinus.

of the posterior table of the frontal sinus or the fovea ethmoidalis. On MR imaging, mucosal enhancement is seen although no solid mass is identified. Adjacent dural enhancement may be seen. The signal of the contents of the mucocele is variable due to the protein concentration, and its effect on T1-weighted and T2-weighted images. The presence of proteinaceous concretions may be seen as having no signal intensity within the sinuses, which may be mistaken for air, although the sinuses will be expanded. CT will demonstrate the high attenuation material within the sinuses.

NEUROVASCULAR COMPRESSION DISORDERS

Neurovascular compression disorders include motor and sensory disorders caused by compression of the CN by vascular structures including arteries and veins. Compression of CN V and CN XI can result in headaches.[68]

Trigeminal neuralgia (TN) is recognized as the most common of these disorders and can be extremely painful and difficult to control with medications. In many classic TN cases, MRI and MRA can demonstrate a vessel contacting and compressing the trigeminal nerve (CNV), most frequently at the root entry zone at the midpontine level. The offending vessel is frequently determined to be superior cerebellar artery (SCA);

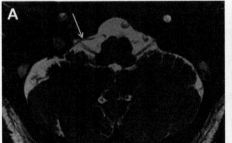
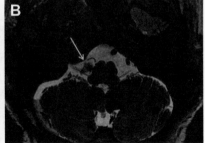

Fig. 12. Axial MR cisternography image (*A*) demonstrates AICA branch (*arrow*) compressing and displacing CN IX cisternal segment in a patient with glossopharyngeal neuralgia. Axial MR cisternography image after microvascular decompression (*B*) demonstrates placement of pledget (*arrow*) separating the AICA branch from CN IX.

however, anterior inferior cerebellar artery (AICA), tortuous basilar and vertebral arteries, and even venous structures may cause neurovascular compression in TN[69,70] (**Figs. 9** and **10**). Multiple sclerosis plaques, tumors, and vascular malformations involving or adjacent to the trigeminal nerve may also present as TN (**Fig. 11**).[71]

Glossopharyngeal neuralgia usually causes tongue, throat, and floor of the mouth pain. Vascular compression of the glossopharyngeal nerve may be caused by AICA, posterior inferior cerebellar artery, and vertebral artery[68] (**Fig. 12**). Chiari type 1 malformation and Eagle syndrome may also cause this disorder. MRI can also be useful for the evaluation of TN and glossopharyngeal neuralgia postmicrovascular decompression and can show the position of the Teflon pledget in relation to the vascular loop and the cranial nerve[68,72](see **Fig. 12**B).

High-quality MRI has shown to be reliable in identifying and characterizing neurovascular compression.[73] Dedicated imaging protocol is critical for accurate diagnosis of neurovascular compression disorders because high-resolution optimized MRI and MRA sequences are required to resolve the small cranial nerve structures and vascular loops while minimizing CSF pulsation artifacts. This protocol should include small field of view sequences centered on the skull base. These should include thin slice T1-weighted images with and without contrast, 3D MR cisternography sequence–high resolution, heavy T2-weighted sequence with CSF suppression (FIESTA, CISS, FRFSE), and a 3D MRA sequence.[73,74] 3T imaging is preferred because the higher resolution may allow for increased sensitivity in the detection of neurovascular compression.[75] 3D fusion software can be used to demonstrate neurovascular compression and help with preoperative planning by coregistering the MR cisternography images with MRA images. Color coding can be used to designate vessels showing arterial flow on MRA (see **Fig. 10**).[68,72,76]

CLINICS CARE POINTS

- Care should be taken to distinguish primary empty sella from secondary empty sella and normal variation which are not associated with IIH.
- Unilateral or bilateral stenosis of transverse sinuses has been reported in most of the patients with IIH, which is best assessed on MRV or CTV.
- Severe cases of ICH may result in subdural hematomas.
- A variety of intracranial and skull base tumors may cause headaches due to dural involvement.
- Dedicated high-resolution MR cisternography and MR angiography imaging is necessary to demonstrate vascular compression of CN in neurovascular compression disorders.

DISCLOSURE

The authors have nothing to disclose.

REFERENCES

1. Osborn RE, Alder DC, Mitchell CS. MR imaging of the brain in patients with migraine headaches. AJNR Am J Neuroradiol 1991;12:521–4.
2. Evans RW. Diagnostic testing for migraine and other primary headaches. Neurol Clin 2009;27:393–415.
3. Sempere AP, Porta-Etessam J, Medrano V, et al. Neuroimaging in the evaluation of patients with non-acute headache. Cephalalgia 2005;25:30–5.

4. Agostoni E. Headache in cerebral venous thrombosis. Neurol Sci 2004;25(Suppl 3):S206–10.

5. May A. A review of diagnostic and functional imaging in headache. J Headache Pain 2006;7:174–84.

6. Medina LS, D'Souza B, Vasconcellos E. Adults and children with headache: evidence-based diagnostic evaluation. Neuroimaging Clin N Am 2003;13:225–35.

7. Yuh WT, Zhu M, Taoka T, et al. MR imaging of pituitary morphology in idiopathic intracranial hypertension. J Magn Reson Imaging 2000;12:808–13.

8. Rohr AC, Riedel C, Fruehauf MC, et al. MR imaging findings in patients with secondary intracranial hypertension. AJNR Am J Neuroradiol 2011;32:1021–9.

9. Sage MR, Blumbergs PC. Primary empty sella turcica: a radiological-anatomical correlation. Australas Radiol 2000;44:341–8.

10. Ranganathan S, Lee SH, Checkver A, et al. Magnetic resonance imaging finding of empty sella in obesity related idiopathic intracranial hypertension is associated with enlarged sella turcica. Neuroradiology 2013;55:955–61.

11. Batur Caglayan HZ, Ucar M, Hasanreisoglu M, et al. Magnetic resonance imaging of idiopathic intracranial hypertension: before and after treatment. J Neuroophthalmol 2019;39:324–9.

12. Evans RW. Incidental findings and normal anatomical variants on MRI of the brain in adults for primary headaches. Headache 2017;57:780–91.

13. Guitelman M, Garcia Basavilbaso N, Vitale M, et al. Primary empty sella (PES): a review of 175 cases. Pituitary 2013;16:270–4.

14. Kyung SE, Botelho JV, Horton JC. Enlargement of the sella turcica in pseudotumor cerebri. J Neurosurg 2014;120:538–42.

15. Chang RO, Marshall BK, Yahyavi N, et al. Neuroimaging features of idiopathic intracranial hypertension persist after resolution of papilloedema. Neuroophthalmology 2016;40:165–70.

16. Zagardo MT, Cail WS, Kelman SE, et al. Reversible empty sella in idiopathic intracranial hypertension: an indicator of successful therapy? AJNR Am J Neuroradiol 1996;17:1953–6.

17. Brodsky MC, Vaphiades M. Magnetic resonance imaging in pseudotumor cerebri. Ophthalmology 1998;105:1686–93.

18. Saindane AM, Lim PP, Aiken A, et al. Factors determining the clinical significance of an "empty" sella turcica. AJR Am J Roentgenol 2013;200:1125–31.

19. Bidot S, Saindane AM, Peragallo JH, et al. Brain imaging in idiopathic intracranial hypertension. J Neuroophthalmol 2015;35:400–11.

20. Ridha MA, Saindane AM, Bruce BB, et al. MRI findings of elevated intracranial pressure in cerebral venous thrombosis versus idiopathic intracranial hypertension with transverse sinus stenosis. Neuroophthalmology 2013;37:1–6.

21. Agid R, Farb RI, Willinsky RA, et al. Idiopathic intracranial hypertension: the validity of cross-sectional neuroimaging signs. Neuroradiology 2006;48:521–7.

22. Degnan AJ, Levy LM. Pseudotumor cerebri: brief review of clinical syndrome and imaging findings. AJNR Am J Neuroradiol 2011;32:1986–93.

23. Jacobson DM. Intracranial hypertension and the syndrome of acquired hyperopia with choroidal folds. J Neuroophthalmol 1995;15:178–85.

24. Maralani PJ, Hassanlou M, Torres C, et al. Accuracy of brain imaging in the diagnosis of idiopathic intracranial hypertension. Clin Radiol 2012;67:656–63.

25. Brodsky MC. Flattening of the posterior sclera: hypotony or elevated intracranial pressure? Am J Ophthalmol 2004;138:511, author reply 511-512.

26. Viets R, Parsons M, Van Stavern G, et al. Hyperintense optic nerve heads on diffusion-weighted imaging: a potential imaging sign of papilledema. AJNR Am J Neuroradiol 2013;34:1438–42.

27. Salvay DM, Padhye LV, Huecker JB, et al. Correlation between papilledema grade and diffusion-weighted magnetic resonance imaging in idiopathic intracranial hypertension. J Neuroophthalmol 2014;34:331–5.

28. Brodsky MC, Glasier CM. Magnetic resonance visualization of the swollen optic disc in papilledema. J Neuroophthalmol 1995;15:122–4.

29. Hoffmann J, Schmidt C, Kunte H, et al. Volumetric assessment of optic nerve sheath and hypophysis in idiopathic intracranial hypertension. AJNR Am J Neuroradiol 2014;35:513–8.

30. Kamali A, Aein A, Naderi N, et al. Neuroimaging Features of Intracranial Hypertension in Pediatric Patients With New-Onset Idiopathic Seizures, a Comparison With Patients with Confirmed Diagnosis of Idiopathic Intracranial Hypertension: A Preliminary Study. J Child Neurol 2021;36:1103–10.

31. Passi N, Degnan AJ, Levy LM. MR imaging of papilledema and visual pathways: effects of increased intracranial pressure and pathophysiologic mechanisms. AJNR Am J Neuroradiol 2013;34:919–24.

32. Gorkem SB, Doganay S, Canpolat M, et al. MR imaging findings in children with pseudotumor cerebri and comparison with healthy controls. Childs Nerv Syst 2015;31:373–80.

33. Farb RI, Vanek I, Scott JN, et al. Idiopathic intracranial hypertension: the prevalence and morphology of sinovenous stenosis. Neurology 2003;60:1418–24.

34. Johnston I, Kollar C, Dunkley S, et al. Cranial venous outflow obstruction in the pseudotumour syndrome: incidence, nature and relevance. J Clin Neurosci 2002;9:273–8.

35. Bono F, Messina D, Giliberto C, et al. Bilateral transverse sinus stenosis predicts IIH without papilledema in patients with migraine. Neurology 2006;67:419–23.

36. Riggeal BD, Bruce BB, Saindane AM, et al. Clinical course of idiopathic intracranial hypertension with transverse sinus stenosis. Neurology 2013;80:289–95.

37. Rohr A, Bindeballe J, Riedel C, et al. The entire dural sinus tree is compressed in patients with idiopathic intracranial hypertension: a longitudinal, volumetric magnetic resonance imaging study. Neuroradiology 2012;54:25–33.

38. Fraser C, Plant GT. The syndrome of pseudotumour cerebri and idiopathic intracranial hypertension. Curr Opin Neurol 2011;24:12–7.

39. Nicholson P, Brinjikji W, Radovanovic I, et al. Venous sinus stenting for idiopathic intracranial hypertension: a systematic review and meta-analysis. J Neurointerv Surg 2019;11:380–5.

40. Aiken AH, Hoots JA, Saindane AM, et al. Incidence of cerebellar tonsillar ectopia in idiopathic intracranial hypertension: a mimic of the Chiari I malformation. AJNR Am J Neuroradiol 2012;33:1901–6.

41. Kellie G. An account of the appearances observed in the dissection of two of three individuals presumed to have perished in the storm of the 3d, and whose bodies were discovered in the vicinity of leith on the morning of the 4th, November 1821; with some reflections on the pathology of the brain: part I. Trans Med Chir Soc Edinb 1824;1:84–122.

42. Ferris EB. The effect of high intracranial venous pressure upon the cerebral circulation and its relation to cerebral symptoms. J Clin Invest 1939;18:19–24.

43. Mokri B. The Monro-Kellie hypothesis: applications in CSF volume depletion. Neurology 2001;56:1746–8.

44. Leep Hunderfund AN, Mokri B. Second-half-of-the-day headache as a manifestation of spontaneous CSF leak. J Neurol 2012;259:306–10.
45. Mokri B. Spontaneous cerebrospinal fluid leaks: from intracranial hypotension to cerebrospinal fluid hypovolemia–evolution of a concept. Mayo Clin Proc 1999;74: 1113–23.
46. Kranz PG, Tanpitukpongse TP, Choudhury KR, et al. Imaging signs in spontaneous intracranial hypotension: prevalence and relationship to CSF pressure. AJNR Am J Neuroradiol 2016;37:1374–8.
47. Farb RI, Forghani R, Lee SK, et al. The venous distension sign: a diagnostic sign of intracranial hypotension at MR imaging of the brain. AJNR Am J Neuroradiol 2007;28:1489–93.
48. Shah LM, McLean LA, Heilbrun ME, et al. Intracranial hypotension: improved MRI detection with diagnostic intracranial angles. AJR Am J Roentgenol 2013;200: 400–7.
49. Schievink WI. Spontaneous spinal cerebrospinal fluid leaks and intracranial hypotension. JAMA 2006;295:2286–96.
50. Stone JA, Castillo M, Neelon B, et al. Evaluation of CSF leaks: high-resolution CT compared with contrast-enhanced CT and radionuclide cisternography. AJNR Am J Neuroradiol 1999;20:706–12.
51. Eljamel MS, Pidgeon CN. Localization of inactive cerebrospinal fluid fistulas. J Neurosurg 1995;83:795–8.
52. Mostafa BE, Khafagi A. Combined HRCT and MRI in the detection of CSF rhinorrhea. Skull Base 2004;14:157–62 [discussion: 162].
53. Zuckerman JD, DelGaudio JM. Utility of preoperative high-resolution CT and intraoperative image guidance in identification of cerebrospinal fluid leaks for endoscopic repair. Am J Rhinol 2008;22:151–4.
54. Oakley GM, Alt JA, Schlosser RJ, et al. Diagnosis of cerebrospinal fluid rhinorrhea: an evidence-based review with recommendations. Int Forum Allergy Rhinol 2016;6:8–16.
55. Zapalac JS, Marple BF, Schwade ND. Skull base cerebrospinal fluid fistulas: a comprehensive diagnostic algorithm. Otolaryngol Head Neck Surg 2002;126: 669–76.
56. Algin O, Hakyemez B, Gokalp G, et al. The contribution of 3D-CISS and contrast-enhanced MR cisternography in detecting cerebrospinal fluid leak in patients with rhinorrhoea. Br J Radiol 2010;83:225–32.
57. Shetty PG, Shroff MM, Sahani DV, et al. Evaluation of high-resolution CT and MR cisternography in the diagnosis of cerebrospinal fluid fistula. AJNR Am J Neuroradiol 1998;19:633–9.
58. Keerl R, Weber RK, Draf W, et al. Use of sodium fluorescein solution for detection of cerebrospinal fluid fistulas: an analysis of 420 administrations and reported complications in Europe and the United States. Laryngoscope 2004;114:266–72.
59. Dammann F, Pereira P, Laniado M, et al. Inverted papilloma of the nasal cavity and the paranasal sinuses: using CT for primary diagnosis and follow-up. AJR Am J Roentgenol 1999;172:543–8.
60. Ojiri H, Ujita M, Tada S, et al. Potentially distinctive features of sinonasal inverted papilloma on MR imaging. AJR Am J Roentgenol 2000;175:465–8.
61. Som PMB-GM, Kassel EE, Genden EM. Tumors and tumor-like conditions of the sinonasal cavities. In: Som PMCH, editor. Head and neck imaging. 5th edition. St. Louis: Elsevier; 2011.
62. Derdeyn CP, Moran CJ, Wippold FJ 2nd, et al. MRI of esthesioneuroblastoma. J Comput Assist Tomogr 1994;18:16–21.

63. Som PM, Lidov M, Brandwein M, et al. Sinonasal esthesioneuroblastoma with intracranial extension: marginal tumor cysts as a diagnostic MR finding. AJNR Am J Neuroradiol 1994;15:1259–62.
64. Batsakis JG. Tumors of the head and neck : clinical and pathological considerations. 2d edition. Baltimore: Williams & Wilkins; 1979.
65. MF M. Imaging of the nasal cavity and paranasal sinuses. In: Mafee MFVG, Becker M, editors. Imaging of the head and neck. 2nd edition. Sttutgart: Thieme; 2005. p. 412–66.
66. Sigal R, Monnet O, de Baere T, et al. Adenoid cystic carcinoma of the head and neck: evaluation with MR imaging and clinical-pathologic correlation in 27 patients. Radiology 1992;184:95–101.
67. Hansen FS, van der Poel NA, Freling NJM, et al. Mucocele formation after frontal sinus obliteration. Rhinology 2018;56:106–10.
68. Haller S, Etienne L, Kovari E, et al. Imaging of neurovascular compression syndromes: trigeminal neuralgia, hemifacial spasm, vestibular paroxysmia, and glossopharyngeal neuralgia. AJNR Am J Neuroradiol 2016;37:1384–92.
69. Tash RR, Sze G, Leslie DR. Trigeminal neuralgia: MR imaging features. Radiology 1989;172:767–70.
70. Lorenzoni J, David P, Levivier M. Patterns of neurovascular compression in patients with classic trigeminal neuralgia: a high-resolution MRI-based study. Eur J Radiol 2012;81:1851–7.
71. Becker M, Kohler R, Vargas MI, et al. Pathology of the trigeminal nerve. Neuroimaging Clin N Am 2008;18:283–307, x.
72. Casselman J, Mermuys K, Delanote J, et al. MRI of the cranial nerves–more than meets the eye: technical considerations and advanced anatomy. Neuroimaging Clin N Am 2008;18:197–231, preceding x.
73. Leal PR, Hermier M, Souza MA, et al. Visualization of vascular compression of the trigeminal nerve with high-resolution 3T MRI: a prospective study comparing preoperative imaging analysis to surgical findings in 40 consecutive patients who underwent microvascular decompression for trigeminal neuralgia. Neurosurgery 2011;69:15–25 [discussion: 26].
74. Yoshino N, Akimoto H, Yamada I, et al. Trigeminal neuralgia: evaluation of neuralgic manifestation and site of neurovascular compression with 3D CISS MR imaging and MR angiography. Radiology 2003;228:539–45.
75. Garcia M, Naraghi R, Zumbrunn T, et al. High-resolution 3D-constructive interference in steady-state MR imaging and 3D time-of-flight MR angiography in neurovascular compression: a comparison between 3T and 1.5T. AJNR Am J Neuroradiol 2012;33:1251–6.
76. Satoh T, Omi M, Nabeshima M, et al. Severity analysis of neurovascular contact in patients with trigeminal neuralgia: assessment with the inner view of the 3D MR cisternogram and angiogram fusion imaging. AJNR Am J Neuroradiol 2009;30:603–7.

Idiopathic Intracranial Hypertension
Implications for the Otolaryngologist

Dorothy W. Pan, MD, PhD[a],*, Erik Vanstrum, BA[b], Joni K. Doherty, MD, PhD[a]

KEYWORDS

- Idiopathic intracranial hypertension • Headache • Papilledema
- Cerebrospinal fluid leak

KEY POINTS

- Idiopathic intracranial hypertension presents as a triad of headaches, visual changes, and papilledema in the absence of a secondary cause for elevated intracranial pressure.
- There is an association between obesity and idiopathic intracranial hypertension.
- Diagnosis of idiopathic intracranial hypertension uses the modified Dandy criteria or the Friedman diagnostic criteria. A lumbar puncture with opening pressure and neuroimaging to rule out other causes of intracranial hypertension is required.
- The major goals of treatment for idiopathic intracranial hypertension are to prevent vision loss and improve the patient's headaches.
- Cerebrospinal fluid (CSF) opening pressure may be elevated or falsely normal in the presence of an active CSF leak. Consideration of the diagnosis of idiopathic intracranial hypertension and management of elevated intracranial pressure before CSF leak repair and perioperatively are crucial to success of the repair. Sometimes a ventriculoperitoneal shunt is necessary for control of intracranial pressures.

INTRODUCTION
Nomenclature

Idiopathic intracranial hypertension (IIH), benign intracranial hypertension, and pseudotumor cerebri syndrome (PTCS) are all terms that have been used interchangeably to describe a syndrome characterized by the triad of elevated intracranial pressure (ICP) along with headache and papilledema in the setting of normal ventricular architecture with no clear cause. Although benign intracranial hypertension has been used

[a] Caruso Department of Otolaryngology–Head and Neck Surgery, Keck School of Medicine, University of Southern California, 1537 Norfolk Street, Suite 5800, Los Angeles, CA 90033, USA; [b] Keck School of Medicine, University of Southern California, 1537 Norfolk Street, Suite 5800, Los Angeles, CA 90033, USA
* Corresponding author.
E-mail address: dorothy.pan@med.usc.edu

Otolaryngol Clin N Am 55 (2022) 579–594
https://doi.org/10.1016/j.otc.2022.02.005
0030-6665/22/© 2022 Elsevier Inc. All rights reserved.
oto.theclinics.com

as a label for these symptoms, this disease process is not "benign" and is associated with significant morbidity. Most patients have debilitating headaches, and an estimated 1% to 2% of new IIH cases present with blindness annually.[1,2] The name pseudotumor cerebri syndrome was formerly used to describe this syndrome in the literature, which has more recently been revived. Some investigators suggest that primary PTCS and IIH are equivalent terms and should be defined by their idiopathic nature. Cases with identifiable causes (eg, thrombosis or medications) should be termed secondary PTCS.[3] However, there is not yet widespread agreement or use of this terminology.

Epidemiology

IIH has an incidence of 0.9 to 2.4 per 100,000 in the general population; however, this rate is increasing in parallel with the ongoing obesity epidemic in the United States.[4] In obese women of childbearing age, the incidence of IIH is 20 times this level.[5,6] IIH can occur in pediatric populations and shows similar predilection for male and female patients before the age of 7 years.[7] After the first decade of life, IIH predominately affects female-to-male patients at a ratio of 6 to 10:1.[8,9]

Although patients with IIH are typically cared for by an interdisciplinary team, otolaryngologists increasingly play an important role in the initial diagnosis and management of IIH complications, particularly spontaneous cerebrospinal fluid (CSF) leak. This review surveys the recent literature on the topic of IIH with a focus on areas of interest to the otolaryngologist.

PATHOPHYSIOLOGY

There remains significant controversy surrounding the underlying mechanism of disease in IIH. It is generally agreed that cerebral venous hypertension is fundamental to the pathologic state in IIH, but why this occurs is unclear. Multiple theories exist to explain such hypertension, with many involving altered CSF flow dynamics, which itself is an incompletely understood concept.

Cerebrospinal Fluid Overproduction

Although overproduction of CSF has been proposed as the underlying cause in IIH, it is likely no more than a contributing factor in IIH. Patients with choroid plexus hyperplasia develop hydrocephalus, whereas patients with IIH retain normal ventricular architecture on neuroimaging.[10] Aquaporins are a family of water transport channels widely expressed in the membranes of the choroid plexus and ependymal cells of the ventricles as well as astrocytic foot processes along the blood-brain barrier and brain-CSF interfaces. Research in animal models has shown that alterations in aquaporins can result in excess CSF; however, there is no clear association with IIH in humans.[10]

Impaired Cerebrospinal Fluid Resorption

Impaired CSF resorption has also been posited as an underlying cause and is supported by the commonly identified neuroimaging finding of venous stenosis, often in the bilateral or dominant transverse sinuses.[11] Although transverse sinus stent placement relieves patient symptoms, the stenosis can recur.[12] Patients that undergo CSF diversion, such as a ventriculoperitoneal shunt (VPS), demonstrate improved sinus patency, suggesting that stenosis is a result of extrinsic compression and not the cause of IIH.[13,14] Although CSF drainage was previously thought to occur primarily at the arachnoid villi and granulations, burgeoning evidence suggests alternative drainage mechanisms, including through the glymphatic system, the central nervous system (CNS) lymphatics drainage system.[15]

Obesity, Inflammation, and Obstructive Sleep Apnea

Seventy percent to 80% of patients with IIH are obese; however, the pathophysiologic mechanism linking obesity and IIH is unclear.[16] It is thought that central adipose accumulation may support elevated intra-abdominal pressures by compression, extending these pressures across the pleural and cardiac spaces, resulting in decreased venous return from the brain and therefore decreased CSF absorption.[17] Indeed, bariatric surgery is an effective treatment for IIH, even in cases that are resistant to other methods of intervention.[18] However, not all patients with IIH are obese, and for this reason, it is thought that obesity is only a contributory factor to existing IIH.[19] CSF leptin is significantly elevated in patients with IIH, regardless of obesity status, suggesting a potential role of hypothalamic leptin resistance in the pathogenesis of IIH.[20]

There appears to be a link between IIH and an obesity-associated elevation of inflammatory molecules. It is well documented that obesity is consistent with a low-grade proinflammatory state.[21,22] Oligoclonal bands and elevated CSF cytokines can be elevated in patients with IIH.[23] However, how a proinflammatory state might contribute to the pathogenesis of IIH remains unclear. In addition, early studies showed increased vitamin A and its metabolites in the CSF of patients with IIH.[24] However, more recent analyses with improved methods of measuring these substances suggest vitamin levels are not causing a direct toxic effect.[25]

The increased incidence of IIH seen in women of childbearing age and the lack of gender predilection in pediatric populations suggest that sex steroids may play a role in disease development. Although no discrete hormonal signature has been identified, there is building evidence that steroid dysregulation at the cellular level may be contributing to raised ICP.[26] About 10% of IIH cases occur in men, and important differences in associated comorbidities exist between sexes.[9] For example, men with IIH are significantly more likely to have associated obstructive sleep apnea (OSA) than women.[9] It is thought that OSA might contribute to IIH with nocturnal hypoxia and hypercapnia, raising venous cerebral pressures.[27] In a cohort of 721 IIH patients, nearly a quarter of men were found to have concomitant OSA, as compared with only 4% of women.[9] During extended CSF pressure monitoring in asleep men with OSA, ICPs were noted to increase as high as 750 mm H_2O following apneic episodes.[28]

It is likely that a combination of factors that contribute to IIH, and a new hypothesis into the origins of IIH should favor multifactorial mechanisms.

CLINICAL PRESENTATION
Headache

Because of the heterogeneity of presenting symptoms, patients with IIH might first be evaluated by numerous specialists, including neurologists, ophthalmologists, or otolaryngologists. Headache is the most common presenting symptom in IIH (84%–100%), is constant or daily in about half of cases, and severely impacts the quality of life.[29–32] In a review of 165 patients participating in the Idiopathic Intracranial Hypertension Treatment Trial (IIHTT), the largest prospective cohort of untreated patients, headache was associated with substantial disability.[29] Furthermore, most patients with headache (85%) reported it to be pulsatile and progressively painful, often associated with vomiting.[30] Headache in IIH has originally been thought of as distinct from migraine, but with significant overlap of symptoms, including visual disturbances, migraine has emerged as a common phenotypic descriptor. Several case series that include descriptions of headache symptoms suggest that migraine is the most common headache phenotype seen in IIH.[33]

Visual Disturbance

Changes in vision are a hallmark symptom of IIH. Transient visual obscurations lasting less than 30 seconds are reported in most patients (68% of the IIHTT cohort), although they are notably not specific to IIH.[29] The spectrum of visual change extends from floaters and diplopia to complete visual loss, a complication of advanced disease that can occur in about 10% of patients, although rates may be higher in male and pediatric patients.[9,29,30,34,35] Patients with IIH do not present with focal neurologic deficits; however, the exception is an isolated abducens nerve palsy.[29] Bilateral papilledema is another common finding on fundoscopic examination and arises because of increased ICP expanding the subarachnoid compartment of the optic nerve, although such edema can arise asymmetrically and is not always present.[36]

Otologic Manifestations

The above hallmark manifestations of IIH are relatively nonspecific, and it is important for the otolaryngologist to be aware of them in circumstances during which patients present primarily with neurotologic complaints, such as tinnitus. Pulsatile tinnitus is reported in one-half to three-quarters of IIH patients, often bilaterally, and they are consistently found to have sigmoid sinus wall abnormalities on neuroimaging.[29,37,38] Venous sinus stenting relieves pulsatile tinnitus, suggesting that a combination of raised ICP and turbulent flow may be the underlying mechanism.[39] Of note, tinnitus can also occur unilaterally (one-third of the IIHTT cohort) or continuously.[37]

An often-cited comorbidity is dizziness, with some reports suggesting that most patients experience vestibular disturbance.[29] The mechanism remains unclear, although it has been suggested that increased ICP could cause compressive effects of the cochleovestibular nerves or the brainstem.[40] The similarity in presentation and demographic profile between Meniere's, vestibular migraine, and IIH are striking and have been noted throughout the literature.[41] Although further research is required to reliably differentiate these conditions, a detailed history with a particular focus on visual obscurations may help to elucidate the underlying pathologic condition.

Spontaneous Cerebrospinal Fluid Leak

Spontaneous CSF leak is a known complication of IIH, and on initial presentation, patients may complain of rhinorrhea, otorrhea, meningitis, hearing loss, or postural headache.[42] There is extensive overlap between the demographic, clinical, and radiographic profiles of patients with these 2 disorders (ie, obese premenopausal women), and for this reason, it is suspected that many patients with CSF leak have underlying IIH.[43] However, CSF outflow effectively reduces ICP, thus providing relief from compression damage, masking symptoms, and obscuring or postponing IIH diagnosis. For this reason, it is unsurprising that those with CSF leak present with similar symptoms to those with IIH, such as headache, tinnitus, and diplopia, however, at significantly lower rates.[44]

Spontaneous CSF leak is an increasingly recognized condition, which is reflected in the increasing number of referrals and craniotomies performed each year.[44,45] Case series have identified that in patients presenting with spontaneous CSF leak, 28% to as high as 72% have verifiable underlying IIH.[46,47] Often rhinorrhea (67%) is the most common presentation with leak occurring from the temporal bone (39%), followed by the ethmoid (28%) and sphenoid (28%) bones.[46] Interestingly, patients with CSF leak present at an older age than IIH patients (eg, 50 years), presumably because of interval calvarium thinning, with otherwise similar baseline clinicodemographic characteristics.[46]

Although it is unclear how many patients with spontaneous CSF leak have underlying IIH, this further supports the notion that IIH is a contributory mechanism in that patients with CSF leak at the level of the skull base rarely develop symptoms of hypotension, suggesting a state of pressure equilibrium is reached.[48]

Other

Other otolaryngologic manifestations in IIH include aural fullness, low-frequency sensorineural hearing loss, and sensitivity to loudness.[37,40] Hemifacial spasm, or unilateral facial nerve hyperexcitability resulting in involuntary contraction of facial musculature, has also been reported in rare instances.[49]

DIAGNOSIS AND TESTING
Key Consults and Testing

Patients may present initially to an otolaryngologist with symptoms such as pulsatile tinnitus or dizziness. They may present with sleep apnea. Sometimes, patients will present with spontaneous CSF leaks, such as CSF rhinorrhea or otorrhea, from the anterior or lateral skull base, respectively.[41] It is important to get a history, including these associated symptoms of headaches and visual changes. These patients need neurology and ophthalmology consult for further testing and evaluation. Other consults to be considered include neurosurgery, bariatric surgery, nutritionist, or sleep specialist, as many of these patients are obese and may have sleep apnea. Referral to the ophthalmologist is important for a funduscopic examination and visual fields testing to determine whether papilledema is present and if there is visual compromise. Neuroimaging with an MRI of the brain is preferred to rule out any mass lesions; however, a computed tomographic (CT) scan of the head can be a more rapid imaging technique if MRI is not immediately or readily available. A lumbar puncture with opening pressure is necessary in patients suspected of having IIH, although the pressure may be falsely normal in the event of an active CSF leak. Other confounders that can have an effect on lumbar puncture opening pressure include body position, emotions such as crying and anxiety, or pain.[41]

Modified Dandy Criteria

The criteria for the diagnosis of IIH are the modified Dandy criteria described in 1985, listed in **Box 1**. These criteria include (1) the signs and symptoms of increased ICP, including headache, transient visual obscurations, tinnitus, papilledema, and visual loss; (2) no impaired consciousness or localizing neurologic deficits on examination except possibly cranial nerve VI palsies; (3) increases in lumbar puncture opening

---

Box 1
Modified Dandy criteria

The modified Dandy diagnostic criteria for idiopathic intracranial hypertension
1. Signs and symptoms of increased intracranial pressure, including headache, visual changes, papilledema
2. Absence of localizing neurologic signs except unilateral or bilateral abducens nerve palsy
3. Elevated CSF opening pressure greater than 25 cm H_2O with normal CSF composition
4. Normal or small symmetric ventricles on imaging with no intracranial mass or venous obstruction
5. No other cause of increased intracranial pressure

pressure greater than 250 mm H2O or 25 cm H2O with normal CSF composition on analysis; (4) imaging showing no other cause for elevated ICP; and (5) no other reason for elevated ICP is found.[8,17,30,41]

Friedman Diagnostic Criteria

These criteria were updated by Freidman in 2013 with criteria for patients with and without papilledema, as shown in **Box 2**. The criteria usually required for diagnosis include (A) papilledema, (B) normal neurologic examination except for cranial nerve abnormalities, (C) normal neuroimaging without hydrocephalus or mass lesion, (D) normal CSF composition, and (E) elevated lumbar puncture opening pressure greater than 250 mm H2O in adults and greater than 280 mm H2O in children. For patients without papilledema, a diagnosis of IIH can be made if criteria B–E are met, the patient has at least 1 CN VI palsy, and 3 of 4 possible neuroimaging criteria are met. These neuroimaging criteria include (1) empty sella, (2) flattening of the posterior aspect of the globe, (3) distention or perioptic subarachnoid space with or without a tortuous optic nerve, and (4) transverse venous sinus stenosis. Freidman splits patients into 2 groups, those with and those without papilledema. If the measured CSF pressure is lower than 350 mm H2O, but all other criteria are met, then the diagnosis is considered probable IIH.[3,17,41]

Idiopathic Intracranial Hypertension Treatment Trial

The IIHTT developed an algorithm in 2014, which essentially is identical to the modified Dandy criteria except that the threshold for elevated CSF opening pressure is

---

Box 2
Friedman diagnostic criteria for idiopathic intracranial hypertension

1. Required for diagnosis:
   A. Papilledema
   B. Normal neurologic examination except for cranial nerve 6 abnormalities
   C. Neuroimaging: Normal brain parenchyma without evidence of hydrocephalus, mass, or structural lesion and no abnormal meningeal enhancement on MRI, with and without gadolinium, for typical patients (female and obese), and MRI, with and without gadolinium, and magnetic resonance venography for others; if MRI is unavailable or contraindicated, contrast-enhanced CT may be used
   D. Normal CSF composition
   E. Elevated lumbar puncture opening pressure (>25 cm H2O in adults and >28 cm H2O in children [25 cm H2O if the child is not sedated and not obese])

2. Diagnosis without papilledema:
   A. Diagnosis made if B–E from above are satisfied, and the patient has a unilateral or bilateral abducens nerve palsy
   B. Suggested diagnosis if B–E from above are satisfied, and in addition at least 3 of the following neuroimaging criteria are satisfied:
      i. Empty sella
      i. Flattening of the posterior aspect of the globe
      i. Distention of the perioptic subarachnoid space with or without a tortuous optic nerve
      i. Transverse venous sinus stenosis
         A diagnosis is definite if the patient fulfills criteria A–E. The diagnosis is probable if criteria A–D are met but the measured CSF pressure is lower than specified for a definite diagnosis

Data from Friedman DI, Liu GT, Digre KB. Revised diagnostic criteria for the pseudotumor cerebri syndrome in adults and children. *Neurology.* 2013;81(13):1159-1165. https://doi.org/10.1212/WNL.0b013e3182a55f17

lowered to 20 cm H_2O in certain instances.[17] If the opening pressure is 20 to 25 cm H_2O, the patient also needs to have at least one of these criteria: (1) pulse-synchronous tinnitus, (2) abducens nerve palsy, (3) grade II papilledema, (4) no evidence of pseudo-papilledema, (5) lateral sinus stenosis or collapse on magnetic resonance venography (MRV), and (6) partially empty sella with unfolded perioptic nerve CSF spaces.[50] Given that the IIHTT study sought to determine the effectiveness of weight loss and acetazolamide on vision, the study also had bilateral papilledema and visual field loss in their inclusion criteria.[50]

Secondary Causes of Elevated Intracranial Pressure to Rule Out

Table 1 shows several conditions to consider that may cause secondary intracranial hypertension. As previously mentioned, neuroimaging with an MRI of the brain and a lumbar puncture with opening pressure are key in the diagnosis of IIH. MRI of the brain is required to rule out any mass lesions, cerebral venous sinus thromboses, bilateral jugular vein thrombosis, obstructive hydrocephalus, middle ear, or mastoid infection. In addition, one should ensure that there has not been surgical ligation of bilateral jugular veins, no previous intracranial infection, or subarachnoid hemorrhage causing decreased CSF absorption. Systemic venous abnormalities, including elevated right heart pressure, superior vena cava syndrome, and arteriovenous fistulas, should be excluded.[3,10,34]

A comprehensive review of the patient's medication list and supplements should be performed, as certain medications can elevate ICP. These include antibiotics, including tetracycline, minocycline, doxycycline, nalidixic acid, and sulfa drugs. Vitamins, including vitamin A, and retinoids, such as isotretinoin and all-trans retinoic acid, used in the treatment of promyelocytic leukemia have been implicated in elevated ICP. Hormones and hormone modulators, including human growth hormone, thyroxine (in children), leuprorelin acetate, levonorgestrel (Norplant system), danazol, and other contraceptive drugs, as well as anabolic steroids and withdrawal from chronic corticosteroids can elevate ICP. Other drugs and exposures, including lithium, chlordecone, carbidopa/levodopa, cyclosporin, and phenytoin, have been implicated in elevated ICP.[3,17,41]

Elevated ICPs can also be a secondary effect of other diagnoses. These other diagnoses include endocrine disorders, such as Addison disease and hypoparathyroidism, and genetic syndromes, such as Turner syndrome or Down syndrome. Hypercapnia from sleep apnea and Pickwickian syndrome, as well as other medical conditions, can also elevate ICPs.[3] Although some consider OSA to be a secondary cause of elevated ICPs, it is an important entity to consider in the treatment of intracranial hypertension, and thus, the authors discuss it as part of treatment in their review.[3,10,34]

THERAPEUTIC OPTIONS

The major goals for the treatment of IIH are to relieve the patient's headache and to protect vision.[41] If vision is imminently threatened, this is termed fulminant IIH, and more invasive treatment, such as surgery, should be considered immediately to preserve vision, as shown in **Fig. 1**. If the patient has a diagnosis of IIH and vision is stable, medical management can be considered first. In the event of an active CSF leak, repair of the leak to prevent meningitis with adjunct medical therapies should be considered.

Weight Loss

Particularly in obese patients, an initial step in treatment includes lifestyle modification and weight loss.[29,41] Studies have shown that a 5% to 10% reduction in body weight

Table 1
Secondary causes for elevated intracranial pressure

Venous drainage obstruction	Cerebral venous sinus thrombosis Bilateral jugular vein thrombosis or surgical ligation Superior vena cava syndrome Increased right heart pressure Arteriovenous fistulas Previous infection (eg, intracranial, mastoid) Previous subarachnoid hemorrhage
Medications and exposures	Antibiotics • Fluoroquinolones • Tetracycline • Minocycline • Doxycycline • Nalidixic acid • Sulfa Vitamin A derivatives • Isotretinoin • All-trans retinoic acid Steroids • Corticosteroid withdrawal • Anabolic steroids Hormones (modulators) • Danazol • Levonorgestrel implant • Growth hormone • Leuprorelin acetate • Levothyroxine (in children) • Tamoxifen Cyclosporin Lithium Indomethacin Cimetidine Carbidopa/levodopa Phenytoin Chlordecone
Endocrine	Addison's disease Adrenal insufficiency Cushing syndrome Hypoparathyroidism Hypothyroidism Hyperthyroidism
Other medical conditions	Chronic kidney disease/renal failure Hematologic • Anemia • Polycythemia vera Hypercapnia • Obstructive sleep apnea • Pickwickian syndrome • Chronic obstructive pulmonary disease Systemic lupus erythematosus Psittacosis
Syndromic	Down syndrome Craniosynostosis Turner syndrome

Data from Friedman DI, Liu GT, Digre KB. Revised diagnostic criteria for the pseudotumor cerebri syndrome in adults and children. *Neurology.* 2013;81(13):1159-1165. https://doi.org/10.1212/WNL.0b013e3182a55f17 and intracranial hypertension: Pathophysiology and management. *J Neurol Neurosurg Psychiatry.* 2016;87(9):982-992. https://doi.org/10.1136/jnnp-2015-311302

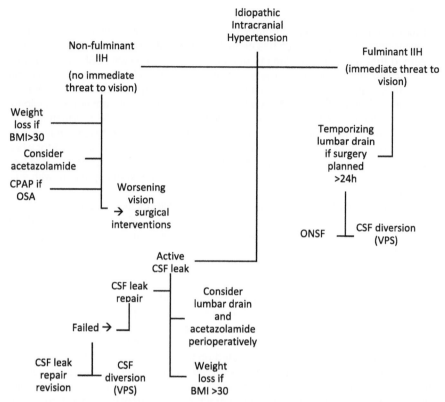

Fig. 1. IIH treatment algorithm. Treatment algorithm for IIH when vision is not immediately threatened, starting with medical management. When vision is threatened, often surgical approaches are necessary to preserve vision. In the event of an active CSF leak, the leak should be repaired surgically, with medical management perioperatively, and consideration of surgical management such as CSF diversion should there be recurrent CSF leak. BMI, body mass inde. (*Data from* Mukherjee N, Bhatti MT. Update on the surgical management of idiopathic intracranial hypertension. Curr Neurol Neurosci Rep. 2014;14:438. doi:10.1007/s11910-014-0438-8 and Mollan SP, Ali F, Hassan-Smith G, Botfield H, Friedman DI, Sinclair AJ. Evolving evidence in adult idiopathic intracranial hypertension: Pathophysiology and management. J Neurol Neurosurg Psychiatry. 2016;87(9):982-992. doi:10.1136/jnnp-2015-311302)

is associated with improvement or resolution of papilledema.[16,17,51,52] In addition, CSF opening pressure can decrease up to 8 cm H_2O with improvement in headaches.[16] A community weight loss program can be an initial step to result in weight loss achievement and can result in success, although some patients will require bariatric surgery.[18,53]

Continuous Positive Airway Pressure

For patients with OSA, an important initial step in treatment is to initiate continuous positive airway pressure (CPAP) at the appropriate titrated dose to decrease apneas while asleep. This can lead to normalization of ICPs and significant symptom improvement.[41]

Diuretics

Diuretics are a mainstay in the treatment of intracranial hypertension. The most used diuretic is acetazolamide, which has been the subject of clinical trials. The IIHTT study confirmed that using acetazolamide does improve visual fields, CSF opening pressure, papilledema by objective measures, and quality of life as compared with placebo. Study patients were given high doses of up to 4 g per day with no safety or tolerability concerns.[17,29,33,41,54] Acetazolamide is a carbonic anhydrase inhibitor, and the mechanism of action to decrease ICP is to decrease CSF production in the choroid plexus. The recommended dosing is to start at 500 mg twice a day and increase the dosage to up to 4 g per day as appropriate. The major side effect for which patients should be counseled is significant paresthesia in the hands. It can also be a photosensitizer and is a sulfa drug so would be contraindicated in patients with sulfa allergies.

Other diuretics that can be used in the treatment of IIH include furosemide, alone or in combination with other diuretics, such as acetazolamide. Furosemide has a side effect of hypokalemia. Chlorthalidone can also be used as a diuretic alone or in combination.[17,30]

Other Medications

Second-line medications for IIH include topiramate and corticosteroids. Topiramate is a medication commonly used for migraine prophylaxis and has mild carbonic anhydrase inhibitor activity. This medication is an appetite suppressant and often has the beneficial side effect of weight loss for the patients taking topiramate. Dosage usually starts at 25 mg daily and can be titrated up to 100 mg twice a day as tolerated.[55]

Corticosteroids are not used as a direct treatment modality for IIH, but rather they are used in the short term for acute visual loss. Furthermore, with corticosteroid withdrawal, patients can develop rebound intracranial hypertension. Therefore, a prolonged corticosteroid taper is recommended.[30,41]

Lumbar Puncture and Lumbar Drain

Historically, serial lumbar punctures have been used to drain CSF from the CNS and decrease ICP.[30,41] However, given that CSF is constantly being produced and reaccumulates within 6 hours after CSF drainage, this method is not effective or practical. In the short term, a lumbar drain is placed to relieve ICP and decrease stress on the skull base after a CSF leak repair, as will be discussed later.

SURGICAL MANAGEMENT
Cerebrospinal Fluid Leak Repair

Patients with IIH can develop spontaneous CSF leaks and encephaloceles owing to the ICP, causing pressure points at the skull base leading to chronic bone resorption. Sometimes, there may be multiple areas of bone defects in 10% to 20% of these patients, resulting in multifocal location for CSF leak.[56] Patients can have an anterior skull base CSF leak or a middle cranial fossa CSF leak, or sometimes a combination of the 2 locations. Both can present with CSF rhinorrhea, as a middle cranial fossa tegmen defect can lead to CSF collecting in the middle ear and draining into the nasopharynx via the Eustachian tube in the absence of tympanic membrane perforation. This can additionally result in conductive hearing loss. With a tympanic membrane perforation, there can be CSF otorrhea. Collecting fluid from CSF rhinorrhea or otorrhea and sending the fluid for a beta-2 transferrin assay confirms that the fluid is indeed CSF.

Nasal endoscopy and otomicroscopy, as well as CT scans, can aid in the diagnosis of the location for the CSF leakage.

The indication for the repair of these CSF leaks is the theory that patients are at increased risk of developing meningitis with an active CSF leak, with CSF rhinorrhea thought to be at higher risk than CSF otorrhea.[42,57] Perioperative antibiotics for CSF leak repair should cover pneumococcus and staphylococcus, as well as consideration for pseudomonas in lateral skull base repairs.[56]

Anterior skull base spontaneous CSF leaks most commonly develop in the cribriform plate and sphenoid sinus. These can additionally span more than 1 sinus or be multifocal.[57] The mainstay of repair of these CSF leaks is an endoscopic approach with multilayer closure of the leak. The multilayer closure can involve a combination of abdominal fat, temporalis fascia versus acellular dermis versus fascia lata, and a free mucosa graft or nasoseptal flap. Occasionally, a bone graft is used.[57] After repair, these CSF leaks have a high recurrence rate of 25% to 87%.[42,57] To decrease the possibility of a recurrence, a lumbar drain and bedrest are often used to help drain CSF to decrease ICP. In addition, some patients are placed on acetazolamide perioperatively, whether in the hospital or after discharge as an outpatient to decrease ICP; however, this has not been shown to reduce the recurrence of CSF leak.[57] Active management of elevated ICP, however, does increase the success rate of CSF leak closure at 92.8% compared with 81.9% for patients who did not undergo active management of elevated ICP.[58] Recurrent CSF leaks after repair are often due to unrecognized elevated ICP or the inability to control the elevated ICP with medications, therefore requiring a VPS.[42,57]

Temporal bone spontaneous CSF leaks are most commonly present in the tegmen tympani and tegmen mastoideum.[59] Similar to anterior skull base CSF leaks, multiple defects can be present, up to two-thirds of the time with temporal bone CSF leaks.[59] Similar to anterior skull base defects, multilayer closure with 2 to 3 layers of material is necessary for the success of defect closure. The materials used include a soft tissue seal, such as temporalis fascia, abdominal fat, or dural regeneration matrix, and resurfacing with bone graft, bone cement, or cartilage.[59] The most common surgical approach for temporal bone CSF leak repair is the middle fossa craniotomy. This approach exposes the entire tegmen mastoideum and tegmen tympani without disturbing the ossicles. The disadvantages of the middle fossa craniotomy include intensive care unit monitoring, temporal lobe injury, seizures, transient aphasia, and intracranial hematoma. An alternative approach to the tegmen mastoideum that avoids a craniotomy is the transmastoid approach; however, defects in the tegmen tympanicum may cause disturbance of the ossicular chain. This approach has the advantage of being able to repair a posterior fossa defect, however.[59]

Other lateral skull base issues resulting from chronic IIH include superior semicircular canal dehiscence.

Cerebrospinal Fluid Shunting

When conservative management and medications to control elevated ICP fail, a VPS can be placed by the neurosurgical team. This results in a fast and sustained reduction in ICP. Major indications for a VPS include advancing vision loss, debilitating headaches, and recurrent CSF leaks. The complications of this procedure include infection rates of 5% to 7%, shunt obstruction leading to recurrent elevated ICP, and revision procedures. The rate of revision procedures is quoted to be as high as 30% for VPS. However, VPS have fewer complications compared with lumboperitoneal shunts, which can require revision procedures 60% of the time and are infrequently used today.[17,30,41]

Transverse Sinus Shunting

When transverse sinus stenosis is seen in neuroimaging, such as MRV or CT venography (CTV), stenting of the sinus with an endovascular procedure can be considered. This corrects the venous outflow obstruction at the stenosed dural sinus. The complications of this procedure include subdural hematoma, venous thrombosis, and need for long-term antiplatelet medication use owing to the stent. The procedure has a failure rate of 10%, with restenosis of the venous sinus commonly occurring, suggesting this is not a primary mechanism for elevated ICP, but rather the elevated ICP causing the dural sinus stenosis.[17,41]

Optic Nerve Sheath Fenestration

Optic nerve sheath fenestration (ONSF) is a procedure performed primarily by ophthalmologists in the setting of visual loss with papilledema for which medical therapy has been ineffective. This procedure leads to improvement with the optic nerve but has no effect on ICP, as it does not alter the CNS. The patients selected for this procedure often have poor preoperative visual acuity, although studies have shown a similar magnitude of vision improvement is achieved with VPS.[17,30,41,60,61]

DISCUSSION

IIH typically presents as a triad of headaches, visual changes, and papilledema, although patients can present initially to an otolaryngologist with complaints such as tinnitus, dizziness, hearing loss, and CSF otorrhea or rhinorrhea. Appropriate diagnosis of this condition with the modified Dandy criteria or the Friedman diagnostic criteria with appropriate referral to neurology and ophthalmology colleagues, as well as neuroimaging and lumbar puncture with opening pressure is necessary. Treatment goals are to relieve headaches, prevent visual loss, and close any CSF leak. Management can be conservative with weight loss in obese patients, treatment of OSA, including diuretics, most commonly acetazolamide, or other medications, such as topiramate. Surgical treatment is indicated for active CSF leaks to prevent meningitis. CSF shunting is often successful in decreasing ICP and preventing vision loss. Transverse sinus stenting can be considered, although restenosis can occur. ONSF procedures are often performed by ophthalmologists when medical treatment has failed to prevent worsening vision but does not relieve ICP.

SUMMARY

IIH can play a role in some of the patients that otolaryngologists manage, particularly those with anterior or lateral skull base CSF leaks. It is important to recognize this entity, make appropriate referrals, and appropriately diagnose and treat IIH.

CLINICS CARE POINTS

- Having suspicion for idiopathic intracranial hypertension with appropriate referrals to neurology and ophthalmology and performing neuroimaging and lumbar puncture with opening pressure are key to the diagnosis and management of idiopathic intracranial hypertension.
- The major goals of idiopathic intracranial hypertension treatment are to prevent vision loss, improve headaches, and close an active cerebrospinal fluid leak if present to prevent meningitis.
- Cerebrospinal fluid opening pressure may be elevated or falsely normal in patients with an active cerebrospinal fluid leak. Consideration of the diagnosis of idiopathic intracranial

hypertension and management of elevated intracranial pressure before cerebrospinal fluid leak repair and perioperatively is crucial to the success of the repair.

- In obese patients, 5% to 10% weight loss with lifestyle modification, medical treatment, and bariatric surgery, if necessary, will improve papilledema, decrease cerebrospinal fluid opening pressure, and improve headaches.

- In patients with obstructive sleep apnea, initiation of continuous positive airway pressure can be key to normalization of elevated intracranial pressure and significant symptom improvement.

- Acetazolamide, starting at 500 mg twice a day with dose escalation up to 4 g a day, is a well-tolerated diuretic that improves vision and papilledema and decreases intracranial pressure with symptom improvement.

- Topiramate is a second-line medication for idiopathic intracranial hypertension and has the beneficial side effect of weight loss.

- Sometimes a ventriculoperitoneal shunt placed by neurosurgeons is necessary for control of intracranial pressures and to prevent worsening vision.

- Transverse sinus stenting can be considered when transverse sinus stenosis is seen on neuroimaging; however, it has a high failure and restenosis rate, as it is the elevated intracranial pressures causing the stenosis.

- Optic nerve sheath fenestration is a procedure that can be performed by ophthalmologists in patients with worsening vision when medical therapy for idiopathic intracranial hypertension has failed. This procedure only addresses vision and not the elevated intracranial pressure.

DISCLOSURE

The authors have nothing to disclose.

REFERENCES

1. Best J, Silvestri G, Burton B, et al. The incidence of blindness due to idiopathic intracranial hypertension in the UK. Open Ophthalmol J 2013;7(1):26–9.
2. D'Amico D, Curone M, Ciasca P, et al. Headache prevalence and clinical features in patients with idiopathic intracranial hypertension (IIH). Neurol Sci 2013; 34(SUPPL. 1):147–9.
3. Friedman DI, Liu GT, Digre KB. Revised diagnostic criteria for the pseudotumor cerebri syndrome in adults and children. Neurology 2013;81(13):1159–65.
4. Kilgore KP, Lee MS, Leavitt JA, et al. Re-evaluating the incidence of idiopathic intracranial hypertension in an era of increasing obesity. Ophthalmology 2017; 124(5):697–700.
5. McCluskey G, Mulholland DA, McCarron P, et al. Idiopathic intracranial hypertension in the northwest of Northern Ireland: epidemiology and clinical management. Neuroepidemiology 2015;45:34–9.
6. Durcan FJ, Corbett JJ, Wall M. Population studies in Iowa and Louisiana. Arch Neurol 1988;45:875–7.
7. Matthews YY, Dean F, Lim MJ, et al. Pseudotumor cerebri syndrome in childhood: incidence, clinical profile and risk factors in a national prospective population-based cohort study. Arch Dis Child 2017;102(8):715–21.
8. Sundholm A, Burkill S, Sveinsson O, et al. Population-based incidence and clinical characteristics of idiopathic intracranial hypertension. Acta Neurol Scand 2017;136(5):427–33.

9. Bruce BB, Kedar S, Van Stavern GP, et al. Idiopathic intracranial hypertension in men. Neurology 2009;72:304–9.
10. Baykan B, Ekizoğlu E, Altiokka Uzun G. An update on the pathophysiology of idiopathic intracranial hypertension alias pseudotumor cerebri. Agri 2015;27(2): 63–72.
11. Riggeal BD, Bruce BB, Saindane AM, et al. Clinical course of idiopathic intracranial hypertension with transverse sinus stenosis. Neurology 2013;80(3):289–95.
12. Ahmed RM, Wilkinson M, Parker GD, et al. Transverse sinus stenting for idiopathic intracranial hypertension: a review of 52 patients and of model predictions. Am J Neuroradiol 2011;32(8):1408–14.
13. Rohr A, Dorner L, Stingele R, et al. Reversibility of venous sinus obstruction in idiopathic intracranial hypertension. AJNR 2007;28:656–9.
14. Higgins JNP, Pickard JD. Lateral sinus stenoses in idiopathic intracranial hypertension resolving after CSF diversion. Neurology 2004;62:1907–8.
15. Tamura R, Yoshida K, Toda M. Current understanding of lymphatic vessels in the central nervous system. Neurosurg Rev 2020;43(4):1055–64.
16. Subramaniam S, Fletcher WA. Obesity and weight loss in idiopathic intracranial hypertension: a narrative review. J Neuroophthalmol 2017;37(2):197–205.
17. Burkett JG, Ailani J. An up to date review of pseudotumor cerebri syndrome. Curr Neurol Neurosci Rep 2018;18(6):1–7.
18. Handley JD, Baruah BP, Williams DM, et al. Bariatric surgery as a treatment for idiopathic intracranial hypertension: a systematic review. Surg Obes Relat Dis 2015;11(6):1396–403.
19. Hannerz J, Ericson K. The relationship between idiopathic intracranial hypertension and obesity. Headache 2009;49:178–84.
20. Ball AK, Sinclair AJ, Curnow SJ, et al. Elevated cerebrospinal fluid (CSF) leptin in idiopathic intracranial hypertension (IIH): evidence for hypothalamic leptin resistance. Clin Endocrinol (Oxf) 2009;70:863–9.
21. Panagiotakos DB, Pitsavos C, Yannakoulia M, et al. The implication of obesity and central fat on markers of chronic inflammation: the ATTICA study. Atherosclerosis 2005;183:308–15.
22. Sinclair AJ, Ball AK, Burdon MA, et al. Exploring the pathogenesis of IIH: an inflammatory perspective. J Neuroimmunol 2008;201-202:212–20.
23. Altiokka-Uzun G, Tuzun E, Ekizoglu E, et al. Oligoclonal bands and increased cytokine levels in idiopathic intracranial hypertension. Cephalalgia 2015;35(13): 1153–61.
24. Warner JEA, Larson AJ, Bhosale P, et al. Retinol-binding protein and retinol analysis in cerebrospinal fluid and serum of patients with and without idiopathic intracranial hypertension. J Neuroophthalmol 2007;27(4):258–62.
25. Libien J, Kupersmith MJ, Blaner W, et al. Role of vitamin A metabolism in IIH: results from the idiopathic intracranial hypertension treatment trial. J Neurol Sci 2017;372:78–84.
26. Markey KA, Uldall M, Botfield H, et al. Idiopathic intracranial hypertension, hormones, and 11 β-hydroxysteroid dehydrogenases. J Pain Res 2016;9:223–32.
27. Jennum P, Borgesen SE. Intracranial pressure and obstructive sleep apnea. Chest 1989;95:279–83.
28. Sugita Y, Iijima S, Teshima Y, et al. Marked episodic elevation of cerebrospinal fluid pressure during nocturnal sleep in patients with sleep apnea hypersomnia syndrome. Electroencephalogr Clin Neurophysiol 1985;60:214–9.
29. Wall M, Kupersmith MJ, Kieburtz KD, et al. The idiopathic intracranial hypertension treatment trial clinical profile at baseline. JAMA Neurol 2014;71(6):693–701.

30. Wall M, George D. Idiopathic intracranial hypertension. Brain 1991;114:155–80.
31. Yiangou A, Mitchell J, Markey KA, et al. Therapeutic lumbar puncture for head-ache in idiopathic intracranial hypertension: minimal gain, is it worth the pain? Cephalalgia 2019;39(2):245–53.
32. Sinclair AJ, Kuruvath S, Sen D, et al. Is cerebrospinal fluid shunting in idiopathic intracranial hypertension worthwhile? A 10-year review. Cephalalgia 2011;31(16):1627–33.
33. Mollan SP, Ali F, Hassan-Smith G, et al. Evolving evidence in adult idiopathic intra-cranial hypertension: pathophysiology and management. J Neurol Neurosurg Psychiatry 2016;87(9):982–92.
34. Acheson JF. Idiopathic intracranial hypertension and visual function. Br Med Bull 2006;79-80(1):233–44.
35. Stiebel-Kalish H, Kalish Y, Lusky M, et al. Puberty as a risk factor for less favor-able visual outcome in idiopathic intracranial hypertension. Am J Ophthalmol 2006;142(2):279–84.
36. De Simone R, Ranieri A, Sansone M, et al. Dural sinus collapsibility, idiopathic intracranial hypertension, and the pathogenesis of chronic migraine. Neurol Sci 2019;40:59–70.
37. Ozer S, Ozer PA, Kaya SC, et al. Results of audiological evaluation in patients with idiopathic intracranial hypertension. J Int Adv Otol 2013;9(2):193–202.
38. Kline NL, Angster K, Archer E, et al. Association of pulse synchronous tinnitus and sigmoid sinus wall abnormalities in patients with idiopathic intracranial hyper-tension. Am J Otolaryngol 2020;41(6):102675.
39. Boddu S, Dinkin M, Suurna M, et al. Resolution of pulsatile tinnitus after venous sinus stenting in patients with idiopathic intracranial hypertension. PLoS One 2016;11(10):1–13.
40. Sismanis A. Otologic manifestations of benign intracranial hypertension syn-drome: diagnosis and management. Laryngoscope. 1987 Aug;97(S42):1-17.
41. Stevens SM, Rizk HG, Golnik K, et al. Idiopathic intracranial hypertension: contemporary review and implications for the otolaryngologist. Laryngoscope 2018;128(1):248–56.
42. Pérez MA, Bialer OY, Bruce BB, et al. Primary spontaneous cerebrospinal fluid leaks and idiopathic intracranial hypertension. J Neuroophthalmol 2013;33(4):327–34.
43. Tam EK, Gilbert AL. Spontaneous cerebrospinal fluid leak and idiopathic intracra-nial hypertension. Curr Opin Ophthalmol 2019;30(6):467–71.
44. Bidot S, Levy JM, Saindane AM, et al. Do most patients with a spontaneous ce-rebrospinal fluid leak have idiopathic intracranial hypertension? J Neuroophthalmol 2019;39(4):487–95.
45. Nelson RF, Gantz BJ, Hansen MR. The rising incidence of spontaneous cerebro-spinal fluid leaks in the United States and the association with obesity and obstructive sleep apnea. Otol Neurotol 2015;36(3):476–80.
46. Bidot S, Levy JM, Saindane AM, et al. Spontaneous skull base cerebrospinal fluid leaks and their relationship to idiopathic intracranial hypertension. Am J Rhinol Al-lergy 2021;35(1):36–43.
47. Schlosser RJ, Woodworth BA, Wilensky EM, et al. Spontaneous cerebrospinal fluid leaks: a variant of benign intracranial hypertension. Ann Otol Rhinol Laryngol 2006;115(7):495–500.
48. Schievink WI, Schwartz MS, Maya MM, et al. Lack of causal association between spontaneous intracranial hypotension and cranial cerebrospinal fluid leaks: clin-ical article. J Neurosurg 2012;116(4):749–54.

49. Poff CB, Lipschitz N, Kohlberg GD, et al. Hemifacial spasm as a rare clinical presentation of idiopathic intracranial hypertension: case report and literature review. Ann Otol Rhinol Laryngol 2020;129(8):829–32.

50. Friedman DI, McDermott MP, Kieburtz K, et al. The idiopathic intracranial hypertension treatment trial: design considerations and methods. J Neuroophthalmol 2014;34(2):107–17.

51. Kupersmith MJ, Gamell L, Turbin R, et al. Effects of weight loss on the course of idiopathic intracranial hypertension in women. Neurology 1998;50(4):1094–8.

52. Johnson LN, Krohel GB, Madsen RW, et al. The role of weight loss and acetazolamide in the treatment of idiopathic intracranial (pseudotumor cerebri). Ophthalmology 1998;105:2313–7.

53. Ottridge R, Mollan SP, Botfield H, et al. Randomised controlled trial of bariatric surgery versus a community weight loss programme for the sustained treatment of idiopathic intracranial hypertension: the idiopathic intracranial hypertension weight trial (IIH:WT) protocol. BMJ Open 2017;7(9):e017426.

54. ten Hove MW, Friedman DI, Patel AD, et al. Safety and tolerability of acetazolamide in the idiopathic intracranial hypertension treatment trial. J Neuroophthalmol 2016;36(1):13–9.

55. Thurtell MJ. Idiopathic intracranial hypertension. Contin (Minneap Minn) 2019; 25(5, Neuro-Ophthalmology):1289–309.

56. Stevens SM, Brown LSN, Ezell PC, et al. The mouse round-window approach for ototoxic agent delivery: a rapid and reliable technique for inducing cochlear cell degeneration. J Vis Exp 2015;2015(105):6–8.

57. Jiang ZY, McLean C, Perez C, et al. Surgical outcomes and postoperative management in spontaneous cerebrospinal fluid rhinorrhea. J Neurol Surgery, B Skull Base 2018;79(2):193–9.

58. Teachey W, Grayson J, Cho DY, et al. Intervention for elevated intracranial pressure improves success rate after repair of spontaneous cerebrospinal fluid leaks. Laryngoscope 2017;127(9):2011–6.

59. Kutz JW, Johnson AK, Wick CC. Surgical management of spontaneous cerebrospinal fistulas and encephaloceles of the temporal bone. Laryngoscope 2018; 128(9):2170–7.

60. Mukherjee N, Bhatti MT. Update on the surgical management of idiopathic intracranial hypertension. Curr Neurol Neurosci Rep 2014;14:438.

61. Fonseca PL, Rigamonti D, Miller NR, et al. Visual outcomes of surgical intervention for pseudotumour cerebri: optic nerve sheath fenestration versus cerebrospinal fluid diversion. Br J Ophthalmol 2014;98(10):1360–3.

Neuralgia and Atypical Facial, Ear, and Head Pain

Raffaello M. Cutri, BS[a], Dejan Shakya[b], Seiji B. Shibata, MD, PhD[c],*

KEYWORDS

- Temporomandibular dysfunction • Facial neuralgias
- Myofascial pain dysfunction syndrome • Trigeminal nerve • Glossopharyngeal nerve
- Intermedius nerve

KEY POINTS

- Trigeminal neuralgia (TN) manifests in the facial region innervated by the trigeminal nerve and causes pain in the jaw, teeth, or gums.
- Glossopharyngeal neuralgia (GPN) affects the glossopharyngeal nerve and causes pain in the throat, tongue, and ear canal, while geniculate neuralgia (GN) presents in the distribution of the intermedius nerve.
- Myofascial Pain Dysfunction Syndrome (MPDS) is a stress-related disorder characterized by pain that is often described as dull, radiating, unilateral, and aching.
- Diagnosis of MPDS requires that two of the three criteria be met: the presence of a taut band on palpation, a hypersensitive spot, and the presence of referred pain to a distant area.
- Pharmacologic therapy for TN, GPN, and GN includes anticonvulsants (namely carbamazepine), analgesics, steroids, and antidepressants (TCAs). For those who failed to respond to medications, microvascular decompression is the preferred surgical treatment.

INTRODUCTION

Though there have been considerable strides in the diagnosis and care of orofacial pain disorders, facial neuralgias, and myofascial pain dysfunction syndrome remain incredibly cumbersome for patients and difficult to manage for providers. Cranial neuralgias, myofascial pain syndromes, temporomandibular dysfunction (TMD), dental pain, tumors, neurovascular pain, and psychiatric diseases can all present with similar symptoms.[1] As a result, a patient's quest for the treatment of their orofacial pain often begins on the wrong foot, with a misdiagnosis or unnecessary procedure, which makes it all the more frustrating for them.[2] Understanding the natural history, clinical presentation, and management of facial neuralgias and myofascial pain dysfunction

[a] Keck School of Medicine, University of Southern California, 1537 Norfolk Street, Suite 5800, Los Angeles, CA 90033, USA; [b] Dornsife College of Letters, Arts and Science, University of Southern California, 1537 Norfolk Street, Suite 5800, Los Angeles, CA 90033, USA; [c] Caruso Department of Otolaryngology Head & Neck Surgery, University of Southern California, 1537 Norfolk Street, Suite 5800, Los Angeles, CA 90033, USA
* Corresponding author.
E-mail address: Seiji.Shibata@med.usc.edu

Otolaryngol Clin N Am 55 (2022) 595–606
https://doi.org/10.1016/j.otc.2022.02.006
0030-6665/22/© 2022 Elsevier Inc. All rights reserved.

oto.theclinics.com

syndrome can help clinicians better recognize and treat these conditions. In this article, we review updated knowledge on the pathophysiology, incidence, clinical features, diagnostic criteria, and medical management of TN, GPN, GN, and MPDS.

TRIGEMINAL NEURALGIA

The term *tic douloureux*, French for "painful tic," was first put in text in 1756 by Nicholas André.[4] His documented case studies depicted patients with facial spasms that were caused by agonizing facial pain. Now referred to as trigeminal neuralgia, the condition generally presents as short episodes of lancinating, unilateral pain affecting the jaw, teeth, or gums that last for seconds to minutes at a time. The pain can be triggered easily by everyday activities such as eating or speaking and occurs due to the disruption of the trigeminal nerve.[5,6]

The trigeminal nerve possesses three branches: the ophthalmic nerve (V1), the maxillary nerve (V2), and the mandibular nerve (V3). Trigeminal neuralgia is characterized by pain in at least one of these 3 divisions.[7] Of the three, the maxillary nerve and the mandibular nerve are most commonly affected. The ophthalmic nerve, which gives sensation to the eyes and forehead, is usually spared, and is especially rarely targeted alone.[8] The maxillary nerve gives sensations to the roof of the mouth, the upper lip, and the cheeks, while the mandibular nerve gives sensation to the lower lip and jaw. The mandibular nerve is the only branch with motor function as well as sensory function and is most commonly associated with activities such as mastication and swallowing. The mandibular nerve is also the branch of the trigeminal nerve that most correlates with pain within trigeminal neuralgia, which explains why eating can trigger pain spells.[9] TN is most common in elderly populations, with a general incidence rate of 4.3 per 100,000 people in the United States.[10] The condition more commonly affects women compared to men in a 1.6:1 ratio.[11]

TN is classified into 3 categories: classic, secondary, or idiopathic. The cause of classic TN is suspected to be the result of neurovascular compression of the trigeminal nerve at the root entry zone (REZ).[12,13] This is supported by the fact that microvascular decompression (MVD) has shown strong improvement in the conduction of the trigeminal nerve via intraoperative electrode recordings.[14] Injury to the nerve root can also result in demyelination in the immediate and adjacent areas of the REZ, which can also play a part in the pathophysiology of trigeminal neuralgia.[15] Secondary TN occurs due to intracranial lesions including tumors, infarction, and multiple sclerosis, and idiopathic TN is whereby no cause is apparent.[16]

According to the International Classification of Headache Disorders (ICHD, 3rd edition, 2018), the diagnostic criteria for TN include recurrent attacks of unilateral facial pain, occurring in one or more divisions of the trigeminal nerve and not radiating beyond the distribution of the trigeminal nerve. The pain should also possess all of the following characteristics: the pain is severe, electric-shock-like, shooting, or stabbing in quality, the attacks last seconds to 2 minutes, and the onset of pain is triggered by innocuous stimuli, such as brushing the teeth. Additionally, the pain must not be better accounted for by another ICHD-3 diagnosis and should not be able to be traced back to any sort of neurologic deficit. It is important to note that neurologic examination may occasionally demonstrate sensory loss in the patient, and in those patients neuroimaging should be conducted to assess for other possible causes.[17] In general, it is recommended to include neuroimaging studies in the work up of trigeminal neuralgia to distinguish between classic and secondary TN. MRI or CT can identify intracranial lesions causing secondary TN, while MRI is useful to identify neurovascular compression in classic TN.[18,19]

The first step in treating TN is using pharmacologic agents such as carbamazepine, gabapentin, topiramate, and pregabalin.[5] Around 80% of patients with TN are able to manage their pain using such medications, but in the case whereby the medication is unsuccessful or unable to be used due to allergy or intolerable side effects, there are a number of surgical options that are readily available.[20] As mentioned previously, microvascular decompression is the favored procedure for patients that do not respond to medications. The procedure involves identifying the offending vessel that's compressing the trigeminal nerve root, moving it from under the nerve to over the nerve, and inserting a small sponge (eg, Teflon) to keep the artery separated from the nerve. Meta-analyses have shown that MVD is the most successful intervention in the treatment of classic trigeminal neuralgia, demonstrating low recurrence rates of pain. The most common complications of the procedure include CSF leak (2%), sensory loss in the distribution of the trigeminal nerve (2.9%), and ipsilateral hearing loss (1.8%).[21] Other procedural options include gamma knife radiosurgery, neurectomy, trigeminal rhizotomy, and peripheral nerve blocks.[22]

GLOSSOPHARYNGEAL NEURALGIA

Glossopharyngeal neuralgia (GPN) is often misdiagnosed as trigeminal neuralgia (TN). GPN consists of recurrent pain paroxysms that last seconds to minutes and are triggered by chewing, coughing, yawning, talking, and swallowing. However, GPN occurs in the distribution of the glossopharyngeal nerve and pharyngeal and auricular branches of the vagus nerve, affecting the back of the throat, base of the tongue, tonsillar fossa, ear canal, and the angle of the mandible.[23] Like TN, the pain has been described as sharp, stabbing, "electric shock-like," and "needle-like." The pain nearly always manifests unilaterally and more frequently on the left side. Clusters of pain attacks can last for weeks to months with the time between paroxysms ranging from minutes to hours. GPN is relapsing and remitting in nature and intervals between clusters are irregular, ranging from days to years.[24] In approximately 10% of cases, patients may experience profound vagal effects causing bradycardia, syncope, hypotension, seizures, and cardiac arrest.[25,26] This is known as vagoglossopharyngeal neuralgia and arises due to the communication between the carotid sinus nerve (a branch of cranial nerve IX) and the vagus nerve. Activation of the carotid sinus nerve can stimulate the vagus nerve and trigger a vagal reaction (ie, arrhythmia, hypotension, syncope).[27]

Knowing the anatomy of the glossopharyngeal nerve is important to understand the triggers of GPN as well as its surgical management. The glossopharyngeal nerve possesses somatosensory, visceral sensory, efferent motor, and parasympathetic fibers. Its branches include the tympanic nerve, stylopharyngeal nerve, tonsillar nerve, carotid sinus nerve, branches to the posterior third of the tongue, lingual branches, and a communicating branch to the vagus nerve. It provides somatosensory information from the inner surface of the tympanic membrane, upper pharynx, and posterior one-third of the tongue, and carries visceral sensory information from the carotid body and carotid sinus. The glossopharyngeal nerve exits from the upper medulla of the brain stem, anterior to the vagus nerve, and subsequently exits the skull through the jugular foramen. It continues inferiorly, running between the carotid artery and internal jugular vein and passes under the styloid process. The nerve then arches around the side of the neck, courses beneath the hyoglossus muscle, and distributes to the palatine tonsils, mucous membrane of the fauces and base of the tongue, and glands of the mouth.[28–30]

Most of the GPN cases are caused by compression of the nerve root entry zone, but in many others, the etiology is unknown.[31,32] Idiopathic GPN is suspected to arise from the demyelination and axon-degeneration of cranial nerves IX and X.[33] In the cases of neurovascular conflict, the cause may stem from compression of the glossopharyngeal nerve by vascular structures (most common cause), intracranial tumors (medullary tumors and those originating from the cerebellopontine angle), laryngeal, oropharyngeal, and nasopharyngeal carcinomas, eagle syndrome, parapharyngeal infections, occipital cervical malformations, and inflammatory and autoimmune diseases such as multiple sclerosis and Sjogren's syndrome. Neurovascular compression induced GPN is typically caused by the posterior inferior cerebellar artery.[34] Compared with TN, GPN is rare. The prevalence of GPN is about 0.8 in 100,000, while the prevalence of TN is 4.7 in 100,000.[35]

A diagnosis of GPN is made clinically. The 2018 ICHD diagnostic criteria of GPN include recurring attacks of unilateral pain located in glossopharyngeal distribution and pain that has all of the following 4 characteristics: recurring paroxysmal attacks lasting a few seconds to 2 minutes, severe in intensity, shooting, stabbing, or sharp in quality, and precipitated by swallowing, coughing, talking or yawning. Additionally, the patient's presentation should not be better accounted for by another ICHD-3 diagnosis.[17] The differential diagnoses of GPN include TN, superior laryngeal neuralgia, geniculate neuralgia, Jacob's neuralgia, temporal arteritis, and temporomandibular dysfunction.[36] When evaluating a patient with GPN, laboratory tests including erythrocyte sedimentation rate, basal metabolic pane, complete blood count, and antinuclear antibody (ANA) should be obtained to rule out underlying inflammatory, autoimmune, infectious, and neoplastic etiologies. Although GPN is a clinical diagnosis, magnetic resonance imaging (MRI), 3D CT-angiography, and magnetic resonance angiography (MRA) are useful to detect cases caused by glossopharyngeal nerve demyelination and compression by tumors, vessels, or bony prominences.[20,37]

Pharmacologic treatment of GPN is similar to other facial neuralgias and consists of anticonvulsants, analgesics, steroids, and antidepressants. Carbamazepine and oxcarbazepine demonstrate good response rates, but efficacy may decline over time.[38] When patients are refractory to medication, microvascular decompression is the most commonly performed procedure. One review reported a long-term pain freedom post-MVD in 84.7% of patients.[39] Other intracranial interventions include rhizotomy or intracranial root resection of the glossopharyngeal and vagus nerves; however, these procedures can lead to persistent dysphagia and vocal cord paralysis. For those patients who fail pharmacologic management and who cannot tolerate intracranial surgery, percutaneous radiofrequency rhizotomy may be considered.[33] The prognosis for GPN is variable depending on patient symptoms. Most patients will only have a single episode of symptoms with an annual recurrence rate of 3.6%. Approximately 25% of patients will require surgery, and the rest can be managed medically.[30,40]

GENICULATE NEURALGIA

Geniculate, or nervus intermedius, neuralgia, is another rare form of facial neuralgia that affects the intermedius nerve, and commonly manifests as episodes of deep inner ear pain, lasting minutes to seconds. Dr Ramsay Hunt was the first to describe the condition in 1907. The famed neurologist noted the cutaneous manifestation of herpes zoster oticus and identified its subsequent pathology as "tic douloureux of the ear."[41] Now known as Geniculate neuralgia (GN), the disorder is characterized as recurring pain paroxysms at the posterior wall of the external ear canal that are triggered by mechanical or sensory stimuli such as swallowing, touch, noise, and cold. The condition may be associated with disorders of lacrimation, salivation, and taste disturbance, and on physical examination, the external ear canal is free of structural lesions.[17,42]

The affected intermedius nerve carries parasympathetic and sensory nerve fibers that are responsible for taste in the anterior two-thirds of the tongue, palate, floor of the mouth, and sensation of the external auditory meatus as well as the mucous membranes of the nose and nasopharynx. The anatomy of the intermedius nerve cutaneous fibers is particularly important in the surgical treatment of GN. After leaving the brainstem, the intermedius nerve's 3 segments take various paths before reaching the geniculate ganglion. The proximal segment closely adheres to the VIII nerve, the intermediate segment runs between the motor root of the facial nerve and the VIII, and the distal segment joins the motor root of the facial nerve.[41,43]

It is suspected that vascular compression of root entry zones of cranial nerves VII and VIII is an important factor in the pathogenesis of GN. Arteries such as the anterior inferior cerebellar artery (AICA), posterior inferior cerebellar artery (PICA), arteria vertebralis branches, and vena petrosum may all exert pressure on the acousticofacial bundle, although the AICA is typically the offending vessel. This additional strain on the nerve or the root entry zones may lead to nerve demyelination. A local inflammatory response may accompany this demyelination and subsequently increase nerve excitability and pain perception. In cases without vascular compression, the etiology of GN pain remains unclear.[44]

Because of the rarity of GN, there are limited data on the incidence, prevalence, and risk factors of the condition. In a systematic search conducted by Tang and colleagues using PubMed, Embase, the Cumulative Index to Nursing and Allied Health Literature, there were fewer than 150 cases of GN reported up until 2012.[45] Before considering GN as a potential diagnosis, a thorough neuro-otological examination should be conducted to rule out more common causes of ear pain. Otitis externa or media, temporomandibular dysfunction, dental lesions, carcinoma of the larynx or nasopharynx, vascular lesions such as temporal arteritis, herpes zoster oticus, and rare syndromes such as Eagle's syndrome should be included in the differential diagnosis for referred otalgia. Once neuralgia is suspected, it is important to distinguish GN from trigeminal neuralgia and glossopharyngeal neuralgia. Cranial nerves V, VII, IX, and X all provide somatosensory innervation to the ear. Therefore, trigeminal and glossopharyngeal neuralgia may also manifest as ear pain. Differentiation among the 3 is possible only by pain distribution and location. TN will localize in maxillary (V2) and mandibular (V3) nerve distributions, while GPN will predominantly present in the base of the tongue, soft palate, and tonsillar fossa.[46] When clinical suspicion of GN is high, MRI of the cerebellopontine angle is vital to assess for neurovascular compression. Virtually all symptomatic patients and occasionally asymptomatic patients will show neurovascular contact. Thus, MRA is highly sensitive, but may possess poor specificity.[44,47]

Medical therapy is attempted first in the treatment of GN; however, medical treatment often fails. For those who do not respond to medication, surgery may be considered. Medical treatment of GN, like other forms of facial neuralgia, includes medications such as carbamazepine, gabapentin, lamotrigine, and tricyclic antidepressants.[48] Surgical options include microvascular decompression (MVD) or sectioning of the nervus intermedius (NI). Both have shown optimistic results in the treatment of GN. In a published series of 8 patients with GN, Goulin Lippi Fernandes, and colleagues[49] demonstrate favorable outcomes at a median of 35 months in 7 of the patients after isolated MVD. Prophylactic MVD of cranial nerves V, IX, and X in addition to nervus intermedius sectioning may be considered due to the high risk of an alternative diagnosis causing the patient's pain.[50] In a recent series, Link and colleagues performed NI sectioning in 9 patients and MVD in 2 others, with additional cranial-nerve treatments in most of the patients, including MVD or rhizotomy of CN

V, IX, or X. All of their patients experienced relief in symptoms, and 8 of them had complete resolution of pain.[38,45,51–54]

MYOFASCIAL PAIN DYSFUNCTION SYNDROME

Myofascial pain dysfunction syndrome (MPDS) is another orofacial pain disorder that affects the muscles of mastication. Its presentation in the maxillofacial region can make it difficult to distinguish from similarly presenting facial neuralgias, so a well-conducted history and physical examination are imperative for accurate diagnosis. The pain from MPDS is derived from the presence of 2 to 5 mm trigger points within muscle or fascia, and is thus termed "myofascial pain." MPDS is characterized by myofascial pain with the presence of temporomandibular joint (TMJ) dysfunction. As a result, patients may complain of tenderness around the TMJ as well as clicking or popping noises with jaw movement. The pain associated with MPDS is often described as dull, radiating, unilateral, and aching.[55] MPDS is believed to be a stress-related disorder. Stress can increase tension in muscles and eventually lead to fatigue and spasms. Risk factors can be degenerative (aging and breakdown of skeletal structure), structural (due to conditions like scoliosis or spondylosis), trauma-based, or systemic (iron or Vitamin D deficiency). Chronic overuse of certain muscles or poor posture can also lead to the aching pain of MPDS.[20]

Diagnosing myofascial pain (MFP) can be challenging due to the variability of patient presentation. Most patients (67%) display the tenderness of the elevator muscles during palpation, while 40% complain of pain during mastication and 30% have myalgia with bruxism.[56] An important diagnostic feature of MFP includes eliciting pain or tenderness on the palpation of myofascial trigger points (MTrPs). In the past, there was no consensus among clinicians and researchers regarding the diagnostic criteria for myofascial trigger points. In 2017, a multi-national Delphi survey yielded an expert-based standardized method for trigger point diagnosis. The method requires that 2 of the 3 criteria be met: the presence of a taut band on palpation, a hypersensitive spot, and the presence of referred pain to a distant area.[57] A thorough history and physical should be followed with laboratory studies including a complete blood count as well as serum calcium, phosphorus, uric acid, creatinine, phosphokinase, alkaline phosphatase, and ESR. These tests will help rule out infection, bone disorders, muscular disorders, and inflammatory processes such as rheumatoid arthritis. [20]. Several imaging studies and diagnostic tools can help in the diagnosis of MFP. When MFP is associated with TMJ dysfunction, in the case of MPDS, an MRI is indicated to view the disc position of temporomandibular joint and condyle.[58] Additionally, ultrasound can assess for myofascial trigger points, which appear as focal, hypoechoic nodules, with decreased vibration amplitude and increased stiffness. Electromyography (EMG) may also be used, as MTrPs will demonstrate increased EMG activity at rest.[59]

After identifying MPDS as the cause of a patient's pain, it is important to explain the psychophysiologic nature of their illness. Stress can be an underlying provocation of MPDS, so patient counseling on exercise, deep breathing, and relaxation techniques may help improve symptoms. Other than lifestyle modifications, there are several pharmacologic and nonpharmacologic treatments that can relieve myofascial pain. Antidepressants (SSRIs, SNRIs, TCAs) may be prescribed in the presence of mood disorders, and amitriptyline, in particular, has been shown to be effective in several trials. Benzodiazepines may improve symptoms, but should not be used for long-term treatment due to their side effect profile. Botulinum toxin has an off-label use in the treatment of myofascial pain, but literature on its effectiveness is mixed. Therapeutic ultrasound is a newer technique that can help treat myofascial pain through applying

Table 1
Medical and surgical treatments for geniculate, trigeminal, and glossopharyngeal neuralgias[1-5]

Class	Treatment	Neuralgias Treated	Dosage (mg/d)	Potential Side Effects[2]
First Line Medical - Anticonvulsants	Carbamazepine	TN, GPN, GN	200–300	Dizziness, sedation, ataxia, hyponatremia
First Line Medical - Anticonvulsants	Oxcarbazepine	TN, GPN, GN	1200–2400	Dizziness, sedation, ataxia, hyponatremia
Second Line Medical - Skeletal Muscle Relaxants	Baclofen	TN, GPN, GN	60–80	Dizziness, drowsiness, nausea, hypotension, constipation, can cause withdrawal
Second Line Medical - Anticonvulsants	Lamotrigine	TN, GPN, GN	200–400	Dizziness, headaches, vertigo, ataxia, skin rash
Third Line Medical - Anticonvulsants	Pregabalin	TN, GPN, GN	150–600	Dizziness, sleepiness
Third Line Medical - Anticonvulsants	Gabapentin	TN, GPN, GN	300–1800	Dizziness, headaches, nausea, ankle edema, hyperlipidemia
Third Line Medical - Anticonvulsants	Topiramate	TN, GPN, GN	100–400	Dizziness, drowsiness, cognitive impairment, weight loss
Third Line Medical	Botulinum Toxin A	TN	20–75 units delivered transcutaneously	Only mild side effects seen - local swelling at administration site, temporary muscle weakness
Surgical	Microvascular Decompression	TN, GPN, GN		Postoperative trigeminal nerve deficit (1.6% to 22%), hearing loss (1.2% to 6.8%), leaking of cerebrospinal fluid (1.5%–4%)
Surgical - Percutaneous	Glycerol Rhizotomy	TN, GPN, GN		Aseptic meningitis (0.12% to 3%), bacterial meningitis (1.5% to 1.7%), hypesthesia (23.3% to 72%)
Surgical - Percutaneous	Radiofrequency Rhizotomy	TN, GPN, GN		Decreased sensation in cornea (5.7% to 17.3%), hypesthesia (3.3%), masseter weakness (4%)

(continued on next page)

Table 1
(continued)

Class	Treatment	Neuralgias Treated	Dosage (mg/d)	Potential Side Effects[2]
Surgical	Gamma Knife Radiosurgery	TN, GPN, GN		Hypesthesia (6% to 42%), decreased sensation in cornea (0% to 3.1%), anesthesia dolorosa (0.2%)
Surgical - Percutaneous	Balloon Compression	TN, GPN, GN		Hypesthesia (89% to 100%), hearing loss (2.4% to 6.3%), masseter weakness (1.2% to 12%)
Surgical	Internal Neurolysis	TN, GPN, GN		Hypesthesia, anesthesia dolorosa, facial dysesthesia

mechanical and thermal energy to connective tissues, improving circulation, metabolism, and tissue pliability.[60] Dry needling, also referred to as intramuscular stimulation, has been shown to be an effective treatment for pain relief. It involves the insertion of needles directly into the trigger point which damages the motor-end plate, resulting in the denervation of muscles and relaxation of trigger points.[61] Other less studied treatments include NSAIDs, muscle relaxants (cyclobenzaprine, tizanidine), lidocaine patches, and manipulative therapy (OMT). Myofascial pain syndrome typically resolves with continued treatment; however, many patients may suffer from the condition for decades. Outcomes are best when patients are treated by a multidisciplinary team consisting of physicians, nurses, and physiotherapists.[62]

SUMMARY

Facial neuralgias and myofascial pain dysfunction syndrome can have complex, overlapping presentations that can make them difficult to distinguish. Additionally, these conditions may have idiopathic presentations, adding to the complexity of diagnosis and treatment. The regularity of misdiagnoses related to maxillofacial pain can lead to unnecessary procedures and even surgeries. Understanding the presentations and diagnostic criteria of TN, GPN, GN, and MPDS will equip health care workers with the knowledge to facilitate an accurate diagnosis and frame treatment. Nevertheless, there remains a need for further research into the distinct etiologies and ideal treatments for facial neuralgias and myofascial pain dysfunction syndrome.

CLINICS CARE POINTS

- Facial neuralgias are characterized by recurrent electric-shock-like pain attacks that occur in the distribution of various cranial nerves.

- Trigeminal neuralgia (TN) is the most common of the facial neuralgias and presents with pain in the distribution of the trigeminal nerve, commonly in maxillary (V2) and mandibular (V3) nerve distributions

- Glossopharyngeal neuralgia (GPN) and geniculate neuralgia (GN) are rarer and cause pain via the glossopharyngeal and intermedius nerves typically affecting the posterior wall of the external ear canal.[3]

- Myofascial pain dysfunction syndrome (MPDS) is characterized by chronic pain in various trigger points, fascial constrictions, and pressure sensitivities.

- Neuroimaging including CT and MRI should be included in the initial work up of facial neuralgias to identify causes of possible nerve compression as well as other causes of the patient's facial pain.

- Pharmacologic therapy for TN, GPN, and GN includes anticonvulsants (namely carbamazepine), analgesics, steroids, and antidepressants (TCAs) listed in **Table1**.

- Surgical management includes microvascular decompression, rhizotomy, gamma knife radiosurgery, balloon compression, and internal neurolysis.

REFERENCES

1. Siqueira JT, Lin HC, et al. Clinical study of patients with persistent orofacial pain. Arq Neuropsiquiatr 2004;62(4):988–96.
2. Christoforou J. Neuropathic orofacial pain. Dent Clin North Am 2018;62(4): 565–84.
3. Katta-Charles SD. Craniofacial neuralgias. NeuroRehabilitation 2020;47(3): 299–314.

4. Brown JA, Coursaget C, Preul MC, et al. Mercury water and cauterizing stones: nicolas Andre and tic douloureux. J Neurosurg 1999;90(5):977–81.
5. Zakrzewska JM, Linskey ME. Trigeminal neuralgia. BMJ 2014;348:g474.
6. Eller JL, Raslan AM, Burchiel KJ. Trigeminal neuralgia: definition and classification. Neurosurg Focus 2005;18(5):1–3.
7. Gietzen L. Trigeminal neuralgia. J Am Acad PAs 2017;30(1):46–7.
8. Katusic S, Beard CM, Bergstralth E, et al. Incidence and clinical features of trigeminal neuralgia, Rochester, Minnesota, 1945–1984. Ann Neurol 1990;27(1): 89–95.
9. Loh HS, Ling SY, Shanmuhasuntharam P, et al. Trigeminal neuraligia. A retrospective survey of a sample of patients in Singapore and Malaysia. Aust Dent J 1998; 43(3):188–91.
10. Nurmikko TJ, Eldridge PR. Trigeminal neuralgia - Pathophysiology, diagnosis and current treatment. Br J Anaesth 2001;87(1):117–32.
11. Bennetto L, Patel NK, Fuller G. Trigeminal neuralgia and its management. BMJ 2007;334(7586):201–5.
12. Haines SJ, Jannetta PJ, Zorub DS. Microvascular relations of the trigeminal nerve: an anatomical study with clinical correlation. J Neurosurg 1980;52(3): 381–6.
13. Jannetta PJ. Arterial compression of the trigeminal nerve at the pons in patients with trigeminal neuralgia. J Neurosurg 1967;26(1part2):159–62.
14. Barker FG, Jannetta PJ, Bissonette DJ, et al. The long-term outcome of microvascular decompression for trigeminal neuralgia. N Engl J Med 1996;334(17): 1077–84.
15. Hilton DA, Love S, Gradidge T, et al. Pathological findings associated with trigeminal neuralgia caused by vascular compression. Neurosurgery 1994;35(2): 299–303.
16. Toda K. Etiology of Trigeminal Neuralgia. Oral Sci Int 2007;4(1):10–8.
17. Headache classification committee of the international headache society (IHS) The International classification of headache disorders. 3rd edition. Cephalalgia 2018;38(1):1–211.
18. Borges A, Casselman J. Imaging the trigeminal nerve. Eur J Radiol 2010;74(2): 323–40.
19. Antonini G, Di Pasquale A, Cruccu G, et al. Magnetic resonance imaging contribution for diagnosing symptomatic neurovascular contact in classical trigeminal neuralgia: a blinded case-control study and meta-analysis. Pain 2014;155(8): 1464–71.
20. Khan M, Nishi SE, Hassan SN, et al. Trigeminal neuralgia, glossopharyngeal neuralgia, and myofascial pain dysfunction syndrome: an update. Pain Res Manag 2017;2017:7438326. https://doi.org/10.1155/2017/7438326.
21. Cruccu G, Di Stefano G, Truini A. Trigeminal Neuralgia. N Engl J Med 2020; 383(8):754–62.
22. Shankar Kikkeri N, Nagalli S. Trigeminal Neuralgia. In: StatPearls. Treasure Island (FL): StatPearls Publishing; 2021.
23. Blumenfeld A, Nikolskaya G. Glossopharyngeal neuralgia. Curr Pain Headache Rep 2013;17(7):343.
24. KONG Y, HEYMAN A, ENTMAN ML, et al. Glossopharyngeal neuralgia associated with bradycardia, syncope, and seizures. Circulation 1964;30:109–13.
25. Esaki T, Osada H, Nakao Y, et al. Surgical management for glossopharyngeal neuralgia associated with cardiac syncope: two case reports. Br J Neurosurg 2007;21(6):599–602.

26. Bruyn GW. Glossopharyngeal neuralgia. Cephalalgia 1983;3(3):143–57.
27. Antherieu P, Vassal F, Sindou M. Vagoglossopharyngeal neuralgia revealed through predominant digestive vagal manifestations. Case report and literature review. Neurochirurgie 2016;62(3):174–7.
28. Singh O, M Das J. Anatomy, head and neck, jugular foramen. In: StatPearls. Treasure Island (FL): StatPearls Publishing; 2021.
29. Walker HK, Hall WD, Hurst JW, editors. Clinical methods: the history, physical, and laboratory examinations. 3rd ed. Boston: Butterworths; 1990.
30. Shah RJ, Padalia D. Glossopharyngeal Neuralgia. In: StatPearls. Treasure Island (FL): StatPearls Publishing; 2021.
31. Spina A, Boari N, Gagliardi F, et al. The emerging role of gamma knife radiosurgery in the management of glossopharyngeal neuralgia. Neurosurg Rev 2019; 42(1):31–8.
32. Kano H, Urgosik D, Liscak R, et al. Stereotactic radiosurgery for idiopathic glossopharyngeal neuralgia: an international multicenter study. J Neurosurg 2016; 125(Suppl 1):147–53.
33. Rey-Dios R, Cohen-Gadol AA. Current neurosurgical management of glossopharyngeal neuralgia and technical nuances for microvascular decompression surgery. Neurosurg Focus 2013;34(3):E8.
34. Singh PM, Kaur M, Trikha A. An uncommonly common: glossopharyngeal neuralgia. Ann Indian Acad Neurol 2013;16(1):1–8.
35. Koopman JS, Dieleman JP, Huygen FJ, et al. Incidence of facial pain in the general population. Pain 2009;147(1–3):122–7.
36. Teixeira MJ, de Siqueira SR, Bor-Seng-Shu E. Glossopharyngeal neuralgia: neurosurgical treatment and differential diagnosis. Acta Neurochir (Wien) 2008; 150(5):471–5.
37. Gaul C, Hastreiter P, Duncker A, et al. Diagnosis and neurosurgical treatment of glossopharyngeal neuralgia: clinical findings and 3-D visualization of neurovascular compression in 19 consecutive patients. J Headache Pain 2011;12(5): 527–34.
38. Franzini A, Messina G, Franzini A, et al. Treatments of glossopharyngeal neuralgia: towards standard procedures. Neurol Sci 2017;38(S1):51–5.
39. O'Neill F, Nurmikko T, Sommer C. Other facial neuralgias. Cephalalgia 2017; 37(7):658–69.
40. Katusic S, Williams DB, Beard CM, et al. Incidence and clinical features of glossopharyngeal neuralgia, Rochester, Minnesota, 1945-1984. Neuroepidemiology 1991;10(5–6):266–75.
41. Alfieri A, Strauss C, Prell J, et al. History of the nervus intermedius of Wrisberg. Ann Anat 2010;192(3):139–44.
42. Bruyn GW. Nervus intermedius neuralgia (Hunt). Cephalalgia 1984;4(1):71–8.
43. Rhoton AL Jr, Kobayashi S, Hollinshead WH. Nervus intermedius. J Neurosurg 1968;29(6):609–18.
44. Saers SJF. Microvascular decompression may be an effective treatment for nervus intermedius neuralgia. J Laryngol Otol 2011;125(5):520–2.
45. Tang IP, Freeman SR, Kontorinis G, et al. Geniculate neuralgia: a systematic review. J Laryngol Otol 2014;128(5):394–9.
46. Siccoli MM, Bassetti CL, Sándor PS. Facial pain: clinical differential diagnosis. Lancet Neurol 2006;5(3):257–67.
47. Yap L, Pothula VB, Lesser T. Microvascular decompression of cochleovestibular nerve. Eur Arch Otorhinolaryngol 2008;265(8):861–9.

48. McQuay H, Carroll D, Jadad AR, et al. Anticonvulsant drugs for management of pain: a systematic review. BMJ 1995;311(7012):1047–52.
49. Goulin Lippi Fernandes E, van Doormaal T, de Ru S, et al. Microvascular Decompression of the VII/VIII Cranial Nerve Complex for the Treatment of Intermediate Nerve Neuralgia: a retrospective case series [published correction appears in Oper Neurosurg (Hagerstown). Oper Neurosurg (Hagerstown) 2018;15(4): 378–85.
50. Lovely TJ, Jannetta PJ. Surgical management of geniculate neuralgia. Am J Otol 1997;18(4):512–7.
51. Peris-Celda M, Oushy S, Perry A, et al. Nervus intermedius and the surgical management of geniculate neuralgia. J Neurosurg 2018;131(2):343–51.
52. Jones MR, Urits I, Ehrhardt KP, et al. A comprehensive review of trigeminal neuralgia. Curr Pain Headache Rep 2019;23(10):74.
53. Al-Quliti KW. Update on neuropathic pain treatment for trigeminal neuralgia. The pharmacological and surgical options. Neurosciences (Riyadh) 2015;20(2): 107–14.
54. Bick SKB. Surgical Treatment of Trigeminal Neuralgia. Neurosurg Clin N Am 2017; 28(3):429–38.
55. Tantanatip A, Chang KV. Myofascial Pain Syndrome. In: StatPearls. Treasure Island (FL): StatPearls Publishing; 2021.
56. Winocur E, Gavish A, Emodi-Perlman A, et al. Hypnorelaxation as treatment for myofascial pain disorder: a comparative study. Oral Surg Oral Med Oral Pathol Oral Radiol Endod 2002;93(4):429–34.
57. Fernández-De-Las-Peñas C, Dommerholt J. International consensus on diagnostic criteria and clinical considerations of myofascial trigger points: a delphi study. Pain Med 2018;19(1):142–50.
58. Ingawalé S, Goswami T. Temporomandibular joint: disorders, treatments, and biomechanics. Ann Biomed Eng 2009;37(5):976–96.
59. Do TP, Heldarskard GF, Kolding LT, et al. Myofascial trigger points in migraine and tension-type headache. J Headache Pain 2018;19(1):84.
60. Borg-Stein J, Iaccarino MA. Myofascial pain syndrome treatments. Phys Med Rehabil Clin N Am 2014;25(2):357–74.
61. Kütük SG, Özkan Y, Kütük M, et al. Comparison of the efficacies of dry needling and botox methods in the treatment of myofascial pain syndrome affecting the temporomandibular joint. J Craniofac Surg 2019;30(5):1556–9.
62. Bordoni B, Sugumar K, Varacallo M. Myofascial Pain. In: StatPearls. Treasure Island (FL): StatPearls Publishing; 2021.

A Review of Medical and Surgical Options for the Treatment of Facial Pain

Marisa C. Penn, BS[a], Wooseong Choi, BS[a], Kaevon Brasfield, BS[a],
Kevin Wu, BS[a], Robert G. Briggs, MD[b],*,
Robert Dallapiazza, MD, PhD[c], Jonathan J. Russin, MD[b,d],
Steven L. Giannotta, MD[b], Darrin J. Lee, MD, PhD[b,d]

KEYWORDS

- Facial pain • Trigeminal neuralgia • Microvascular decompression • Radiotherapy
- Rhizotomy • Neuromodulation

KEY POINTS

- Facial pain is a common medical problem with multiple etiologies making proper diagnosis difficult.
- A multitude of pharmacologic options are available in the initial management of facial pain.
- In patients who fail medical management of their facial pain, second-line surgical options are available, each with its own risk/benefit profile.
- Future areas of research will focus on neuromodulation in the treatment/management of facial pain.

INTRODUCTION TO FACIAL PAIN

Facial pain occurs primarily under the orbitomeatal line, anterior to the pinnae, and above the neck.[1] The trigeminal nerve is most commonly implicated in facial pain syndromes, as its second and third divisions innervate much of the face. However, there is significant overlap with facial pain syndromes and headache disorders owing to the involvement of the trigeminal nerve and other adjacent anatomic structures, including the eyes, ears, nose, paranasal sinuses, and oral cavity.[2] Differentiating pain

[a] Keck School of Medicine, University of Southern California, 1200 North State Street, Suite 3300, Los Angeles, CA 90033, USA; [b] Department of Neurological Surgery, Keck School of Medicine, University of Southern California, 1200 North State Street, Suite 3300, Los Angeles, CA 90033, USA; [c] Department of Neurological Surgery, Tulane School of Medicine, Tulane University, 131 South Robertson Street, Suite 1300, New Orleans, LA 70112, USA; [d] Neurorestoration Center, Keck School of Medicine, University of Southern California, 1200 North State Street, Suite 3300, Los Angeles, CA 90033, USA
* Corresponding author. Department of Neurological Surgery, Keck School of Medicine, University of Southern California, 1200 North State Street, Suite 3300, Los Angeles, CA 90033.
E-mail address: gbriggs023@gmail.com

Otolaryngol Clin N Am 55 (2022) 607–632
https://doi.org/10.1016/j.otc.2022.03.001
0030-6665/22/© 2022 Elsevier Inc. All rights reserved.

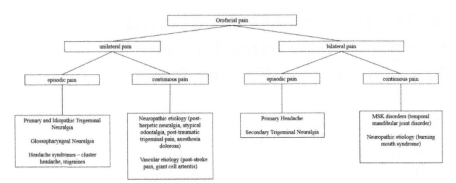

Fig. 1. The differential diagnosis of facial pain. Proper diagnosis depends on the presenting symptoms, including laterality of the pain, continuous nature of the pain, and its distribution.

generated across these various structures can be difficult. As such, a thorough understanding of how facial pain is generated is critical to guide treatment.

Overall, facial pain is relatively common within the general population, with the prevalence estimated between 15.1% and 33.2%.[2-7] The differential diagnosis of chronic orofacial pain is broad and can better be distinguished from primary headache disorders based on the duration and quality of the pain (**Fig. 1**).[8] Unilateral, continuous orofacial pain can have a neuropathic cause, such as in postherpetic neuralgia, atypical odontalgia, or posttraumatic trigeminal pain, sometimes referred to as anesthesia dolorosa. It may also be caused by vascular diseases, such as poststroke pain or giant cell arteritis. Nonunilateral, continuous orofacial pain can be caused by musculoskeletal disorders, such as those involving the temporomandibular joint, neuropathic causes, such as burning mouth syndrome, or may occur owing to persistent, idiopathic facial pain.[8] Unilateral orofacial pain that presents episodically may be due to trigeminal or glossopharyngeal neuralgias or headache syndromes.[8] Nonunilateral, episodic orofacial pain is often a primary headache diagnosis, such as tension or medication-overuse headaches.

An important component in understanding facial pain involves identifying where the pain is generated across the face, especially as it relates to the trigeminal nerve. This pain, called trigeminal neuralgia (TN), has been studied extensively within the literature and can arise from any or all 3 branches of the trigeminal nerve, although it most frequently involves the maxillary (V2) or mandibular (V3) divisions of the nerve (**Fig. 2**).[9] TN classically occurs as paroxysmal pain that is intense, stabbing, or electrical in nature, involving one side of the face. The pain can be debilitating and occur spontaneously without trigger or evoked by various stimuli, such as talking, chewing, or brushing one's teeth.[9]

In 2018, a new classification system of TN was described by the International Headache Society and the International Association for the Study of Pain.[1] Under these guidelines, TN is classified into 3 categories based on cause: classical, secondary, or idiopathic. Classical TN results from neurovascular compression with morphologic changes to the trigeminal root. Secondary TN occurs as a complication of other neurologic diseases, such as in multiple sclerosis or from mass effect from tumors of the cerebellopontine angle. Patients with secondary TN tend to be younger and are more likely to present with sensory deficits as well as bilateral facial pain compared with those with classical TN. The absence of these features does not rule out secondary TN, however, and MRI is recommended to distinguish classical and secondary variants of TN.[10] When

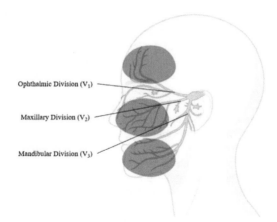

Ophthalmic Division (V₁)

Maxillary Division (V₂)

Mandibular Division (V₃)

Fig. 2. Anatomic divisions of the trigeminal nerve (*V*). Pain elicited along this nerve is called trigeminal neuralgia (TN). In primary TN, the pain is unilateral, episodic, and commonly triggered by activities of daily living. The pain may occur across multiple divisions of the nerve.

there is no evidence of a mass lesion or underlying pathologic condition that can explain a patient's facial pain, a diagnosis of idiopathic TN is made.[10]

Medication is the first-line treatment for orofacial pain, and a patient is considered to have medically refractory pain if he or she has a poor response to or cannot tolerate these medications.[11] For some of these patients, different surgical and neuromodulatory options can be considered to treat this pain. These include microvascular decompression (MVD), percutaneous rhizotomy, gamma knife radiosurgery (GKRS), peripheral nerve stimulation (PNS), deep brain stimulation (DBS), and motor cortex stimulation (MCS). These differing techniques have different success rates, duration of pain relief, and risk profiles, so selecting the appropriate option for a patient with facial pain is critical. The decision to intervene surgically should take into account multiple factors, such as the patient's age, the presence of neurovascular compression, medical comorbidities, and surgical tolerance.[12] The goal of this review is to evaluate these different interventions to better understand how different surgical modalities can be used to treat or control facial pain.

MEDICAL MANAGEMENT OF FACIAL PAIN
Sodium Channel Blockers

Pharmacologic management is considered first-line intervention for facial pain, particularly TN.[13] Dosages can vary and often require slow up-titration and tapering depending on a patient's tolerance for the medication.[14] Sodium channel blockers are most often used. These medications work by blocking voltage-gated sodium channels in a frequency-dependent manner. The anticonvulsive drug, carbamazepine (CBZ), is often the first drug of choice in patients with orofacial pain. In a cross-over study of patients with TN, 90.5% of patients reported pain relief with CBZ monotherapy, although only 21% reported complete resolution of pain.[15] Several studies have estimated the number needed to treat for adequate pain control with CBZ to be 1.7 to 1.8.[16,17] However, this drug can cause considerable side effects, such as drowsiness, slowed cognitive processing, and in rare cases, blood dyscrasias, such as aplastic anemia or agranulocytosis.[18] CBZ can also have significant interactions with the metabolic processing of other medications given its ability to induce the cytochrome p450 enzyme system in the liver. In addition, not all orofacial pain is adequately treated with

CBZ. Some studies have estimated the number needed to harm as 2.6 to 3.7 for minor adverse events when using CBZ, although these results were not statistically significant when compared with the use of a placebo.[19–23] Other facial pain syndromes, such as trigeminal trophic syndrome, a rare form of facial pain that can occur following injury to the trigeminal nerve, have been adequately controlled with CBZ therapy.[24–26]

Oxcarbazepine (OXC), a prodrug to CBZ, is used when patients fail CBZ therapy. Compared with CBZ, OXC has a lower risk profile, including fewer drug-to-drug interactions and fewer side effects.[27] Studies have estimated the number needed to treat for OXC to be 1.7,[22,28,29] although higher doses of the medication are often necessary to achieve adequate pain control. Studies have also demonstrated that OXC has comparable efficacy to CBZ for the treatment of facial pain.[30,31] However, some retrospective studies show CBZ is more highly effective in treating classical TN, with 98% achieving pain control on CBZ monotherapy compared with 94% on OXC monotherapy.[27]

Other novel sodium channel blockers, such as BIIB074, are being evaluated for safety and efficacy in the treatment of TN for patients who are unable to tolerate CBZ or OXC.[32] In one double-blind, multicenter, placebo-controlled, randomized phase 2A clinical trial of 29 patients, 77% of patients were able to achieve relief of pain with this drug.[32] Patients reported similar side effects to other sodium-channel blocker treatments, including headache, dizziness, pyrexia, nasopharyngitis, sleep disturbances, and tremor.[32] Other pharmacologic investigations are underway to find alternative medications that may prove more effective and safer than these other drugs.[33]

Treatment failure with sodium channel blockers usually occurs owing to patients experiencing side effects from the medications rather than analgesic insufficiency. One study found as many as 57% of patients treated with CBZ experienced some form of a pharmacologic side effect.[15] Typical side effects include somnolence, drowsiness, dizziness, rash, or tremor.[14] This class of drug has also been associated with hyponatremia. It is contraindicated in patients with comorbid cardiac disease, such as heart block, hepatic disease, or renal disease, owing to this electrolyte effect. These drugs are also associated with fetal anomalies and therefore are contraindicated in pregnant patients. One study estimated the number needed to harm for patients treated with CBZ to be 24 for severe side effects, but only 3.4 for minor side effects.[17]

Other Anticonvulsants

Some guidelines suggest that patients who fail treatment on a sodium channel blocker should be considered for surgical intervention for further management of their facial pain. However, there is reasonable evidence to attempt either a combination of medications or other monotherapies before considering surgery.[14] Beyond sodium channel blockers, other anticonvulsant medications have demonstrated some efficacy in the treatment of orofacial pain.

Lamotrigine has been shown to be similarly effective in treating TN compared with CBZ. In one study comparing the efficacy of lamotrigine to CBZ in patients with TN, 62% to 63% of patients benefited from lamotrigine treatment, with 77% of these patients reporting complete pain relief and 84% achieving significant pain relief.[15] Similarly to CBZ, lamotrigine has a significant side-effect profile with some 67% of patients reporting side effects while taking the medication.[15] In patients who might benefit or prefer trialing polytherapy before more invasive methods, lamotrigine has demonstrated moderate improvements in combination with CBZ compared with placebo.[34,35]

Other anticonvulsants, such as gabapentin and pregabalin, have also been used to treat facial pain. Randomized controlled clinical trials of patients with chronic masticatory myalgia found that gabapentin, compared with placebo, led to clinically and statistically reduced pain scores and improved quality of life.[36] Gabapentin, which has been used to treat neuropathic pain, has been demonstrated in randomized controlled trials to reduce the perception of pain after oculofacial plastic surgery.[37] Gabapentin's effects can be bolstered with the inclusion of a ropivacaine analgesic block of facial trigger points, for significant, long-lasting reductions in pain that can translate to lower gabapentin dose requirements and improvement in functional well-being.[38] Pregabalin has also shown efficacy in reducing TN symptoms in 59% to 74% of patients in observational and open-label studies.[39–41] Pregabalin also has some efficacy in treating other forms of facial pain, including postherpetic neuralgia. In a study of 25 patients with postherpetic neuralgia treated with pregabalin, 60% achieved at least 50% improvement in pain level at 4 weeks of treatment.[42] Use of pregabalin has also been associated with positive medication side effects, including improved mood, sleep, and reported physical function.[40,41]

Small case series reports investigating other anticonvulsant medications, such as topiramate and levetiracetam, have also demonstrated encouraging results. Topiramate was associated with reduced pain in 75% of patients in a small series of 8 patients with TN.[43] A small case series using levetiracetam also demonstrated improvement in pain scores by greater than 50% in 40% of patients taking the medication and that it reduced daily pain attacks by 62.7% in patients with refractory TN.[44]

Other Medical Therapies

Other medications have also been used to manage facial pain. Drugs such as baclofen, a GABA-B receptor agonist, which is frequently used to treat muscle spasticity, have shown some efficacy in treating TN.[45] One study investigated the efficacy of baclofen as a therapy for orofacial pain in a clinical trial of 25 patients (16 with TN, 9 with other facial pain syndromes, 5 of whom were refractory to CBZ).[46] In this trial, baclofen was found to significantly improve reported pain levels by 68.1%. Similar results using baclofen have been demonstrated in patients experiencing/refractory TN with 74% of patients reporting improvement in their facial pain when taking the medication, although only 30% of patients remained pain-free by their 5-year follow-up visit and 22% of patients had become refractory to baclofen use by 18 months of therapy.[47] Chimeric baclofen may also be more effective than racemic baclofen in patients with TN, as demonstrated in one double-blind, cross-over trial of 15 patients.[48]

Antidepressants have also been trialed in the treatment of persistent, idiopathic facial pain, although evidence in the literature is mixed regarding their efficacy. In one series of 16 patients with atypical facial pain treated with low-dose amitriptyline, the medication was effective in reducing pain in all patients at up to 12 months of follow-up.[49] Another prospective series of 29 patients treated with duloxetine for chronic facial pain found 51.7% of patients achieved at least a 50% reduction in their pain score with significant reductions appearing 2 weeks after treatment initiation.[50] A randomized controlled study of venlafaxine for atypical facial pain also demonstrated a modest response in pain relief compared with placebo with less pain relief.[51] However, no significant correlation was found between serum concentration of venlafaxine and symptom response. In addition, there was no significant reduction in pain intensity between the maximum tolerated venlafaxine dose and placebo.

At present, little data exist on the number of drugs or the duration of pharmacologic treatment that should be attempted before surgical options for facial pain are considered.[10] However, in general, if patients do not respond to medical treatment, either from lack of response to their medications or because of developing side effects, then surgical evaluation is warranted as a form of second-line therapy. Surgical options to treat facial pain are numerous, including open cranial surgery, stereotactic radiosurgery, ablation via rhizotomy, and various forms of neuromodulation, including peripheral, deep brain, and motor cortex forms of stimulation. Selection of the appropriate intervention should consider all clinical and radiographic factors, as different surgical modalities may be better suited for different patients.

SURGICAL MANAGEMENT OF FACIAL PAIN
Microvascular Decompression

MVD involves the surgical decompression of the cranial nerve causing neuralgia and is often considered in the surgical treatment of TN when medical therapy has failed.[14] It is the only nonablative procedural option for the treatment of TN. Typically, preoperative imaging will demonstrate mass effect from an adjacent structure, such as a blood vessel. The procedure involves performing a retrosigmoid craniotomy to gain access to the posterior fossa to visualize the vascular bundle offending the nerve. A sponge is inserted between the nerve and artery to halt the production of abnormal, dysregulated pain signals (**Fig. 3**).

As the MVD procedure is designed to alleviate orofacial pain caused by a compressive vessel, it has been shown to lead to significant, long-lasting pain relief for a variety of orofacial pain syndromes. In one study, 70% to 74% of patients who underwent an MVD were pain-free at 10 years postprocedure.[52] In a retrospective review of 156 patients at a single center, the probability of a patient being pain-free after an MVD was estimated at 93%.[53] Studies continue to demonstrate strong pain relief in most patients. However, some 10% to 18% of patients may not achieve satisfactory pain relief following the operation.[53,54] For those with continued pain after an MVD, further surgical exploration can be considered. Repeat surgery may elucidate more points of neurovascular contact along the offending nerve or its branches. Decompression of these vessels can lead to resolution of the pain in most cases.[54] Thus, radiographic neurovascular compression with high-resolution MRI is often used to identify potential open surgical candidates.

MVD is generally a well-tolerated procedure. Rates of complications are low, with 0.05% to 7% of patients reporting minor side effects, such as new aching or burning pain, sensory loss, or mild or transient cranial nerve dysfunction following the operation.[8,14,55] The most common complication is postoperative delirium. A review of 912

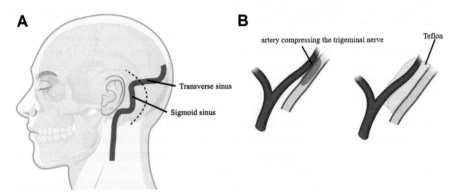

Fig. 3. An MVD. (*A*) A retrosigmoid craniotomy is planned that allows access to the trigeminal nerve and the corresponding compressing vessel. (*B*) During the procedure, a soft Teflon pad is placed between the offending vessel and the trigeminal nerve to prevent further injury to the nerve and treat the patient's underlying TN.

patients who underwent MVD for orofacial pain owing to primary cranial nerve disorders, including TN, found that up to 24.2% of these patients suffered postoperative delirium.[56] A history of hypertension, preoperative CBZ therapy, postoperative sleep disturbance, and postoperative tension pneumocephalus was significantly associated with an increased risk of postoperative delirium.[56]

Major adverse events, such as permanent cranial nerve dysfunction, stroke, or death, occur rarely, at a rate of 0.12% to 2.0%.[8,53,55,57] As the only nonablative surgical technique, it is much less likely to result in significant, permanent morbidity or mortality. Furthermore, data suggest different surgical approaches, such as microscopy or neuroendoscopy, do not lead to differences in cure rates or postsurgical complications.[58] However, in some cases, despite adequate decompression and initial pain relief following the operation, facial pain has been known to recur. In a retrospective review at a single center, pain recurrence occurred in 18% of MVD cases over a 25-year period.[53] The quality of pain recurrence was less severe in 50% of cases, and 30% of patients with recurrent pain experienced it on the contralateral side opposite the initial site of pain.[53] Pain recurrence was more likely to occur within 2 years of the surgery; thereafter, the rate of pain recurrence was estimated at 2% to 3.5% per year.[53]

Radiosurgery

GKRS is a relatively noninvasive, ablative surgical technique that involves the delivery of a single dose of highly focused radiation to a target lesion while sparing nearby clinical structures (**Fig. 4**). As a minimally invasive procedure associated with low rates of complications, GKRS may be preferred over MVD in patients with advanced age, significant medical comorbidities, and preferences against an open craniotomy or percutaneous procedures.

Commonly used targets for GKRS in TN are the retrogasserian and proximal nerve root entry zone portion of the nerve. In the first reported use of GKRS for TN in 1971, Leksell[59] targeted the Gasserian ganglion to treat 2 patients. Other researchers noted that they could achieve better pain reduction when targeting the retrogasserian portion of the trigeminal nerve.[60] Subsequent studies in the 1990s demonstrated pain relief was not adequately achieved in some TN patients receiving radiosurgery ablation to the Gasserian ganglion,[61,62] and instead, found that the proximal portion of the nerve, including the nerve root entry zone, was a more effective target. With the proximal nerve root entry zone targeted, 58% of patients was able to achieve complete pain relief, and some 36% of those who continued to have pain reported at least a 50% reduction in pain.[63]

Data available regarding the use of GKRS for the treatment of various facial pain syndromes are mixed. A retrospective case series of 21 patients treated with GKRS for facial pain secondary to head and neck tumors demonstrated only modest pain relief.[64] Although 81% of patients achieved some form of pain reduction, only 33% of patients experienced significant improvement in their pain, whereas 4.8% of patients saw no improvement in their pain following GKRS.[64] In contrast, other data strongly support the efficacy of GKRS in achieving pain relief in patients with TN. The precise, targeted nature of this treatment modality has led to encouraging outcomes for patients with TN, with various sources reporting that 50% to 52% of patients are pain-free at long-term follow-up following GKRS.[8,45,65] In primary TN, rates of initial pain relief ranged from 81% to 89% of patients in various retrospective studies.[66–75] A prospective, single-center study of 30 patients with medically refractive TN treated with GKRS demonstrated complete improvement in pain following GKRS in 40% of

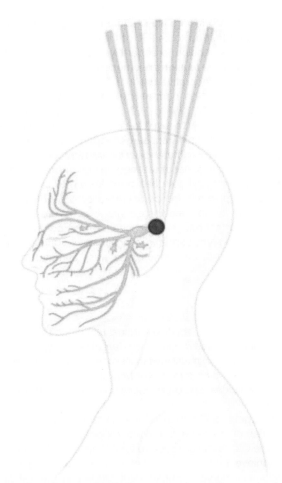

Fig. 4. A GKRS procedure. Beams of radiation converging at the proximal portion of the trigeminal nerve. The retrogasserian portion and proximal root entry zone are the most common targets when using GKRS to treat TN.

participants, whereas 10% and 33% of patients reported good and fair reduction in pain, repsectively.[76]

Although GKRS is relatively well tolerated, side effects of this procedure include transient neuropathic disturbances, including facial numbness, sensory loss, or paresthesia.[66,67,69–71,73–75,77,78] A commonly reported side effect is some degree of facial numbness, which occurs in 8% to 32% of patients.[66,69–71,77,78] Other complications have been rarely experienced by patients after undergoing GKRS. However, one retrospective study reported that 12.9% of patients experienced eye discomfort after GKRS.[71]

Despite its tolerability, a primary complaint of GKRS therapy is the delay and relatively short duration of pain relief. Various studies report complete pain relief in the acute posttreatment period, with or without the use of medication ranging up to 92%.[66,67,69,70,72] The average time to pain relief ranged from 22 to 102 days, indicating that response to GKRS may be delayed compared with other procedures. Moreover, in one single-center, retrospective case review of 112 patients with TN refractory to medical or surgical management treated with GKRS, 77% of patients reported pain relief occurring after a median of 3 weeks.[79] This delay in response may be related to the progression of facial pain, as patients with a shorter history of TN obtained earlier pain relief.[71]

In addition, many studies have found that the analgesic effects of GKRS deteriorate over time.[64,79,80] Compared with MVD, the duration of pain relief is relatively shorter after GKRS. In primary TN, only about half of the initial responders reported good pain control 5 years after undergoing GKRS.[77] Similar results were noted after GKRS for secondary TN. For orofacial pain secondary to head and neck tumors, 47% of patients experienced a relapse of pain within the first 2 years, with a median relapse time of 12 months following radiotherapy.[64] In TN secondary to multiple sclerosis, only 54% of patients reported pain relief 3 years after undergoing GKRS.[73]

CyberKnife radiosurgery (CKRS) is another technique that delivers radiation in conjunction with real-time radiographic guidance and 3-dimensional image correlation, allowing for precise and highly conformal treatment without a stereotactic headframe. It has been shown to have similar efficacy to GKRS in the treatment of facial pain, with a similar side-effect profile. This modality allows for the delivery of fractionated radiation, allowing for it to be given to targets near vulnerable structures. This form of radiotherapy has demonstrated high efficacy in up to 80% to 85% of patients with various forms of TG, including that caused by multiple sclerosis, and allows targeting of the trigeminal nerve root.[81,82] Patients may experience mild facial numbness following this procedure.[82] Similar to GKRS, CKRS's effectiveness wanes over time, with about half of patients continuing to experience adequate pain control at 4 years of follow-up from CKRS treatment.[82] Thus, patients who have typical TN symptoms but either do not have overt evidence of neurovascular compression or are poor surgical candidates are often the target radiosurgery patient population.

Percutaneous Rhizotomy

Percutaneous rhizotomy is a procedure during which the trigeminal ganglion is accessed and lesioned through the foramen ovale using a percutaneous needle leading to the disruption of afferent pain fibers within the trigeminal nerve (**Fig. 5**).[83] It is a less-invasive procedure compared with other surgical and neuromodulatory approaches used in the treatment of facial pain. Percutaneous rhizotomy is preferred over MVD for patients with significant medical comorbidities and those who prefer not to undergo open craniotomy.[12] In contrast to the MVD, use of the percutaneous rhizotomy technique does not require MRI evidence of nerve compression and therefore can be used for most cases of TN.[83] There are 3 types of percutaneous rhizotomy that differ by the mechanism of injury to the underlying nerve fibers: balloon compression rhizotomy (BCR), glycerol rhizotomy (GR), and radiofrequency rhizotomy (RFR). BCR uses mechanical inflation of a balloon to compress the trigeminal ganglion. GR involves injecting glycerol, a nerve irritant, into the trigeminal cistern. RFR uses thermal lesioning by using radiofrequency waves that generate heat to temperatures ranging from 55°C to 70°C.

It is important to consider the different characteristics of each rhizotomy approach when developing a plan to treat a patient's facial pain. For example, BCR specifically damages the large, myelinated fibers of the trigeminal nerve,[84] which may be more advantageous in patients who are experiencing TN of the ophthalmic division of the nerve, as the unmyelinated fibers involved in the corneal reflex are likely to be spared.[84] In addition, unlike GR and RFR, BCR does not require patient cooperation during surgery and can be performed under general anesthesia for patient comfort.[85]

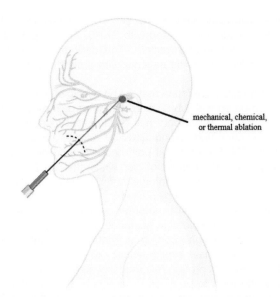

mechanical, chemical, or thermal ablation

Fig. 5. A percutaneous rhizotomy procedure. Under fluoroscopy, the trigeminal ganglion is ablated via a percutaneous approach through the cheek to reach the foramen ovale where the trigeminal ganglion resides. Lesioning is achieved using mechanical, chemical, or thermal ablative techniques.

However, BCR is associated with the trigeminal depressor response more than GR or RFR. This response, which can be seen when the percutaneous needle used during the procedure is introduced through the foramen ovale or during the process of balloon inflation, causes hypotension, bradycardia, apnea, and gastric hypermotility.[86] This autonomic response to BCR must be considered in patients with cardiovascular comorbidities.

For patients with primary TN, the 3 rhizotomy procedures are associated with high rates of initial pain relief. Studies with at least 100 patients that reported rates of complete pain relief, as well as rates and duration of pain recurrence, were selected for comparison of the 3 procedures. After BCR, the percent of patients who reported complete pain relief ranged from 90% to 100% (n = 1061).[87–91] After RFR (n = 3138), rates of pain resolution ranged from 94.8% to 97.6%.[92,93] Outcomes after GR varied the most, with 69% to 90.1% of patients reporting complete pain relief immediately after GR (n = 856).[94–98] These results indicate that all 3 forms of percutaneous rhizotomy can be efficacious in treating TN.[99] The significant variation in the success rate of GR is not well understood but may be attributed to discrepancies or variations in surgical technique. In addition, patients may require multiple GR procedures to achieve adequate pain relief. In one large retrospective study, multiple GR procedures were needed to achieve satisfactory rates and duration of pain relief.[100]

Lower rates of pain recurrence have also been shown in RFR compared with BCR or GR. The recurrence rate after BCR ranges from 20% to 48%,[87–91] whereas the recurrence rate after GR varied significantly from 18.5% to 70%.[94,96–98] After RFR, recurrence rates have been shown to range from 12.8% to 25%.[93,101] One retrospective study reported a recurrence rate of 20% over 9 years of follow-up after RFR.[102] The median time to recurrence after BCR and RFR averaged 2.3 years (n = 100) and 2.1 to 2.7 years (n = 572), respectively.[91,94,97]

Because percutaneous rhizotomy is destructive by nature, it is associated with some degree of postoperative sensory deficit.[91,103] For example, both hypesthesia and dysesthesia are typically transient, but common complications that occur after each of the percutaneous procedures with similar rates of dysesthesia have been shown across multiple studies.[87–94,96–98] In addition, the 3 percutaneous procedures also have slight variations in their postoperative complication profile. For example, BCR is associated with masseter and masticatory muscle weakness owing to disruption of the large, myelinated trigeminal motor fibers innervating the muscles of mastication.[91] Although it is associated with the highest rates of pain relief, RFR can also cause a greater incidence of severe side effects, such as anesthesia dolorosa and corneal anesthesia.[104] Other rare but reported side effects include cranial nerve palsies, herpes labialis, and meningitis.[103,104] As the long-term benefits are not as robust as that of MVD or radiosurgery, rhizotomies are generally reserved for those patients who have severe, acute pain and are not appropriate for surgical decompression or have symptomatic TN (ie, multiple sclerosis).

REFRACTORY PAIN MANAGEMENT
Peripheral Nerve Stimulation

PNS is a common treatment modality for chronic pain management that involves implantation of a small electrode to deliver programmed, regular electrical impulses to a nerve. For a variety of facial pain syndromes, including TN, neuropathic pain, and trigeminal postherpetic neuralgia, PNS is targeted at the trigeminal nerve, but more complex pain may require PNS targeting of the occipital nerve, sphenopalatine ganglion, or Gasserian ganglion.[105] PNS was first explored for pain in 1965, based on Melzack and Wall's Gate Control Theory, which suggested that innocuous sensory input carried by larger nerve fibers disrupts the transmission of nociceptive input carried by smaller nerve fibers.[106] Subsequent studies have demonstrated that nonpainful electrical stimulation of peripheral nerves can suppress pain perception.[107] This modality of pain control typically requires multiple interventions, with stimulation trials occurring before device implantation in order to ensure patient tolerability and response to therapy.[108,109]

Although the literature is scarce, some studies demonstrate efficacy when using PNS in the treatment of various facial pain syndromes. In a small retrospective analysis of 18 patients with herpes zoster ophthalmicus, 83% of patients achieved at least a 50% reduction in pain symptoms.[110] In addition, one small case series of patients with trigeminal neuropathic pain demonstrated sustained, long-term control of pain after PNS therapy.[111] The cases described in the study suggest promising efficacy in the treatment of facial pain secondary to facial trauma and herpes zoster that was otherwise poorly managed with medical therapy.[111]

Compared with other treatment modalities, PNS requires a longer treatment duration to demonstrate efficacy. In one study investigating PNS for the management of occipital neuralgia, there was an average latency period of 8 months of stimulation before patients experienced a 50% reduction in their pain level.[112] Patient response to PNS treatment also demonstrates considerable variability, with some studies reporting freedom from pain in 68% to 75% of patients,[109,113] whereas others suggest a more modest response in 25% to 73% of patients with only partial improvement in pain level.[108,113]

PNS, when selected appropriately for patients with facial pain, carries a low risk of side effects and complications. Stimulation trials before device implantation ensure the lowest tolerable stimulation doses for patients and prevent surgical device implantation in those who cannot otherwise tolerate the device. Trial stimulation involves electrode placement on the day before surgery, with programming on the same day so patients are trained in handling and adjusting stimulation voltage.[109] Some studies reported no immediate postimplantation adverse effects.[112] In a small case series of 10 patients undergoing trial stimulation, 1 (10%) patient experienced contradictory effects (ie, increased pain) and 1 (10%) patient experienced no improvement in pain symptoms.[109] These individuals did not undergo formal device implantation, and the investigators suggested that trail stimulation is essential to identify proper candidates for formal PNS device implantation.[109] Other reports of headache in the absence of facial pain have also been reported with PNS therapy.[111]

Complications of PNS reported in the literature include wound breakdown or skin erosion with hardware exposure (typically necessitating debridement postimplantation and hardware removal), damage to device electrodes, device disconnection, and displacement or migration of the device.[108,109,113,114] Rarely, revision surgeries are required for complete hardware removal owing to inadequate pain relief or loss of device effectiveness. Other rare side effects that have been observed include scalp hypoesthesia, paresthesias, and allergic reactions to device materials.[109,111,112,114,115]

Deep Brain Stimulation

DBS is an approved treatment option for a variety of neurologic and psychiatric diseases, including essential tremor, Parkinson disease, idiopathic dystonia, and obsessive-compulsive disorder.[116,117] It has been explored since the 1970s and 1980s for its potential to treat chronic pain syndromes but has yet to be Food and Drug Administration approved. Evidence for DBS in the treatment of specific pain syndromes and disorders has been mixed, and after the failure of clinical trials for DBS for pain in 2001,[118] less attention has been given to the study of DBS to manage and treat chronic facial pain.[119]

Common DBS targets for chronic pain syndromes include the periaqueductal gray (PAG) region and the ventral posterolateral nucleus of the thalamus (VPL) (Fig. 6).[116,120] The exact process by which pain relief occurs from DBS targeting of these regions is not known, but some theories suggest it may lead to the release of endogenous opioids or to modulation of ascending pain pathways and neural circuitry.[119] DBS of these regions has demonstrated functional changes in regional cerebral blood flow, which may lead to long-term changes in pain perception.[121] As DBS is designed to target neural pathways centrally, its use seems especially relevant for patients with demyelinating pain syndromes refractory to medical management.[117]

Despite the failure of previous trials, recent evidence for DBS in the treatment of chronic facial pain syndromes seems more promising. A prospective study of 56 patients with chronic pain syndromes, including six with trigeminal neuropathic pain, treated with DBS to the PAG and lateral somatosensory thalamus demonstrated mixed results across different syndromes, with the most success seen in patients with chronic low back or leg pain. However, 50% of patients in this study with trigeminal neuropathic pain and/or dysesthesia dolorosa achieved at least a 50% reduction in their pain.[120] A recent trial of 15 patients with poststroke neuropathic pain who underwent DBS of the VPL thalamus and PAG achieved an overall reduction of 48.8% in 80% of patients.[122] For those who continued to require analgesic medications after DBS therapy, all were able to switch to nonopiate pain medications. Similarly, a small case series of 7 patients with unilateral, intractable facial pain found pain scores were significantly decreased at 1-year follow-up after DBS implantation. Another small patient series using DBS for the treatment of facial pain found that 2/5 (40%) of the patients treated were pain-free at 1-year follow-up.[123] The remaining patients experienced some reduction in pain but continued to require analgesic medication

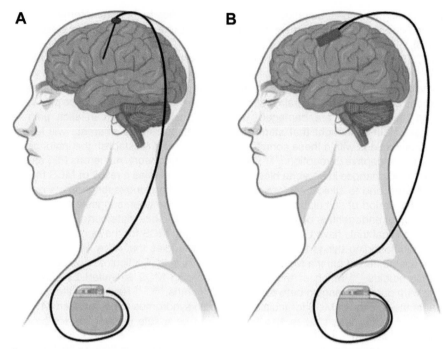

Fig. 6. Forms of neuromodulation used in the treatment of facial pain. (*A*) DBS is one option with electrodes typically implanted in the PAG or VPL. (*B*) MCS involves using array electrodes over the primary sensorimotor cortex.

to control symptoms. Evidence from other small case series suggests that DBS may be more effective in certain pain syndromes, especially posttraumatic facial pain, as these patients experienced higher rates of pain relief after DBS than those patients with poststroke and postherpetic neuralgias.[124] In one small series of 3 patients with intractable neuropathic pain undergoing DBS implantation of the VPL, PAG, or both, patients experienced a 37.3% reduction in pain scores by the 1-year follow-up.[121] Unlike other refractory pain options, DBS offers long-term relief and does not show diminishing effects over time. A longitudinal, small case series of DBS for intractable pain that followed patients for 15 years postimplantation found that DBS was very effective for patients with TN.[125]

Results from DBS therapy are not instantaneous, and patients should consequently be counseled to manage expectations appropriately. Clinical trials have shown that many patients do not experience maximum pain relief until 6 to 9 months after DBS implantation,[117] which may reflect the need for programming adjustments early in the postoperative period to determine appropriate and effective stimulation settings for individual patients. As with the other procedures described here, DBS therapy is not without risk. Side effects reported in the literature include headache and transient diplopia of unclear cause.[117,125]

Motor Cortex Stimulation

MCS is an invasive neuromodulatory technique that has been used for the treatment of intractable pain syndromes for many years. Response rates throughout the literature have varied, but some studies demonstrate encouraging results for the use of MCS warranting its further investigation.[126] This technique involves localization of the motor cortex using functional techniques and imaging studies before craniotomy, followed by paddle electrodes placement over the motor cortex in the epidural space (see **Fig. 6**).[127]

MCS is thought to work in part at the cortical level to alter neural circuitry, as the primary motor cortex is known to inhibit the primary somatosensory cortex, VPL, and spinothalamic tract.[119,128] The highly organized pathways between these structures are responsible for much of the brain's perception and response to nociceptive pain input. When these circuits are damaged, normal nonpainful stimuli can elicit pain responses.[119] It is thought that stimulation of damaged motor afferents will lead to new connections within these somatosensory areas and reestablish the inhibitory inputs on nociceptive perception.[119,129] In support of this theory, numerous PET studies have found changes in cerebral blood flow to these areas as a result of MCS therapy that correspond to clinical analgesic effects, suggesting long-lasting effects beyond the initial period of stimulation.[128,130–134] MCS has also been suggested to increase secretion of endogenous opioids in the anterior middle cingulate cortex and PAG.[135]

Few clinical trials have been performed evaluating MCS for the treatment of facial pain. Confounding things further is the fact that studies that have been completed have used different criteria for patient selection, making it difficult to compare results across studies.[119] Much of the literature regarding MCS is limited by short-term follow-up duration, ranging between 3 and 12 months.[136,137] Reviews of literature estimate the efficacy of MCS for facial chronic pain syndromes to be between 64% and 88%.[127,132,136] These studies also find MCS to be a safe intervention for properly selected candidates.[126] Other small retrospective case series found epidural MCS to lead to meaningful alleviation of greater than 50% of pain in 50% to 80% of facial pain cases and satisfactory pain relief in 52% to 60%.[138–140] In a case series of 8 patients with complex pain syndromes, five of which suffered from intractable facial pain, 54% achieved pain relief.[137] A prospective, double-blinded crossover study evaluating pain relief with MCS in 10 patients during on- and off-stimulation states found that patients with chronic neuropathic pain reported significant pain relief.[141] These patients reported significantly improved scores in pain scales as well as quality-of-life scales, suggestive that MCS causes affective changes in addition to decreasing pain intensity.[141] Another double-blinded crossover study found 100% long-term pain relief in patients undergoing MCS for treatment of thalamic and postherpetic neuralgia facial pain.[142] Of note, 3 patients of the 11 patients reported in this series did not report improvement in the subacute trial period and therefore were excluded from long-term stimulation and analysis.[142]

Although the data on the amount of pain relief are mixed, some studies have identified predictors of significant response to MCS therapy. In one prospective review of 31 patients with medically refractory neuropathic pain treated with MCS, the level of pain relief in the first month after implantation was a strong predictor of long-term pain relief.[140] Decreases in either the dosage or the frequency of analgesic medication use also led to clinically significant improvements in quality of life, even with some lingering pain. In the same study, 52% of patients decreased their intake of analgesic medications following MCS therapy, and 36% completely discontinued their analgesic medications.[140]

Although MCS may provide significant pain relief in some cases, the effect of MCS on pain level has been shown to diminish over time.[126] A retrospective case series of MCS for various causes of facial pain found that all 8 patients who underwent permanent MCS implantation reported satisfactory pain control.[143] However, 38% failed to report continued pain control at 6-month follow-up. Another case series of 14 patients with neuropathic pain, 7 of which had TN, also found a transient response.[144] Of these 14 patients, 5 (35.7%) patients saw an improvement of at least 50% pain reduction, but only 2 of these patients maintained this level of pain control at last follow-up.

MCS is an invasive surgical procedure, but overall appears to be relatively safe based on data across case series. A systematic review of 10 studies including 157 patients who underwent MCS reported few overall complications with MCS procedures.[136] The most common reported complication was an intraoperative seizure, which occurred in 12% of patients. Of note, no patients went on to develop long-term seizures. Other complications that have been reported include infection, hardware complications, transient or long-lasting neurologic defects (including weakness), subdural or epidural hemorrhage, and localized scalp pain or headache.[126,136]

Dorsal Root Entry Zone Ablation Therapy

For patients who fail to respond to other medical and surgical interventions, including MVD or GKRS, dorsal root entry zone (DREZ) ablation therapy may provide pain relief.[145] This procedure involves the lesioning of the DREZ, often via radiofrequency thermocoagulation or mechanical disruption, within targeted spinal levels. It is an invasive process, often involving partial laminectomy and craniectomy, with placement of electrodes for radiofrequency lesioning.[146] For many pain syndromes, including TN, anesthesia dolorosa, postherpetic neuralgia, and trigeminal cancer pain, the specific target is the nucleus caudalis (NC).[145] The NC represents the pain-generating region following deafferentation, thereby leading to inappropriate pain signaling.[147] Linear ablations are generally made 1-mm apart along the axis of the spinal cord from the obex to the C2 level, thereby destroying nociceptive afferents from the ipsilateral face.[145,147,148]

NC DREZ offers substantial pain relief for patients who have failed other modalities. In several studies investigating NC DREZ for pain relief, 77% to 98% of patients who underwent the procedure experienced pain relief immediately following surgery.[145,147,149] At 1-year follow-up, 58% to 71% of these same patients were able to maintain pain relief.[145,147] When queried on the degree of pain relief at 1-year follow-up, 68.9% of patients reported being at least being very satisfied with their pain relief in one study, whereas 67% of patients reported excellent pain relief in another.[145,150] The average duration of pain relief was reported to be 4.3 years in one study.[145]

The most common complication from NC DREZ is transient ataxia immediately following the procedure.[145,148] In addition, transient hemiparesis may also be observed owing to damage to the nearby corticospinal tract.[147] Permanent complications, such as neuropathies and radiculopathies, have been reported as well with an incidence rate of 3.6% (n = 83).[145] In addition, this review identified a 3.6% rate of general medical complications and a 2.5% incidence of persistent incisional site pain.[145]

DISCUSSION

Chronic facial pain is a highly prevalent disorder with a variety of medical and surgical treatment options. The surgical options for the treatment of facial pain vary in their degree of complexity, invasiveness, and risk profile. As a result, when patients fail medical therapy, the task of selecting a surgical plan to treat their refractory facial pain can be difficult. Selection of the appropriate intervention should consider all relevant clinical and radiographic factors, as different surgical modalities may be better suited for different patients (**Fig. 7**).

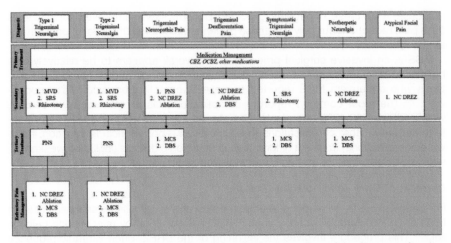

Fig. 7. Proposed treatment algorithm for orofacial pain. Regardless of the diagnosis, first-line management begins with pharmacotherapy, such as with CBZ or OXC. Second-line medications can be tried if the facial pain persists. For pain not adequately managed with medications alone, further treatment may be considered via MVD, stereotactic radiosurgery (SRS), rhizotomy, NC DREZ ablation, or several forms of neuromodulation, including PNS, DBS, or MCS. Further rescue therapies may be attempted should the facial pain recur or remain poorly controlled.

Of all the treatment options, medical management is the least invasive and therefore is considered the first-line therapy. Many providers will not consider more invasive surgical options until patients have demonstrated failure of one or more medications designed to treat their facial pain. One benefit of this treatment modality is that it can be further optimized and tailored to a patient's needs or tolerability, that is, by trialing a combination of medications in the event monotherapy fails to control the pain. As the most common side effects of these medications involve the renal, hepatic, cardiovascular, and hematologic systems, patients with relevant comorbidities may need to consider other treatment options early in their clinical course.

Surgical management of facial pain includes 3 main options: MVD, GKRS/CKRS, or percutaneous rhizotomy. Radiosurgery is the least invasive option and therefore may be preferred in patients who are older or have medical comorbidities that make open surgical modalities unsafe. Furthermore, the precise nature of GKRS can provide considerable pain relief while protecting adjacent neuroanatomic structures. The effect of radiotherapy may however provide only temporary pain relief.

Percutaneous rhizotomy is a less-invasive surgical procedure that is efficacious in the treatment of chronic facial pain. As it involves the use of a percutaneous needle rather than an open craniotomy, it confers similar advantages to radiosurgery for patients who may be poor candidates for general anesthesia because of age, or cardiovascular or respiratory comorbidities. Of the 3 types of percutaneous rhizotomy, BCR is associated with the longest-lasting pain relief. However, all rhizotomy procedures may require repeat procedures to achieve adequate pain relief.

Of all the surgical options, the MVD is the most invasive, as it requires performing a retrosigmoid craniotomy as well as manipulating the underlying cranial nerves and blood vessels arising from and supplying the brainstem, respectively. Despite this, the MVD has been shown to provide significant pain relief. In addition, as the only nonablative surgical technique, the MVD is less likely to result in permanent nerve damage when compared with radiation treatments or rhizotomy.

Despite their differences and similar efficacy profiles in the literature, rhizotomy, radiotherapy, and open surgical options to treat facial pain are not equivocal. A single-center study comparing the use of the MVD and GKRS for the treatment of typical TN found that complete pain relief was achieved in 68% of patients treated with MVD, compared with 48% of patients treated with GKRS.[151] The study reported no permanent complications with either intervention. An additional study found no statistically significant difference in clinical outcome between the use of GR or GKRS for control of facial pain.[152]

In the authors' clinical experience, MVD is the most common surgical approach used for patients with TN given its efficacy and long-term benefits. Although MVD is more invasive than the other techniques mentioned here, the operation is generally well tolerated and provides immediate relief of facial pain with durable long-term results. The GKRS and rhizotomy procedures are reserved for patients who do not have a clear underlying anatomic cause (neurovascular compression) for their pain, do not want open surgery, or have significant medical comorbidities placing them at higher risk of complications from open cranial surgery. The rhizotomy is preferred when immediate pain relief is requested (as opposed to GKRS). GKRS is often chosen in patients who are poor surgical candidates or who do not want open surgery. These treatments can be effective with few side effects but are associated with higher rates of recurrent facial pain that may require additional intervention. Because some patients may undergo multiple radiotherapy treatments for their facial pain, special attention must be given to GKRS planning to avoid excessive radiation exposure to the nerve root entry zone and pons (40 Gy to the 50% isodose lines with specific care to avoid overlap of the entry zone).

For patients who otherwise fail to respond to medical or surgical treatments, DREZ ablation therapy may offer significant pain relief. As an invasive and ablative process, it may not be a viable option for patients who are poor surgical candidates. It may also lead to further complications, including neuropathies or ataxia that may be permanent following the procedure. However, DREZ can help in the treatment of refractory facial pain, with even complete resolution of pain, in those who have failed multiple modalities of pain control.

Several neuromodulation techniques also exist for the treatment of neuropathic facial pain. In contrast to the more common surgical and radiotherapy treatments, neuromodulation usually involves multiple stages of intervention: a trial stage to gauge responses to stimulation followed by formal implantation of the device. Pain response to these neuromodulation techniques is often delayed compared with other interventions, presumably related to the need for prolonged stimulation before pain levels improve. Data on the efficacy of PNS, DBS, and MCS suggest these forms of treatment can achieve modest amounts of pain control. However, these neuromodulatory techniques have been insufficiently studied as they relate to the treatment of facial pain. Much of the data within the literature are limited by small sample sizes, short-term patient follow-up, and a lack of randomized, controlled trials. Despite this, these techniques are nonablative in nature, seem to have low side-effect profiles, and appear to be well-tolerated by patients.

SUMMARY

The causes of facial pain are numerous. Although the differential diagnosis is broad, many pharmacologic options are available for the first-line treatment of facial pain. When pharmacotherapy fails, multiple surgical techniques (including radiosurgery and neuromodulation techniques) are available to control refractory facial pain. These different approaches have variable safety, efficacy, and side-effect profiles as reviewed here, highlighting the difficulty in approach selection when managing a patient's facial pain. Additional research is necessary to better optimize how different surgical options can be used to better control facial pain.

CLINICS CARE POINTS

- Facial pain has many causes for which an accurate diagnosis is critical for the successful management of the pain.

- Pharmacotherapy should be attempted first before considering surgical options to manage facial pain.

- If conservative management fails, surgical intervention in the treatment of facial pain can be considered. Appropriate technique selection, including open surgery, radiotherapy, rhizotomy, or neuromodulatory options, depends on patient clinical and radiographic factors.

DISCLOSURES

The authors do not have any financial or commercial conflicts of interest to report.

REFERENCES

1. Headache Classification Committee of the International Headache Society (IHS): the International Classification of Headache Disorders. Cephalalgia 2018;38(1):1–211, 3rd edition.
2. Ananthan S, Benoliel R. Chronic orofacial pain. J Neural Transm (Vienna) 2020; 127(4):575–88.
3. Horst OV, Cunha-Cruz J, Zhou L, et al. Prevalence of pain in the orofacial regions in patients visiting general dentists in the Northwest Practice-based REsearch Collaborative in Evidence-based DENTistry research network. J Am Dent Assoc 2015;146(10):721–8.e3.
4. de Melo Júnior PC, Aroucha JMCN, Arnaud M, et al. Prevalence of TMD and level of chronic pain in a group of Brazilian adolescents. PLoS One 2019; 14(2):e0205874.
5. McMillan AS, Wong MC, Zheng J, et al. Prevalence of orofacial pain and treatment seeking in Hong Kong Chinese. J Orofac Pain 2006;20(3):218–25.
6. Ng KF, Tsui SL, Chan WS. Prevalence of common chronic pain in Hong Kong adults. Clin J Pain 2002;18(5):275–81.
7. Macfarlane TV, Blinkhorn AS, Davies RM, et al. Oro-facial pain in the community: prevalence and associated impact. Community Dent Oral Epidemiol 2002;30(1): 52–60.
8. Zakrzewska JM. Differential diagnosis of facial pain and guidelines for management. Br J Anaesth 2013;111(1):95–104.
9. Cruccu G, Di Stefano G, Truini A. Trigeminal neuralgia. N Engl J Med 2020; 383(8):754–62.
10. Bendtsen L, Zakrzewska JM, Abbott J, et al. European Academy of Neurology guideline on trigeminal neuralgia. Eur J Neurol 2019;26(6):831–49.
11. Cruccu G, Truini A. Refractory trigeminal neuralgia. Non-surgical treatment options. CNS Drugs 2013;27(2):91–6.
12. Slavin KV, Nersesyan H, Colpan ME, et al. Current algorithm for the surgical treatment of facial pain. Head Face Med 2007;3:30.

13. Brick N. Carbamazepine for acute and chronic pain in adults. Clin J Oncol Nurs 2011;15(3):335–6.
14. Maarbjerg S, Di Stefano G, Bendtsen L, et al. Trigeminal neuralgia - diagnosis and treatment. Cephalalgia 2017;37(7):648–57.
15. Shaikh S, Yaacob HB, Abd Rahman RB. Lamotrigine for trigeminal neuralgia: efficacy and safety in comparison with carbamazepine. J Chin Med Assoc 2011; 74(6):243–9.
16. Sindrup SH, Jensen TS. Pharmacotherapy of trigeminal neuralgia. Clin J Pain 2002;18(1):22–7.
17. Cruccu G, Gronseth G, Alksne J, et al. AAN-EFNS guidelines on trigeminal neuralgia management. Eur J Neurol 2008;15(10):1013–28.
18. Jones MR, Urits I, Ehrhardt KP, et al. A comprehensive review of trigeminal neuralgia. Curr Pain Headache Rep 2019;23(10):74.
19. Wiffen PJ, Collins S, McQuay HJ, et al. WITHDRAWN. Anticonvulsant drugs for acute and chronic pain. Cochrane Database Syst Rev 2010;1:CD001133.
20. Wiffen P, Collins S, McQuay H, et al. Anticonvulsant drugs for acute and chronic pain. Cochrane Database Syst Rev 2005;(3):CD001133.
21. Wiffen PJ, McQuay HJ, Moore RA. Carbamazepine for acute and chronic pain. Cochrane Database Syst Rev 2005;(3):CD005451.
22. Wiffen PJ, Derry S, Moore RA, et al. Carbamazepine for acute and chronic pain in adults. Cochrane Database Syst Rev 2011;(1):CD005451.
23. Wiffen PJ, Derry S, Moore RA, et al. Carbamazepine for chronic neuropathic pain and fibromyalgia in adults. Cochrane Database Syst Rev 2014;(4): CD005451.
24. Sawada T, Asai J, Nomiyama T, et al. Trigeminal trophic syndrome: report of a case and review of the published work. J Dermatol 2014;41(6):525–8.
25. Fruhauf J, Schaider H, Massone C, et al. Carbamazepine as the only effective treatment in a 52-year-old man with trigeminal trophic syndrome. Mayo Clin Proc 2008;83(4):502–4.
26. Luksić I, Sestan-Crnek S, Virag M, et al. Trigeminal trophic syndrome of all three nerve branches: an underrecognized complication after brain surgery. J Neurosurg 2008;108(1):170–3.
27. Di Stefano G, La Cesa S, Truini A, et al. Natural history and outcome of 200 outpatients with classical trigeminal neuralgia treated with carbamazepine or oxcarbazepine in a tertiary centre for neuropathic pain. J Headache Pain 2014; 15:34.
28. Killian JM, Fromm GH. Carbamazepine in the treatment of neuralgia. Use of side effects. Arch Neurol 1968;19(2):129–36.
29. Nicol CF. A four year double-blind study of tegretol in facial pain. Headache 1969;9(1):54–7.
30. Gomez-Arguelles JM, Dorado R, Sepulveda JM, et al. Oxcarbazepine monotherapy in carbamazepine-unresponsive trigeminal neuralgia. J Clin Neurosci 2008;15(5):516–9.
31. Di Stefano G, Truini A. Pharmacological treatment of trigeminal neuralgia. Expert Rev Neurother 2017;17(10):1003–11.
32. Zakrzewska JM, Palmer J, Morisset V, et al. Safety and efficacy of a Nav1.7 selective sodium channel blocker in patients with trigeminal neuralgia: a double-blind, placebo-controlled, randomised withdrawal phase 2a trial. Lancet Neurol 2017;16(4):291–300.
33. Zakrzewska JM, Palmer J, Ettlin DA, et al. Novel design for a phase IIa placebo-controlled, double-blind randomized withdrawal study to evaluate the safety

and efficacy of CNV1014802 in patients with trigeminal neuralgia. Trials 2013; 14:402.

34. Zakrzewska JM, Chaudhry Z, Nurmikko TJ, et al. Lamotrigine (lamictal) in refractory trigeminal neuralgia: results from a double-blind placebo controlled crossover trial. Pain 1997;73(2):223–30.

35. Wiffen PJ, Derry S, Moore RA. Lamotrigine for acute and chronic pain. Cochrane Database Syst Rev 2011;16(2):CD006044.

36. Kimos P, Biggs C, Mah J, et al. Analgesic action of gabapentin on chronic pain in the masticatory muscles: a randomized controlled trial. Pain 2007;127(1–2): 151–60.

37. Wei LA, Davies BW, Hink EM, et al. Perioperative pregabalin for attenuation of postoperative pain after eyelid surgery. Ophthalmic Plast Reconstr Surg 2015; 31(2):132–5.

38. Lemos L, Flores S, Oliveira P, et al. Gabapentin supplemented with ropivacain block of trigger points improves pain control and quality of life in trigeminal neuralgia patients when compared with gabapentin alone. Clin J Pain 2008;24(1): 64–75.

39. Obermann M, Yoon MS, Sensen K, et al. Efficacy of pregabalin in the treatment of trigeminal neuralgia. Cephalalgia 2008;28(2):174–81.

40. Pérez C, Navarro A, Saldaña MT, et al. Patient-reported outcomes in subjects with painful trigeminal neuralgia receiving pregabalin: evidence from medical practice in primary care settings. Cephalalgia 2009;29(7):781–90.

41. Pérez C, Saldaña MT, Navarro A, et al. Trigeminal neuralgia treated with pregabalin in family medicine settings: its effect on pain alleviation and cost reduction. J Clin Pharmacol 2009;49(5):582–90.

42. Achar A, Chakraborty PP, Bisai S, et al. Comparative study of clinical efficacy of amitriptyline and pregabalin in postherpetic neuralgia. Acta Dermatovenerol Croat 2012;20(2):89–94.

43. Domingues RB, Kuster GW, Aquino CC. Treatment of trigeminal neuralgia with low doses of topiramate. Arq Neuropsiquiatr 2007;65(3B):792–4.

44. Jorns TP, Johnston A, Zakrzewska JM. Pilot study to evaluate the efficacy and tolerability of levetiracetam (Keppra) in treatment of patients with trigeminal neuralgia. Eur J Neurol 2009;16(6):740–4.

45. Gronseth G, Cruccu G, Alksne J, et al. Practice parameter: the diagnostic evaluation and treatment of trigeminal neuralgia (an evidence-based review): report of the Quality Standards Subcommittee of the American Academy of Neurology and the European Federation of Neurological Societies. Neurology 2008;71(15): 1183–90.

46. Steardo L, Leo A, Marano E. Efficacy of baclofen in trigeminal neuralgia and some other painful conditions. A clinical trial. Eur Neurol 1984;23(1):51–5.

47. Fromm GH, Terrence CF, Chattha AS. Baclofen in the treatment of trigeminal neuralgia: double-blind study and long-term follow-up. Ann Neurol 1984;15(3): 240–4.

48. Fromm GH, Terrence CF. Comparison of L-baclofen and racemic baclofen in trigeminal neuralgia. Neurology 1987;37(11):1725–8.

49. Güler N, Durmus E, Tuncer S. Long-term follow-up of patients with atypical facial pain treated with amitriptyline. N Y State Dent J 2005;71(4):38–42.

50. Nagashima W, Kimura H, Ito M, et al. Effectiveness of duloxetine for the treatment of chronic nonorganic orofacial pain. Clin Neuropharmacol 2012;35(6): 273–7.

51. Forssell H, Tasmuth T, Tenovuo O, et al. Venlafaxine in the treatment of atypical facial pain: a randomized controlled trial. J Orofac Pain 2004;18(2):131–7.
52. Zakrzewska JM, Coakham HB. Microvascular decompression for trigeminal neuralgia: update. Curr Opin Neurol 2012;25(3):296–301.
53. Olson S, Atkinson L, Weidmann M. Microvascular decompression for trigeminal neuralgia: recurrences and complications. J Clin Neurosci 2005;12(7):787–9.
54. Abdulrauf SI, Urquiaga JF, Patel R, et al. Awake microvascular decompression for trigeminal neuralgia: concept and initial results. World Neurosurg 2018;113:e309–13.
55. Li X, Zheng X, Wang X, et al. Microvascular decompression treatment for post-Bell's palsy hemifacial spasm. Neurol Res 2013;35(2):187–92.
56. He Z, Cheng H, Wu H, et al. Risk factors for postoperative delirium in patients undergoing microvascular decompression. PLoS One 2019;14(4):e0215374.
57. Reddy VK, Parker SL, Patrawala SA, et al. Microvascular decompression for classic trigeminal neuralgia: determination of minimum clinically important difference in pain improvement for patient reported outcomes. Neurosurgery 2013;72(5):749–54 ; discussion 754.
58. Xiang H, Wu G, Ouyang J, et al. Prospective study of neuroendoscopy versus microscopy: 213 cases of microvascular decompression for trigeminal neuralgia performed by one neurosurgeon. World Neurosurg 2018;111:e335–9.
59. Leksell L. Sterotaxic radiosurgery in trigeminal neuralgia. Acta Chir Scand 1971;137(4):311–4.
60. Regis J, Bartolomei F, Metellus P, et al. Radiosurgery for trigeminal neuralgia and epilepsy. Neurosurg Clin N Am 1999;10(2):359–77.
61. Lindquist C, Kihlström L, Hellstrand E. Functional neurosurgery–a future for the gamma knife? Stereotact Funct Neurosurg 1991;57(1–2):72–81.
62. Rand RW, Jacques DB, Melbye RW, et al. Leksell gamma knife treatment of tic douloureux. Stereotact Funct Neurosurg 1993;61(Suppl 1):93–102.
63. Kondziolka D, Flickinger JC, Lunsford LD, et al. Trigeminal neuralgia radiosurgery: the University of Pittsburgh experience. Stereotact Funct Neurosurg 1996;66(Suppl 1):343–8.
64. Squire SE, Chan MD, Furr RM, et al. Gamma knife radiosurgery in the treatment of tumor-related facial pain. Stereotact Funct Neurosurg 2012;90(3):145–50.
65. Al-Quliti KW. Update on neuropathic pain treatment for trigeminal neuralgia. the pharmacological and surgical options. Neurosciences (Riyadh) 2015;20(2):107–14.
66. Maesawa S, Salame C, Flickinger JC, et al. Clinical outcomes after stereotactic radiosurgery for idiopathic trigeminal neuralgia. J Neurosurg 2001;94(1):14–20.
67. Zheng LG, Xu DS, Kang CS, et al. Stereotactic radiosurgery for primary trigeminal neuralgia using the Leksell Gamma unit. Stereotact Funct Neurosurg 2001;76(1):29–35. https://doi.org/10.1159/000056492.
68. Karam SD, Tai A, Wooster M, et al. Trigeminal neuralgia treatment outcomes following gamma knife radiosurgery with a minimum 3-year follow-up. J Radiat Oncol 2014;3:125–30.
69. Martínez Moreno NE, Gutiérrez-Sárraga J, Rey-Portolés G, et al. Long-term outcomes in the treatment of classical trigeminal neuralgia by gamma knife radiosurgery: a retrospective study in patients with minimum 2-year follow-up. Neurosurgery 2016;79(6):879–88.
70. Régis J, Tuleasca C, Resseguier N, et al. Long-term safety and efficacy of gamma knife surgery in classical trigeminal neuralgia: a 497-patient historical cohort study. J Neurosurg 2016;124(4):1079–87.

71. Zhao H, Shen Y, Yao D, et al. Outcomes of two-isocenter gamma knife radiosurgery for patients with typical trigeminal neuralgia: pain response and quality of life. World Neurosurg 2018;109:e531–8.

72. Barzaghi LR, Albano L, Scudieri C, et al. Factors affecting long-lasting pain relief after gamma knife radiosurgery for trigeminal neuralgia: a single institutional analysis and literature review. Neurosurg Rev 2021;44(5):2797–808.

73. Helis CA, McTyre E, Munley MT, et al. Gamma knife radiosurgery for multiple sclerosis-associated trigeminal neuralgia. Neurosurgery 2019;85(5):E933–9.

74. Weller M, Marshall K, Lovato JF, et al. Single-institution retrospective series of gamma knife radiosurgery in the treatment of multiple sclerosis-related trigeminal neuralgia: factors that predict efficacy. Stereotact Funct Neurosurg 2014; 92(1):53–8.

75. Rogers CL, Shetter AG, Ponce FA, et al. Gamma knife radiosurgery for trigeminal neuralgia associated with multiple sclerosis. J Neurosurg 2002;97(5 Suppl): 529–32.

76. Azar M, Yahyavi ST, Bitaraf MA, et al. Gamma knife radiosurgery in patients with trigeminal neuralgia: quality of life, outcomes, and complications. Clin Neurol Neurosurg 2009;111(2):174–8.

77. Barzaghi LR, Albano L, Scudieri C, et al. Factors affecting long-lasting pain relief after gamma knife radiosurgery for trigeminal neuralgia: a single institutional analysis and literature review. Neurosurg Rev 2021;44(5):2797–808.

78. Karam SD, Tai A, Wooster M, et al. Trigeminal neuralgia treatment outcomes following gamma knife radiosurgery with a minimum 3-year follow-up. J Radiat Oncol 2014;3(2):125–30.

79. Petit JH, Herman JM, Nagda S, et al. Radiosurgical treatment of trigeminal neuralgia: evaluating quality of life and treatment outcomes. Int J Radiat Oncol Biol Phys 2003;56(4):1147–53.

80. Riesenburger RI, Hwang SW, Schirmer CM, et al. Outcomes following single-treatment gamma knife surgery for trigeminal neuralgia with a minimum 3-year follow-up. J Neurosurg 2010;112(4):766–71.

81. Bal W, Łabuz-Roszak B, Tarnawski R, et al. Effectiveness and safety of Cyber-Knife radiosurgery in treatment of trigeminalgia - experiences of Polish neurological and oncological centres. Neurol Neurochir Pol 2020;54(1):28–32.

82. Conti A, Pontoriero A, Iatì G, et al. Frameless stereotactic radiosurgery for treatment of multiple sclerosis-related trigeminal neuralgia. World Neurosurg 2017; 103:702–12.

83. Zakrzewska JM, Linskey ME. Trigeminal neuralgia. Am Fam Physician 2016; 94(2):133–5.

84. Brown JA, Gouda JJ. Percutaneous balloon compression of the trigeminal nerve. Neurosurg Clin N Am 1997;8(1):53–62.

85. Kouzounias K, Schechtmann G, Lind G, et al. Factors that influence outcome of percutaneous balloon compression in the treatment of trigeminal neuralgia. Neurosurgery 2010;67(4):925–34 ; discussion 934.

86. Brown JA, Preul MC. Trigeminal depressor response during percutaneous microcompression of the trigeminal ganglion for trigeminal neuralgia. Neurosurgery 1988;23(6):745–8.

87. Lichtor T, Mullan JF. A 10-year follow-up review of percutaneous microcompression of the trigeminal ganglion. J Neurosurg 1990;72(1):49–54.

88. Correa CF, Teixeira MJ. Balloon compression of the Gasserian ganglion for the treatment of trigeminal neuralgia. Stereotact Funct Neurosurg 1998;71(2):83–9.

89. Skirving DJ, Dan NG. A 20-year review of percutaneous balloon compression of the trigeminal ganglion. J Neurosurg 2001;94(6):913–7.

90. Chen JF, Tu PH, Lee ST. Long-term follow-up of patients treated with percutaneous balloon compression for trigeminal neuralgia in Taiwan. World Neurosurg 2011;76(6):586–91.

91. Bergenheim AT, Asplund P, Linderoth B. Percutaneous retrogasserian balloon compression for trigeminal neuralgia: review of critical technical details and outcomes. World Neurosurg 2013;79(2):359–68.

92. Kanpolat Y, Savas A, Bekar A, et al. Percutaneous controlled radiofrequency trigeminal rhizotomy for the treatment of idiopathic trigeminal neuralgia: 25-year experience with 1,600 patients. Neurosurgery 2001;48(3):524–32 ; discussion 532-4.

93. Broggi G, Franzini A, Lasio G, et al. Long-term results of percutaneous retrogasserian thermorhizotomy for "essential" trigeminal neuralgia: considerations in 1000 consecutive patients. Neurosurgery 1990;26(5):783–6 ; discussion 786-7.

94. Bender MT, Pradilla G, Batra S, et al. Glycerol rhizotomy and radiofrequency thermocoagulation for trigeminal neuralgia in multiple sclerosis. J Neurosurg 2013;118(2):329–36.

95. Slettebo H, Hirschberg H, Lindegaard KF. Long-term results after percutaneous retrogasserian glycerol rhizotomy in patients with trigeminal neuralgia. Acta Neurochir (Wien) 1993;122(3–4):231–5.

96. Steiger HJ. Prognostic factors in the treatment of trigeminal neuralgia. Analysis of a differential therapeutic approach. Acta Neurochir (Wien) 1991; 113(1–2):11–7.

97. Fujimaki T, Fukushima T, Miyazaki S. Percutaneous retrogasserian glycerol injection in the management of trigeminal neuralgia: long-term follow-up results. J Neurosurg 1990;73(2):212–6.

98. Young RF. Glycerol rhizolysis for treatment of trigeminal neuralgia. J Neurosurg 1988;69(1):39–45.

99. Bick SKB, Eskandar EN. Surgical treatment of trigeminal neuralgia. Neurosurg Clin N Am 2017;28(3):429–38.

100. Bender M, Pradilla G, Batra S, et al. Effectiveness of repeat glycerol rhizotomy in treating recurrent trigeminal neuralgia. Neurosurgery 2012;70(5):1125–33 ; discussion 1133-4.

101. Frank F, Fabrizi AP. Percutaneous surgical treatment of trigeminal neuralgia. Acta Neurochir (Wien) 1989;97(3–4):128–30.

102. Taha JM, Tew JM. Comparison of surgical treatments for trigeminal neuralgia: reevaluation of radiofrequency rhizotomy. Neurosurgery 1996;38(5):865–71.

103. Cheng JS, Lim DA, Chang EF, et al. A review of percutaneous treatments for trigeminal neuralgia. Neurosurgery 2014;10(Suppl 1):25–33 ; discussion 33.

104. Wang JY, Bender MT, Bettegowda C. Percutaneous procedures for the treatment of trigeminal neuralgia. Neurosurg Clin N Am 2016;27(3):277–95.

105. Winfree CJ. Peripheral nerve stimulation for facial pain using conventional devices: indications and results. Prog Neurol Surg 2020;35:60–7.

106. Melzack R, Wall PD. Pain mechanisms: a new theory. Science 1965;150(3699): 971–9.

107. Wall PD, Sweet WH. Temporary abolition of pain in man. Science 1967; 155(3758):108–9.

108. Ellis JA, Mejia Munne JC, Winfree CJ. Trigeminal branch stimulation for the treatment of intractable craniofacial pain. J Neurosurg 2015;123(1):283–8.

109. Klein J, Sandi-Gahun S, Schackert G, et al. Peripheral nerve field stimulation for trigeminal neuralgia, trigeminal neuropathic pain, and persistent idiopathic facial pain. Cephalalgia 2016;36(5):445–53.

110. Han R, Guo G, Ni Y, et al. Clinical efficacy of short-term peripheral nerve stimulation in management of facial pain associated with herpes zoster ophthalmicus. Front Neurosci 2020;14:574713.

111. Stidd DA, Wuollet AL, Bowden K, et al. Peripheral nerve stimulation for trigeminal neuropathic pain. Pain Physician 2012;15(1):27–33.

112. Salmasi V, Olatoye OO, Terkawi AS, et al. Peripheral nerve stimulation for occipital neuralgia. Pain Med 2020;21(Suppl 1):S13–7.

113. Slavin KV, Colpan ME, Munawar N, et al. Trigeminal and occipital peripheral nerve stimulation for craniofacial pain: a single-institution experience and review of the literature. Neurosurg Focus 2006;21(6):E5.

114. Slavin KV. Peripheral nerve stimulation for neuropathic pain. Neurotherapeutics 2008;5(1):100–6.

115. de Leon-Casasola OA. Spinal cord and peripheral nerve stimulation techniques for neuropathic pain. J Pain Symptom Manage 2009;38(2 Suppl):S28–38.

116. Aum DJ, Tierney TS. Deep brain stimulation: foundations and future trends. Front Biosci (Landmark Ed) 2018;23:162–82.

117. Ben-Haim S, Mirzadeh Z, Rosenberg WS. Deep brain stimulation for intractable neuropathic facial pain. Neurosurg Focus 2018;45(2):E15.

118. Coffey RJ. Deep brain stimulation for chronic pain: results of two multicenter trials and a structured review. Pain Med 2001;2(3):183–92.

119. Thomas L, Bledsoe JM, Stead M, et al. Motor cortex and deep brain stimulation for the treatment of intractable neuropathic face pain. Curr Neurol Neurosci Rep 2009;9(2):120–6.

120. Rasche D, Rinaldi PC, Young RF, et al. Deep brain stimulation for the treatment of various chronic pain syndromes. Neurosurg Focus 2006;21(6):E8.

121. Pereira EA, Green AL, Bradley KM, et al. Regional cerebral perfusion differences between periventricular grey, thalamic and dual target deep brain stimulation for chronic neuropathic pain. Stereotact Funct Neurosurg 2007;85(4):175–83.

122. Owen SLF, Green AL, Stein JF, et al. Deep brain stimulation for the alleviation of post-stroke neuropathic pain. Pain 2006;120(1–2):202–6.

123. Franzini A, Leone M, Messina G, et al. Neuromodulation in treatment of refractory headaches. Neurol Sci 2008;29(Suppl 1):S65–8.

124. Kashanian A, DiCesare JAT, Rohatgi P, et al. Case series: deep brain stimulation for facial pain. Oper Neurosurg (Hagerstown) 2020;19(5):510–7.

125. Kumar K, Toth C, Nath RK. Deep brain stimulation for intractable pain: a 15-year experience. Neurosurg 1997;40(4):736–46 ; discussion 746-7.

126. Teton ZE, Raslan AM. Motor cortex stimulation for facial pain. Prog Neurol Surg 2020;35:162–9.

127. Senatus P, Zurek S, Deogaonkar M. Deep brain stimulation and motor cortex stimulation for chronic pain. Neurol India 2020;68(Supplement):S235–40.

128. Canavero S, Bonicalzi V. Therapeutic extradural cortical stimulation for central and neuropathic pain: a review. Clin J Pain 2002;18(1):48–55.

129. Tsubokawa T, Katayama Y, Yamamoto T, et al. Chronic motor cortex stimulation in patients with thalamic pain. J Neurosurg 1993;78(3):393–401.

130. Loeser JD, Ward AA, White LE. Chronic deafferentation of human spinal cord neurons. J Neurosurg 1968;29(1):48–50.

131. Brown JA, Lutsep HL, Weinand M, et al. Motor cortex stimulation for the enhancement of recovery from stroke: a prospective, multicenter safety study. Neurosurgery 2006;58(3):464–73.

132. Henderson JM, Lad SP. Motor cortex stimulation and neuropathic facial pain. Neurosurg Focus 2006;21(6):E6.

133. Mertens P, Nuti C, Sindou M, et al. Precentral cortex stimulation for the treatment of central neuropathic pain: results of a prospective study in a 20-patient series. Stereotact Funct Neurosurg 1999;73(1–4):122–5.

134. Peyron R, Garcia-Larrea L, Deiber MP, et al. Electrical stimulation of precentral cortical area in the treatment of central pain: electrophysiological and PET study. Pain 1995;62(3):275–86.

135. Maarrawi J, Peyron R, Mertens P, et al. Motor cortex stimulation for pain control induces changes in the endogenous opioid system. Neurology 2007;69(9): 827–34.

136. Fontaine D, Hamani C, Lozano A. Efficacy and safety of motor cortex stimulation for chronic neuropathic pain: critical review of the literature. J Neurosurg 2009; 110(2):251–6.

137. Buchanan RJ, Darrow D, Monsivais D, et al. Motor cortex stimulation for neuropathic pain syndromes: a case series experience. Neuroreport 2014;25(9): 715–7.

138. Sharma M, Shaw A, Deogaonkar M. Surgical options for complex craniofacial pain. Neurosurg Clin N Am 2014;25(4):763–75.

139. Brown JA, Pilitsis JG. Motor cortex stimulation for central and neuropathic facial pain: a prospective study of 10 patients and observations of enhanced sensory and motor function during stimulation. Neurosurgery 2005;56(2):290–7 ; discussion 290-7.

140. Nuti C, Peyron R, Garcia-Larrea L, et al. Motor cortex stimulation for refractory neuropathic pain: four year outcome and predictors of efficacy. Pain 2005; 118(1–2):43–52.

141. Nguyen JP, Velasco F, Brugières P, et al. Treatment of chronic neuropathic pain by motor cortex stimulation: results of a bicentric controlled crossover trial. Brain Stimul 2008;1(2):89–96.

142. Velasco F, Argüelles C, Carrillo-Ruiz JD, et al. Efficacy of motor cortex stimulation in the treatment of neuropathic pain: a randomized double-blind trial. J Neurosurg 2008;108(4):698–706.

143. Raslan AM, Nasseri M, Bahgat D, et al. Motor cortex stimulation for trigeminal neuropathic or deafferentation pain: an institutional case series experience. Stereotact Funct Neurosurg 2011;89(2):83–8.

144. Sachs AJ, Babu H, Su YF, et al. Lack of efficacy of motor cortex stimulation for the treatment of neuropathic pain in 14 patients. Neuromodulation 2014;17(4): 303–10 ; discussion 310-1.

145. Chivukula S, Tempel ZJ, Chen CJ, et al. Spinal and nucleus caudalis dorsal root entry zone lesioning for chronic pain: efficacy and outcomes. World Neurosurg 2015;84(2):494–504.

146. Sampson JH, Nashold BS. Facial pain due to vascular lesions of the brain stem relieved by dorsal root entry zone lesions in the nucleus caudalis. Report of two cases. J Neurosurg 1992;77(3):473–5.

147. Kanpolat Y, Tuna H, Bozkurt M, et al. Spinal and nucleus caudalis dorsal root entry zone operations for chronic pain. Neurosurgery 2008;62(3 Suppl 1): 235–42 ; discussion 242-4.

148. Husain AM, Elliott SL, Gorecki JP. Neurophysiological monitoring for the nucleus caudalis dorsal root entry zone operation. Neurosurgery 2002;50(4):822–7, discussion 827-8.
149. Bernard EJ, Nashold BS, Caputi F, et al. Nucleus caudalis DREZ lesions for facial pain. Br J Neurosurg 1987;1(1):81–91.
150. Bullard DE, Nashold BS. The caudalis DREZ for facial pain. Stereotact Funct Neurosurg 1997;68(1–4 Pt 1):168–74.
151. Brisman R. Microvascular decompression vs. gamma knife radiosurgery for typical trigeminal neuralgia: preliminary findings. Stereotact Funct Neurosurg 2007;85(2–3):94–8.
152. Pollock BE, Ecker RD. A prospective cost-effectiveness study of trigeminal neuralgia surgery. Clin J Pain 2005;21(4):317–22.

Headache Diagnosis in Children and Adolescents

Vijay A. Patel, MD[a],*, Jeffrey Liaw, MD[b], Robert A. Saadi, MD[c], Huseyin Isildak, MD[d], Christopher L. Kalmar, MD, MBA[e], Sean P. Polster, MD[f]

KEYWORDS

- Headache • Migraines • Pediatric • Primary headache • Rhinogenic headache
- Secondary headache

KEY POINTS

- Primary headaches represent a disease state in themselves, whereas secondary headaches are directly caused or exacerbated by an underlying etiology
- A comprehensive history and physical examination remain critical steps in the evaluation of pediatric headache
- The presence of red flag signs & symptoms should warrant ancillary radiographic imaging
- Pediatric headache and migraine management follows a multifaceted approach including lifestyle modifications, abortive agents, preventive medications, and complementary therapies

INTRODUCTION

Described and categorized since antiquity, written references to headache trace back to Ebers Papyrus in Ancient Egypt at approximately 1550 BC.[1] In modern times, headache continues to persist as a common chief complaint, with a prevalence of up to 80% in children and stands as one of the most frequent reasons for urgent care and ambulatory visits.[2] A comprehensive history and physical examination remain critical; in most situations, it allows the clinician to distinguish between primary and secondary headaches. Referral to an otolaryngologist is often deemed necessary to evaluate for a potential underlying otologic or rhinogenic etiology. Compared with

Funding Source: None.
[a] Division of Otolaryngology - Head & Neck Surgery, Children's Hospital Los Angeles, 4650 Sunset Boulevard MS #58, Los Angeles, CA 90027, USA; [b] Department of Otolaryngology - Head & Neck Surgery, University of Missouri, Columbia, MO 65211 USA; [c] Department of Otolaryngology - Head & Neck Surgery, University of Arkansas, 2801 S University Avenue, Little Rock, AR 72204, USA; [d] Department of Otolaryngology - Head & Neck Surgery, Stony Brook University, 101 Nicolls Road, Stony Brook, NY 11794, USA; [e] Department of Plastic Surgery, Vanderbilt University Medical Center, 1161 Medical Center Drive, Nashville, TN 37212, USA; [f] Department of Neurological Surgery, University of Pittsburgh Medical Center, 200 Lothrop Street, Pittsburgh, PA 15213, USA
* Corresponding author.
E-mail address: vijayapatel@live.com

Otolaryngol Clin N Am 55 (2022) 633–647
https://doi.org/10.1016/j.otc.2022.02.007
0030-6665/22/© 2022 Elsevier Inc. All rights reserved.

adults, headache phenotypes tend to differ in pediatric patients as childhood and adolescence are active periods of brain development and myelination.[3] Furthermore, persistent head pain in children may result in significant impairment, resulting in missed school days and extracurricular events as well as suboptimal participation in regular daily activities. As these changes often lead to significant anxiety and worry for parents and families, it is essential for all health care practitioners to accurately approach pediatric headaches and offer timely therapeutic options.[4] In this article, key elements include identifying distinct types of headache disorders affecting the pediatric population and their associated management.

PRIMARY HEADACHE

Primary headaches are defined as a headache not caused by an underlying disease or condition. Migraines are the most common cause of recurrent headaches in the pediatric population, occurring most frequently in childhood, whereas tension-type headaches (TTH) stand as the most common cause of adolescent headaches.[5]

PEDIATRIC MIGRAINES

Pediatric migraines are defined as recurrent, moderate to severe headaches lasting 2 to 72 hours in duration. The mean age of onset of migraines is 11 years for females and 7 years for males. These headaches are typically unilateral, pulsatile in quality, and aggravated by physical activity. Migraine attacks may also be associated with symptoms such as nausea/vomiting as well as photophobia/phonophobia. In children, 8% of individuals experience headaches consistent with migraines, with a prevalence that increases with age. The prevalence is initially equal across genders during childhood; however, by adolescence, migraines increase proportionally among women to a ratio similarly observed in adults.[6] The International Classification of Headache Disorders 3rd Edition (ICHD-3) subdivides migraines into 3 primary groups:

1. Migraines without aura
2. Migraine with aura
3. Childhood "periodic syndromes"

The ICHD-3 also makes several distinctions when comparing pediatric to adult migraines. Adult migraines last at least 4 to 72 hours, whereas pediatric migraines can be as short as 2 hours and lasts as long as 72 hours (**Table 1**). Additionally, adults typically develop unilateral migraines, yet most of the children (80%) experience bilateral symptoms.

Pediatric Migraine Stages

Migraines typically progress through 4 stages: prodrome, aura (if present), attack, and postdrome. Prodromes may begin a day or 2 before a migraine episode, with up to 70% of pediatric migraineurs experiencing premonitory symptoms such as blurred vision, constipation, fatigue, food craving, frequent yawning, increased urination, mood changes, neck stiffness, and photophobia.[7] Postdromal symptoms are also common in children, with 82% of individuals experiencing symptoms such as food craving, ocular pain, paraesthesias, somnolence, thirst, and visual disturbance.[8]

An aura is defined as a transient focal neurologic phenomenon that occurs before or during a migraine episode. Symptoms can be visual, sensory, or motor and usually occur over several minutes to an hour. The most common auras in the pediatric population are visual and sensory. The best-known visual aura is the fortification spectrum, which is the perception of bright, shimmering, zig-zag lines which spread

Table 1
International Classification of Headache Disorders 3rd Edition, Migraines

	1.1 Migraine without Aura	1.2 Migraine with Aura

Diagnostic Criteria	A. At least 5 attacks fulfilling criteria B and D
	B. Headache attacks lasting 4–72 h (untreated or unsuccessfully treated)
		A. At least 2 attacks fulfilling criteria B and C
		B. One or more of the following fully reversible aura symptoms:
		  1. Visual
		  2. Sensory
		  3. Speech and/or language
		  4. Motor
		  5. Brainstem
		  6. Retinal

	C. Headache has at least 2 of the following 4 characteristics:
	  1. Unilateral location
	  2. Pulsating quality
	  3. Moderate or severe pain intensity
	  4. Aggravation by or causing avoidance of routine physical activity (eg, walking or climbing stairs)
		C. At least 3 of the following 6 characteristics:
		  1. At least one aura symptom spreads gradually over ≥5 min
		  2. Two or more aura symptoms occur in succession
		  3. Each individual aura symptom lasts 5–60 minutes
		  4. At least one aura symptom is unilateral
		  5. At least one aura symptom is positive
		  6. The aura is accompanied, or followed within 60 min, by headache

	D. During headache at least one of the following:
	  1. Nausea and/or vomiting
	  2. Photophobia and phonophobia
	E. Not better accounted for by another ICHD-3 diagnosis
		D. Not better accounted for by another ICHD-3 diagnosis

From Headache Classification Committee of the International Headache Society (IHS) The International Classification of Headache Disorders, 3rd edition. Cephalalgia. 2018;38(1):1-211.

across one's visual field. Sensory auras are often reported as paraesthesias, dysphagia, or hemiplegia.

Otologic Manifestations of Pediatric Migraines

In addition to classic migraine symptoms, children may experience vestibular symptoms related to their disease. Unlike adults, children with vertigo may not have the capability to articulate vertiginous phenomena. Symptoms of vertigo may manifest as expressions of diaphoresis, fear, loss of balance, pallor, staggering, and vomiting. It is, therefore, essential for the clinician to recognize subtle manifestations of vertigo in the pediatric population.

Benign Paroxysmal Vertigo of Childhood

Benign paroxysmal vertigo of childhood (BPVC) is a rare, peripheral vestibular disorder in children manifested as episodes of spontaneous vertigo, lasting minutes to hours without loss of consciousness (**Table 2**). Neurologic, audiometric, and vestibular examinations between attacks are typically normal.[9] Although its pathophysiology and etiology are unknown, it is theorized to be a precursor syndrome to migraines as children with BPVC often have a family history of migraines and develop migraines more frequently when compared with the general population.[10] And while BPVC is an accepted clinical diagnosis within ICHD-3, its treatment is relatively absent from the literature. Although protocols exist on balance training in children, few have been validated.[9]

Benign Paroxysmal Torticollis

Benign paroxysmal torticollis (BPT) is a similarly rare and self-limited disorder characterized by sudden stereotypical head-tilting episodes that remit spontaneously within minutes to days. These episodes can be associated with agitation, emesis, nystagmus, and pallor. Episodes can be provoked by positional changes, suggesting a vestibular etiology. BPT is also thought to be a precursor to BPVC and migraines.

Vestibular Migraines

Vestibular migraines are episodes of vertigo lasting from 5 minutes to 72 hours, with at least half of these events occurring in association with migraine symptoms (see **Table 2**). An age limit is not a criterion of vestibular migraines; therefore, it may be diagnosed in a child who meets diagnostic criteria. Symptoms of vestibular migraines frequently overlap with Ménière's disease; although rare in children, many patients with features of both Ménière's disease and vestibular migraines have been reported.[7] Hearing loss differentiates Ménière's disease from vestibular migraines as individuals with vestibular migraines do not have progressive, fluctuating, sensorineural hearing loss, particularly in the low frequencies.

Pediatric Migraine Therapies

Migraine treatment includes both behavioral and pharmacologic modifications. Prevention strategies include the management of triggers such as addressing underlying stressors, school problems, and modification of lifestyle habits including appropriate nutritional intake and sleep hygiene. Dietary modification may also be necessary to avoid triggers as some foods such as caffeinated beverages, cheeses, chocolate, and ice cream may exacerbate migraines.[11] Pharmacologic therapies are divided into prophylactic and abortive medications; patients with frequent attacks usually require both treatments. Abortive medications are used only during a migraine attack to mitigate symptoms; triptans are first-line drugs in aborting a migraine attack. Nonsteroidal anti-inflammatory drugs (ibuprofen) and acetaminophen have also been used in the pediatric population and found to be effective in controlling pain.[12] Preventative medications are also recommended when migraine attacks are particularly debilitating or occur at least once a week. Preventative medications typically administered in the pediatric population include amitriptyline, divalproex, flunarizine, and topiramate. Cognitive-behavioral therapy, in combination with preventive medication, also serves as an important adjunct and has been shown to help adolescents with chronic migraines improve more when compared with sole medical therapy plus headache education.[13]

PEDIATRIC TENSION-TYPE HEADACHE

TTH are bilateral, nonthrobbing head pain episodes of mild to moderate activity lasting 30 minutes to a week.[7] Unlike migraines, TTH is not typically accompanied by

Table 2 International Classification of Headache Disorders 3rd Edition, Otologic Headaches		
	1.6.2 Benign Paroxysmal Vertigo	**A1.6.6 Vestibular Migraine**
Diagnostic Criteria	A. At least 5 attacks fulfilling criteria B and C	A. At least 5 episodes fulfilling criteria C and D
	B. Vertigo occurring without warning, maximal at onset and resolving spontaneously after minutes to hours without loss of consciousness	B. A current or past history of migraine without aura or migraine with aura
	C. At least one of the following 5 associated symptoms or signs: 1. Nystagmus 2. Ataxia 3. Vomiting 4. Pallor 5. Fearfulness	C. Vestibular symptoms of moderate or severe intensity, lasting between 5 min and 72 h
	D. Normal neurologic examination and audiometric and vestibular functions between attacks	D. At least half of episodes are associated with at least one of the following 3 migrainous features: 1. Headache with at least 2 of the following 4 characteristics: a. Unilateral location b. Pulsating quality c. Moderate or severe intensity d. Aggravation by routine physical activity 2. Photophobia and phonophobia 3. Visual aura
	E. Not attributed to another disorder	E. Not better accounted for by another ICHD-3 diagnosis or by another vestibular disorder

From Headache Classification Committee of the International Headache Society (IHS) The International Classification of Headache Disorders, 3rd edition. Cephalalgia. 2018;38(1):1211.

photophobia or phonophobia, nausea or vomiting, and is not aggravated by physical activity. Symptoms are typically characterized as a bifrontal, band-like, or temporal pain that is continuous. TTH is confirmed based on a detailed history obtained from the child with symptoms fulfilling diagnostic criteria. Similar to migraines, treatment of TTH includes the management of both acute attacks as well preventative therapies. Lifestyle modification, proper sleep hygiene, and avoidance of stressors are also recommended in TTH prevention. During acute attacks, acetaminophen or nonsteroidal anti-inflammatory drugs are commonly used to treat TTH. Aspirin should be avoided in children due to its association with Reye Syndrome.[14]

PEDIATRIC TRIGEMINAL AUTONOMIC CEPHALALGIAS

Trigeminal autonomic cephalalgias (TACs) include cluster headache and paroxysmal hemicrania, which are rarely reported in the pediatric population with a prevalence of <1%.[15] TACs share clinical features of a unilateral headache, with the addition of ipsilateral cranial parasympathetic autonomic features, suggesting that these entities activate the trigeminal-parasympathetic reflex.[7]

Cluster Headache

Cluster headaches are defined as attacks of severe, strictly unilateral pain in the orbital, supraorbital, or temporal region lasting 15 minutes to 3 hours, occurring up to eight times a day. Although the age of onset is usually in the second and third decade of life, onset in the first decade of life is recognized, occurring at a median age of 8.5 years in children with a male predominance, similar to the adult population.[16] As with TACs, autonomic parasympathetic symptoms often manifest including facial sweating, lacrimation, ptosis, and rhinorrhea. Cluster headaches are also associated with migraine symptoms such as nausea, vomiting, phonophobia, and photophobia. These associated symptoms often lead to a misdiagnosis of migraines, particularly in children.[17] The pharmacologic treatment of childhood-onset cluster headaches is not well described in the literature.[18] This is largely due to a long intercluster interval in the pediatric population, making continuous pharmacologic therapy undesirable. The traditional abortive treatment of cluster headaches involves the inhalation of 100% oxygen via a nonrebreathing facial mask, with 70% of patients achieving pain relief within 15 minutes.[19]

Paroxysmal Hemicrania

Paroxysmal hemicrania is defined as attacks of severe, strictly unilateral pain in the orbital, supraorbital, or temporal region lasting 2 to 30 minutes and occurring several times a day. Similar to cluster headaches, attacks are associated with autonomic symptoms which include facial sweating, lacrimation, ptosis, and rhinorrhea. Although primarily observed in adults, childhood-onset paroxysmal hemicrania has been described in the literature.[20] As with the adult population, the defining feature of paroxysmal hemicrania is an absolute response to indomethacin, which represents both a therapeutic and diagnostic parameter (ie, indotest).

PEDIATRIC RHINOGENIC HEADACHE

Pediatric rhinogenic headaches are an important etiology of secondary headache disorders. As a diagnostic group, this mainly includes sinonasal and mucosal contact point pathologies. Given the relative frequency neurologists, otolaryngologists, and pediatricians comanage children with a constellation of symptoms concerning an underlying headache disorder, a comprehensive understanding of inherent diagnostic challenges and management principles surrounding rhinogenic conditions remains essential.

Rhinosinusitis and Headaches

The ICHD-3 provides succinct criteria to assist in the diagnosis of headache secondary to sinonasal pathology[7] (**Table 3**). Acute and chronic pediatric rhinosinusitis are well-described entities supported by evidence-based management guidelines as outlined in the American Academy of Pediatrics, American Academy of Otolaryngology–Head and Neck Surgery, American Rhinologic Society, and European Rhinologic Society.[21–24] Unique elements of interest in ICHD-3 include the fact that the term "sinus headache" is no longer recognized as an accepted clinical diagnosis, the sinonasal disease may exacerbate migraines, and the absence of age parameters potentially restricts its relevance to the pediatric population.[25] Fortunately, a panel of pediatric headache experts recently published a series of recommendations regarding ICHD-

3 and concluded the segment on rhinogenic headache is, indeed, suitable as it stands for pediatric application.[26]

Cranial Autonomic Symptoms

Given the natural overlap with rhinosinusitis manifestations and cranial autonomic symptoms, it often makes it difficult for clinicians to arrive at the appropriate diagnosis. Two recent studies attempted to identify the frequency of cranial autonomic symptoms in pediatric patients with migraines. In a prospective, cross-sectional study of 125 patients by Gelfand and colleagues, 73% exhibited at least 1 cranial autonomic symptom; specifically, 24% of children had nasal congestion or rhinorrhea, with an odds ratio for simultaneous sinonasal symptoms of 16.2 (95% CI, 3.4–84.7).[27] In a retrospective, observational study of 230 children with primary headache, 55%, 25%, and 41% of children exhibited at least 1, 2, or 3 cranial autonomic symptoms, respectively.[28] Given the high prevalence of cranial autonomic symptoms in pediatric patients with primary headache disorders, familiarity with these manifestations is necessary.

Mucosal Contact Point Headaches

One of the most hotly debated etiologies of rhinogenic headache revolves around the significance of symptomatic mucosal contact points.[29] This type of headache is believed to occur from a contact point between mucosal surfaces due to anatomic variations such as turbinate pneumatization and septal anomalies (ie, deviation and spur) (see **Table 3**). Diagnostic criteria for mucosal contact point headache include an absence of sinonasal disease with headache relief following local anesthetic placement to areas of mucosal contact. At this time, the medical literature reporting this phenomenon in children is limited to case reports and small clinical series. In 3 case reports, headache with associated pain (age range, 11–17 years) was responsive to local anesthesia on mucosal contact points.[29–31] In 2 cases, surgical resection provided symptomatic relief, with a follow-up period ranging from 2 weeks to 12 months.[31,32] Two clinical series also described similar findings in the management of mucosal contact point headaches. In a mixed case series of 2 pediatric patients (mean age, 16 years) with pneumatized superior turbinates observed via nasal endoscopy, local anesthesia applied to contact points reduced headache severity scores, with durable results following surgery at 6 and 13 months, respectively. In a retrospective review of 3 patients (range, 6–17 years) with headaches and mucosal contact points observed on computed tomography (CT), all patients reported decreased headaches following surgical resection, with a follow-up period ranging from 6 months to 1 year.[33] Parsons and colleagues also presented their comprehensive experience with 15 pediatric patients with mucosal contact point headaches. In total, 13 children (87%) reported a reduction in both intensity and frequency of headaches following surgical intervention.[33] However, this study did not use local anesthetic as a diagnostic indicator for the potential treatment effect and is limited in its general applicability by the presence of concomitant sinonasal diseases such as allergic rhinitis and chronic rhinosinusitis. Overall, the current body of information surrounding mucosal contact point headaches is sparse, as such, it should not solely be used to guide primary treatment decisions.[34] Furthermore, it is extremely important to note that the presence of mucosal contact points on nasal endoscopy and/or radiographic imaging does not imply that a child will invariably suffer from rhinogenic headaches. Rather, mucosal contact points should be considered as a possible etiology in otherwise unexplainable pediatric headaches, refractory to standard medical therapy.[25]

Table 3
International Classification of Headache Disorders 3rd Edition, Rhinogenic Headaches

	11.5.1 Headache Attributed to Acute Rhinosinusitis	11.5.2 Headache Attributed to Chronic or Recurring Rhinosinusitis	A11.5.3 Headache Attributed to Disorder of the Nasal Mucosa, Turbinates, or Septum

Diagnostic Criteria	A. Any headache fulfilling criterion C
	B. Clinical, nasal endoscopic, and/or imaging evidence of acute rhinosinusitis
	C. Evidence of causation demonstrated by at least 2 of the following:
	  1. Headache has developed in temporal relation to the onset of rhinosinusitis
	  2. Either or both of the following:
	    a. Headache has significantly worsened in parallel with worsening of the rhinosinusitis
	    b. Headache has significantly improved or resolved in parallel with the improvement in or the resolution of the rhinosinusitis
	  3. Headache is exacerbated by pressure applied over the paranasal sinuses in the case of unilateral rhinosinusitis, headache is localized and ipsilateral to it
	D. Not better accounted for by another ICHD-3 diagnosis
		A. Any headache fulfilling criterion C
		B. Clinical, nasal endoscopic, and/or imaging evidence of current or past infection or other inflammatory processes within the paranasal sinuses
		C. Evidence of causation demonstrated by at least 2 of the following:
		  1. Headache has developed in temporal relation to the onset of chronic rhinosinusitis
		  2. Headache waxes and wanes in parallel with the degree of sinus congestion and other symptoms of the chronic rhinosinusitis
		  3. Headache is exacerbated by pressure applied over the paranasal sinuses in the case of unilateral rhinosinusitis, headache is localized and ipsilateral to it
		D. Not better accounted for by another ICHD-3 diagnosis
			A. Any headache fulfilling criterion C
			B. Clinical, nasal endoscopic, and/or imaging evidence of a hypertrophic or inflammatory process within the nasal cavity[1]
			C. Evidence of causation demonstrated by at least 2 of the following:
			  1. Headache has developed in temporal relation to the onset of the intranasal lesion or led to its discovery
			  2. Headache has significantly improved or significantly worsened in parallel with improvement in (with or without treatment) or worsening of the nasal lesion
			  3. Headache has significantly improved following local anesthesia of the mucosa in the region of the lesion headache is ipsilateral to the site of the lesion
			D. Not better accounted for by another ICHD-3 diagnosis

From Headache Classification Committee of the International Headache Society (IHS) The International Classification of Headache Disorders, 3rd edition. Cephalalgia. 2018;38(1):1-211.

SECONDARY HEADACHE

Secondary headaches are the result of an underlying condition; they can manifest as a change in or exacerbation of a primary headache or in an apoplectic manner with an underlying cause. Secondary headaches can be bilateral; but when are they unilateral, it typically does not switch sides and normally present with other examination findings, which may be discrete. It may be difficult to identify underlying conditions that result in nondescript headaches, but a low threshold should exist if a "red flag" symptom is identified (**Table 4**). In patients who undergo consultation regarding any headache syndrome, education and review should be offered regarding "red flag" symptoms. New-onset headache in a patient without a classic description of a primary headache disorder or any "red flag" symptoms warrants neuroimaging. However, even in the absence of any signs or symptoms beyond a headache, radiographic imaging can be justified in the appropriate setting (ie, family history of tumors/cancer, excessive worry, etc.).

Secondary headaches that require emergent evaluation include:

- Sudden onset "thunderclap" headache
- Acute or subacute neck pain or headache with Horner's syndrome
- Headaches with suspected meningitis or encephalitis
- Headache with global or focal neurologic deficits or papilledema
- Headache with orbital or periorbital symptoms
- Headache with possible carbon monoxide exposure

RADIOGRAPHIC IMAGING

Imaging utilization as a screening method has substantially grown in the last decade. Asymptomatic screening for cranial pathology is unwarranted without justification as identified in a detailed history and physical examination. In general, a headache alone is more likely to fit a primary headache syndrome than to be related to an underlying serious medical condition.[35] If clinical suspicion or any findings listed in **Table 4** are identified, magnetic resonance imaging (MRI) without contrast serves as a first-line screening tool in a nonacute setting. MRI without contrast affords advantages of visualizing central nervous system structures without ionizing radiation or contrast load. Modern MRI sequences can identify urgent findings and contrasted sequences can also be added on at a later time if deemed necessary. Additional sequences, such as magnetic resonance angiogram/venogram can also be considered based on features identified on MRI without contrast and the overall clinical picture. In an acute setting, the standard workhorse remains CT, which has some advantages in the pediatric population (**Fig. 1**). The availability and speed of image acquisition make this modality an ideal screening tool. The disadvantages related to radiation exposure are notable and the fact that more occult or low-grade processes can be missed when using CT as a stand-alone modality. Most of the patients who reach a level of suspicion where a CT is ordered and results reveal no identifiable pathology are typically followed up with an MRI. This fact renders CT for screening only in the acute process identification.[36] Outside of an acute, urgent process, MRI is a reasonable first-line modality.[36]

THUNDERCLAP HEADACHE

Thunderclap headaches are severe, unanticipated headaches without prolonged crescendo (peaks within minutes). This presentation typically signals irritation within the subarachnoid space and may be due to various causes such as arterial dissection,

Table 4 Headache "red flags"	
	Signs & Symptoms
Headache Red Flags	Abnormal Neurologic Examination
	Abnormal Visual Examination
	Acute, Severe Headache
	Confusion
	Consistently Worsening Morning Headaches
	Comorbid Seizures
	Duration <6 Months
	Lack of Visual Aura
	Negative Family History of Migraines
	Positional Headaches
	Progressive Course
	Sleep-Related Headaches
	Symptoms of Systemic Illness
	Worsening Headaches with Valsalva Maneuver
	Vomiting

Adapted from Kelly M, Strelzik J, Langdon R, DiSabella M. Pediatric headache: overview. *Curr Opin Pediatr.* 2018;30(6):748 to -754.

posterior reversible encephalopathy syndrome, reversible cerebral vasoconstriction syndrome, subarachnoid hemorrhage, venous sinus thrombosis, and spontaneous intracranial hypotension. In the pediatric population, eliciting headache quality can be quite challenging.

Subarachnoid Hemorrhage

Classically, thunderclap headaches are associated with aneurysmal subarachnoid hemorrhage but can also be "sentinel" in nature from imminent rupture with a small leak of blood into the subarachnoid space. These headaches can also result from pituitary apoplexy, arterial dissection, reversible cerebral vasoconstriction syndrome, posterior reversible encephalopathy syndrome, venous sinus thrombosis, hypertensive crisis, vascular malformations (ie, arteriovenous malformation, cavernous angioma, etc.), and spontaneous intracranial hypotension (ie, cerebrospinal fluid leak). CT and potentially lumbar puncture can be used to confirm or rule out subarachnoid blood and estimate intracranial pressure. The presence of subarachnoid blood should prompt neurosurgical consultation for further evaluation to evaluate the need for additional vascular imaging (angiogram) and possible surgical intervention.

Cervical Artery Dissection

Arterial dissection occurs as a result of luminal blood entering into the arterial wall, leading to occlusion and/or embolism. This is the most common cause of stroke in children from either the carotid or vertebral arteries.[37] Dissection can propagate from the cervical vessels to the intracranial compartment, resulting in a thunderclap headache with associated pain at the site of injury with potentially referred pain. Arterial dissection typically results from a traumatic event with neck stretching.[38] Arterial dissection presents the risk of causing ischemia via embolization; however, if the dissection propagates within the subarachnoid space, the possibility of hemorrhage must be additionally considered. Antiplatelet or anticoagulation is typically indicated unless a direct contraindication is present (intracranial blood). Advanced management

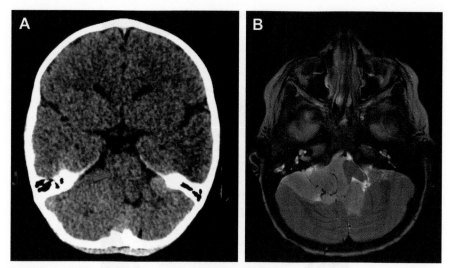

Fig. 1. 3-year-old male who presents with headache as well as new-onset nausea and vomiting. (*A*) Axial CT head reveals midline structures with left shift (*arrow*). (*B*) Subsequent axial MRI head reveals a posterior fossa mass consistent with ependymoma.

should be conducted in concert with neurosurgical consultation and possible endovascular interventions.

Venous Sinus Thrombosis

Most venous sinus thrombosis occurs with an associated headache that is typically insidious over a period of days to weeks. In approximately 10% of cases, the presentation is of thunderclap quality.[39] Typically, it is also accompanied by pain that worsens with Valsalva-type maneuvers and is associated with nausea and/or vomiting. Seizure and stroke-like symptoms also occur in up to 50% of children with venous sinus thrombosis. Underlying hypercoagulopathy from a secondary source should be thoroughly evaluated (ie, medications, illicit drugs, metabolic or genetic abnormality). CT without vascular imaging may miss the diagnosis and a low threshold for MRI and vascular imaging is required to identify venous sinus thrombosis. Typically, with negative screening, second-line imaging would include MRI that would demonstrate associated cerebral changes to alert for the need for dedicated vascular imaging. Venous sinus thrombosis is typically treated with anticoagulation, sometimes this is even conducted in the setting of hemorrhage.[40] Intracranial pressure management and surgical decompression may be necessary, but recovery may be profound even in radiographically severe cases.

Reversible Cerebral Vasoconstrictive Syndrome and Posterior Reversible Encephalopathy Syndrome Spectrum Disorders

These diseases result from the dysregulation of cerebrovascular tone that results in inappropriate vasodilation and constriction. The cause is not entirely clear other than a risk associated with medications or illicit drugs with sympathomimetic activity (ie, cocaine, diet pills, oral contraceptives, pseudoephedrine, selective serotonin reuptake inhibitors, etc.). The presentation is variable and typically associated with an altered level of consciousness as well as neurologic signs/symptoms such as seizures or motor weakness. These cases require advanced neuroimaging with multiple

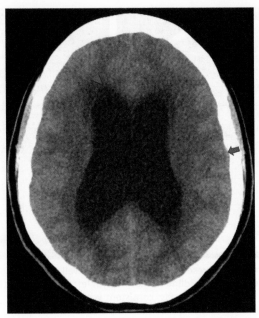

Fig. 2. 14-year-old female who presents with a progressive headache for 1 month, worse in the morning with improvement when lying flat. Axial CT scan reveals ventriculomegaly with loss of cortical sulci (*arrow*) and transependymal flow (*arrowhead*) consistent with obstructive hydrocephalus secondary to aqueductal stenosis.

modalities and potentially cerebrospinal fluid sampling to detect or rule out infectious or autoimmune etiologies. Treatment of an underlying disorder is sought but blood pressure management in the acute setting is the mainstay of treatment.

Intracranial Hypertension

Increased intracranial pressure (ICP) can occur for several reasons or be idiopathic in nature. The presentation of elevated ICP across numerous underlying causes all have similarities on presentation. ICP is the result of pressure from the sum of cranial contents which are the blood, brain, and cerebrospinal fluid. This relationship has been described as the Monro–Kellie doctrine.[40] The symptoms of elevated ICP fit those that make up the "red flag" list in **Table 4**. Common underlying pathologies that occur in the pediatric population include idiopathic intracranial hypertension, cerebral neoplasms, skull base tumors, infection, or outflow obstruction of cerebrospinal fluid (ie, aqueductal stenosis, Chiari malformation, etc.) (**Fig. 2**). The subset of pathologies that lead to elevated intracranial pressure typically presents with crescendo headaches that grow in severity with a march of descending stepwise through the Glasgow Coma Scale. Associated neurologic deficits correlate with pathology location and increased size of the ventricular system. Symptoms from ventriculomegaly typically result in headaches, restriction of upward gaze, abducens nerve palsy, and/or papilledema. Underlying intracranial pathology that produces a headache will likely still respond to traditional headache interventions in a temporizing manner. Specifically, nonsteroidal anti-inflammatory drugs typically produce a noticeable response to secondary headaches[41]; response to treatment should not be a sole exclusion criterion for a more insidious underlying pathology. Infectious etiologies should also be considered when evaluating a patient with acute onset headaches in the setting of systemic illness, fever, and/or altered mental status. Bacterial and viral meningitis can present as a delayed or sudden onset headache, with photophobia and neck stiffness. All clinicians should initiate the proper workup in a timely fashion, particularly when meningitis is suspected.

SUMMARY

Headache is an extremely common neurologic disorder seen in children due to primary and secondary etiologies. Advances in the study of pediatric headache disorders have led to improved recognition of this condition and an increased understanding of underlying mechanisms. A comprehensive evaluation and review of "red flag" signs and symptoms are important to identify the need for radiographic imaging and/or subspecialty care. Fortunately, most children with headaches will fit a primary headache disorder, with migraine being the most common diagnosis. Recognition of otologic and/or rhinologic contributions remains paramount in addressing pediatric headaches refractory to traditional medical therapies. Key management strategies include using developmentally appropriate diagnostic tools, recognizing the unique aspects of a child's life, administering appropriate medications, and incorporating biobehavioral therapies. Future research efforts are necessary to expand treatment options and analyze long-term outcomes in children.

DISCLOSURE

The authors have no disclosures.

REFERENCES

1. Magiorkinis E, Diamantis A, Mitsikostas DD, et al. Headaches in antiquity and during the early scientific era. J Neurol 2009;256(8):1215–20.
2. Antonaci F, Voiticovschi-Iosob C, Di Stefano AL, et al. The evolution of headache from childhood to adulthood: a review of the literature. J Headache Pain 2014; 15:15.
3. Guidetti V, Faedda N. From 0 degrees to 18 degrees : how headache changes over time. Neurol Sci 2017;38(Suppl 1):103–6.
4. Hu S, Helman S, Filip P, et al. The role of the otolaryngologist in the evaluation and management of headaches. Am J Otolaryngol 2019;40(1):115–20.
5. Raieli V, Eliseo M, Pandolfi E, et al. Recurrent and chronic headaches in children below 6 years of age. J Headache Pain 2005;6(3):135–42.
6. Lewis DW. Pediatric migraine. Pediatr Rev 2007;28(2):43–53.
7. Headache Classification Committee of the International Headache Society (IHS) The International Classification of Headache Disorders. 3rd edition. Cephalalgia 2018;38(1):1–211.
8. Mamouri O, Cuvellier JC, Duhamel A, et al. Postdrome symptoms in pediatric migraine: A questionnaire retrospective study by phone in 100 patients. Cephalalgia 2018;38(5):943–8.
9. Batson G. Benign paroxysmal vertigo of childhood: A review of the literature. Paediatr Child Health 2004;9(1):31–4.
10. Lanzi G, Balottin U, Fazzi E, et al. Benign paroxysmal vertigo of childhood: a long-term follow-up. Cephalalgia 1994;14(6):458–60.
11. Teleanu RI, Vladacenco O, Teleanu DM, et al. Treatment of Pediatric Migraine: a Review. Maedica (Bucur) 2016;11(2):136–43.

12. Hamalainen ML, Hoppu K, Valkeila E, et al. Ibuprofen or acetaminophen for the acute treatment of migraine in children: a double-blind, randomized, placebo-controlled, crossover study. Neurology 1997;48(1):103–7.

13. Powers SW, Kashikar-Zuck SM, Allen JR, et al. Cognitive behavioral therapy plus amitriptyline for chronic migraine in children and adolescents: a randomized clinical trial. JAMA 2013;310(24):2622–30.

14. Bonfert M, Straube A, Schroeder AS, et al. Primary headache in children and adolescents: update on pharmacotherapy of migraine and tension-type headache. Neuropediatrics 2013;44(1):3–19.

15. Lambru G, Matharu M. Management of trigeminal autonomic cephalalgias in children and adolescents. Curr Pain Headache Rep 2013;17(4):323.

16. Majumdar A, Ahmed MA, Benton S. Cluster headache in children–experience from a specialist headache clinic. Eur J Paediatr Neurol 2009;13(6):524–9.

17. van Vliet JA, Eekers PJ, Haan J, et al. Features involved in the diagnostic delay of cluster headache. J Neurol Neurosurg Psychiatr 2003;74(8):1123–5.

18. Lampl C. Childhood-onset cluster headache. Pediatr Neurol 2002;27(2):138–40.

19. Kudrow L. Response of cluster headache attacks to oxygen inhalation. Headache 1981;21(1):1–4.

20. Tarantino S, Vollono C, Capuano A, et al. Chronic paroxysmal hemicrania in paediatric age: report of two cases. J Headache Pain 2011;12(2):263–7.

21. Wald ER, Applegate KE, Bordley C, et al. Clinical practice guideline for the diagnosis and management of acute bacterial sinusitis in children aged 1 to 18 years. Pediatrics 2013;132(1):e262–80.

22. Brietzke SE, Shin JJ, Choi S, et al. Clinical consensus statement: pediatric chronic rhinosinusitis. Otolaryngol Head Neck Surg 2014;151(4):542–53.

23. Orlandi RR, Kingdom TT, Smith TL, et al. International consensus statement on allergy and rhinology: rhinosinusitis 2021. Int Forum Allergy Rhinol 2021;11(3):213–739.

24. Fokkens WJ, Lund VJ, Hopkins C, et al. Executive summary of EPOS 2020 including integrated care pathways. Rhinology 2020;58(2):82–111.

25. Barinsky GL, Hanba C, Svider PF. Rhinogenic Headache in Children and Adolescents. Curr Pain Headache Rep 2020;24(3):7.

26. Ozge A, Abu-Arafeh I, Gelfand AA, et al. Experts' opinion about the pediatric secondary headaches diagnostic criteria of the ICHD-3 beta. J Headache Pain 2017;18(1):113.

27. Gelfand AA, Reider AC, Goadsby PJ. Cranial autonomic symptoms in pediatric migraine are the rule, not the exception. Neurology 2013;81(5):431–6.

28. Raieli V, Giordano G, Spitaleri C, et al. Migraine and cranial autonomic symptoms in children and adolescents: a clinical study. J Child Neurol 2015;30(2):182–6.

29. Patel ZM, Kennedy DW, Setzen M, et al. Sinus headache": rhinogenic headache or migraine? An evidence-based guide to diagnosis and treatment. Int Forum Allergy Rhinol 2013;3(3):221–30.

30. Mishra D, Choudhury KK, Gupta A. Headache with autonomic features in a child: cluster headache or contact-point headache? Headache 2008;48(3):473–5.

31. Swain SKSM, Samantray K. An unusual cause of otalgia in a child—a case report. Pediatr Pol 2016;91:480–3.

32. Kim SH. A case of nasal septal deviation-induced rhinogenic contact point otalgia. Am J Otolaryngol 2015;36(3):451–5.

33. Parsons DS, Batra PS. Functional endoscopic sinus surgical outcomes for contact point headaches. Laryngoscope 1998;108(5):696–702.

34. Smith BC, George LC, Svider PF, et al. Rhinogenic headache in pediatric and adolescent patients: an evidence-based review. Int Forum Allergy Rhinol 2019; 9(5):443–51.

35. Dodick DW. Pearls: headache. Semin Neurol 2010;30(1):74–81.

36. Loder E, Weizenbaum E, Frishberg B, et al. Choosing wisely in headache medicine: the American Headache Society's list of five things physicians and patients should question. Headache 2013;53(10):1651–9.

37. Engelter ST, Brandt T, Debette S, et al. Antiplatelets versus anticoagulation in cervical artery dissection. Stroke 2007;38(9):2605–11.

38. Schievink WI. Spontaneous dissection of the carotid and vertebral arteries. N Engl J Med 2001;344(12):898–906.

39. Terazzi E, Mittino D, Ruda R, et al. Cerebral venous thrombosis: a retrospective multicentre study of 48 patients. Neurol Sci 2005;25(6):311–5.

40. Polster SP, Lyne SB, Mansour A. Case Demonstrating the Nuances of Acute Cortical Venous Thrombosis Anticoagulation Guidelines. World Neurosurg 2020;139:215–8.

41. Lee HJ, Phi JH, Kim SK, et al. Papilledema in children with hydrocephalus: incidence and associated factors. J Neurosurg Pediatr 2017;19(6):627–31.

Temporomandibular Joint Syndrome from an Ear Versus Dental-Related Standpoint

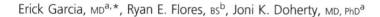

Erick Garcia, MD[a],*, Ryan E. Flores, BS[b], Joni K. Doherty, MD, PhD[a]

KEYWORDS

- Temporomandibular disorder • Headache • Otolaryngology

KEY POINTS

- When evaluating a patient with a suspected temporomandibular disorder with or without headache, a thorough history and physical, including a detailed otologic examination, is imperative to rule out otolaryngologic causes.
- There is a higher prevalence of headaches within the TMD population, which can manifest as primary headache disorders (tension-type headaches and migraines) or secondary headache disorders (headache attributed to TMD).
- TMD symptoms tend to improve with treatment, and therefore prompt recognition and initiation of treatment are essential. The RDC/TMD and ICHD are valuable resources to evaluate this patient population and should be readily available to the otolaryngologist.
- Favorable conservative treatments include NSAIDs, heat therapy, and muscle-stretching exercises. There is mixed literature regarding intraoral occlusive devices, but the decision to refer to a specialist should be made on a case-by-case basis.

INTRODUCTION

Headaches (HAs) are among the most common chief complaints encountered by physicians, with roughly 90% of the population suffering from at least one HA episode per year.[1] HA can incur large costs to society, mostly through loss of work time and can cause disability, suffering, and loss of quality of life on a par with other chronic disorders.[2] Using frequency as a proxy for disability, Stovner and colleagues concluded that although tension-type headaches (TTHs) are less burdensome individually, the societal burden is greater than that of migraines because of their overall higher prevalence. Given the myriad causes and presentations, the third edition of the

[a] Rick and Tina Caruso Department of Otolaryngology - Head & Neck Surgery, Keck Medicine of University of Southern California, Los Angeles, CA, USA; [b] Keck School of Medicine, University of Southern California, Los Angeles, CA, USA
* Corresponding author. USC Caruso Department of Otolaryngology-Head and Neck Surgery, 1450 San Pablo Street, Suite 5100.
E-mail address: erick.garcia@med.usc.edu

Otolaryngol Clin N Am 55 (2022) 649–658
https://doi.org/10.1016/j.otc.2022.02.011
0030-6665/22/© 2022 Elsevier Inc. All rights reserved.

oto.theclinics.com

International Classification of Headache Disorder (ICHD-3) has created a helpful framework to help classify them. Of relevance to this article is the *11.7 headache attributed to temporomandibular disorder (TMD)*, which is temporally located and therefore has significant overlap with TTH and migraines. The diagnostic criteria as defined by the International Headache Society (IHS) can be referred to in **Box 1**. The overlap between TTH and secondary HAs attributed to TMD is further complicated by the increase in HA frequency associated with increased TMD symptoms.[3] In addition, primary HAs such as migraines, episodic tension-type HA, and chronic daily HA are more common in individuals with TMD symptoms than those without.[4] Several studies have established a strong correlation between HA and other dysfunctional symptoms, such as joint noise, pain during mandibular movement, pain in the temporomandibular area, and poor mental health.[5] Patients with HA and TMD reported significantly higher levels of pain and disability compared to patients with only TMD.[6]

The prevalence of HAs in the TMD population varies between 48% and 77%, whereas the prevalence is around 45% in the general population.[4] Thus, TMD is likely an underdiagnosed cause of HAs. Moreover, the myofascial pain subset of TMD can often lead to misinterpretation of symptoms. For instance, Lupoli and colleagues noted that when the lateral pterygoid muscle spasms, deep retro-orbital pain can be felt and as a result be confused with sinus pain. Patients with myofascial pain also experience tenderness to palpation in the muscles of mastication, such as the masseter, temporalis, or pterygoid muscles.[7] In addition, individuals reporting chronic HAs also reported significantly more sites that were painful to palpation when compared with non-HA controls.[6]

In the United States, 40% to 75% of adults are reported to show at least one sign of TMDs, and 33% show at least one symptom.[8,9] It is the second most common musculoskeletal condition, resulting in pain and disability with an annual management cost of $4 billion in the United States.[2] TMDs are most reported in young-to-middle-aged adults (20–50 years of age). The ratio of females to males seeking care has been

---

Box 1
IHS diagnostic criteria for headache attributed to temporomandibular disorder

A. Any headache[1] fulfilling criterion C.

B. Clinical evidence of a painful pathologic process affecting elements of the temporomandibular joints, muscles of mastication, and/or associated structures on one or both sides.

C. Evidence of causation demonstrated by at least 2 of the following:
   a. The headache was developed in temporal relation to the onset of the temporomandibular disorder, or led to its discovery.
   b. The headache is aggravated by jaw motion, jaw function (eg, chewing), and/or jaw parafunction (eg, bruxism).
   c. The headache is provoked on physical examination by temporalis muscle palpation and/or passive movement of the jaw.

D. Not better accounted for by another ICHD-3 diagnosis.[2]

Note
1. Usually temporally located, on one or both sides.
2. There is some overlap between 11.7 *Headache attributed to temporomandibular disorder (TMD)* arising from muscular tension and 2. *Tension-type headache.* When the diagnosis of TMD is uncertain, the headache should be coded as 2. *Tension-type headache* or one of its types or subtypes (presumably with pericranial muscle tenderness).

reported as ranging from 3:1 to 9:1.[8] The International Research Diagnostic Criteria for Temporomandibular Disorders (RDC/TMD) Consortium Network and Orofacial Pain Special Interest Group have established widely used, evidence-based diagnostic criteria for TMD. The classification system was originally based on 2 axes. Axis I represents the physical diagnosis (ie, pain diagnosis, joint diagnosis), whereas axis II represents the psychosocial status (ie, distress and pain disability). The original axis I algorithms have since been updated to meet the target sensitivity and specificity determined by the Validation Project.[10] The diagnostic algorithm for headache attributed to TMD (HATMD) can be seen in **Box 2**. Although TMD is a heterogeneous group of disorders, it is commonly divided into 2 nonmutually exclusive categories: (1) myofascial pain and (2) joint disorders.[11,12] The etiologies of TMD are also broad and can include structural, functional, and even psychological causes. Common symptoms of TMD include HAs, facial pain, and jaw clicking or popping; however, it can also

---

Box 2
Headache attributed to TMD (ICD-9 339.89 and 748.0; ICD-10 G44.89)[§]

Description	Headache in the temple area secondary to pain-related TMD (see Note) that is affected by jaw movement, function, or parafunction, and replication of this headache occurs with provocation testing of the masticatory system.
Criteria History	Positive for both of the following: 1. Headache* of any type in the temple; AND 2. Headache modified by jaw movement, function, and parafunction.
Examination	Positive for both of the following: 1. Confirmation** of headache location in the area of the temporalis muscles; AND 2. Report of familiar headache[†] in the temple area with at least one of the following provocation tests: a. Palpation of the temporalis muscles; OR b. Maximum unassisted or assisted opening, right or left lateral, or protrusive movements.
Validity	Sensitivity 0.89; Specificity 0.87
Comments	The headache is not better accounted for by another headache diagnosis.
Note	A diagnosis of pain-related TMD (eg, myalgia or TMJ arthralgia) must be present and is established using valid diagnostic criteria.
§	The ICD-9 and ICD-10 have not established a specific code for headache attributed to TMD as a secondary cause of headache; ICD-9 339.89 and ICD-10 G44.89 are for "other headache syndrome" and ICD-9784.0 is for "Headache, Facial Pain, Pain in Head NOS (Non-specific)."
*	The timeframe for assessing pain including headaches is in "the last 30 d" because the stated sensitivity and specificity of these criteria were established using this time frame. Although the specific time frame can be dependent on the context in which the pain complaint is being assessed, the validity of this diagnosis based on different time frames has not been established.
**	The examiner must identify with the patient all anatomic locations that they have experienced in the last 30 d. For a given diagnosis, the location of pain produced by the specified provocation tests must be in an anatomic structure consistent with the diagnosis.
†	"Familiar pain" or "familiar headache" is based on patient report that the pain induced by a specific provocation tests has replicated the pain that the patient has experienced in the time frame of interest, which is usually the last 30 d "Familiar pain" is pain that is similar or like the patient's pain complaint. "Familiar headache" is pain that is similar or like the patient's headache complaint.

present with otologic symptoms, such as otalgia, tinnitus, and subjective hearing loss, which can often trigger a referral to otolaryngology. A major source of confusion between the otologic pathway and temporomandibular joint (TMJ) pathology is close anatomic proximity and common sensory innervation via the auriculotemporal nerve.[13] As such, it is imperative that otolaryngologists become familiar with the presentation and management of TMD and/or TMD-associated HAs.

EVALUATION/ASSESSMENT

Evaluation of TMD begins with a thorough history and physical examination. The condition was described by James Costen in 1934, where he concluded that the malocclusion and improper jaw position were the root cause. Therefore, most assessments and treatments are focused on dental repairs.[14] More recently, Cooper and colleagues showed that patients seeking care for TMD presented with facial pain (96%), ear discomfort or dysfunction (82%), HA (79%), and TMJ discomfort or dysfunction (75%).[15] Given the variety of potential ailments with similar presentations, it is important to begin with a broad differential and exclude other serious disorders. Red flag symptoms, such as cervical spine instability, cardiac disease, central neurologic dysfunction, and extreme weight changes must first be ruled out.[12] One approach is to focus on the inclusion of odontogenic causes, such as cavities, versus nonodontogenic causes, like primary or secondary HAs, jaw tumors, trigeminal neuropathic pain syndromes, and systemic diseases.[8] Screening tools have been proposed to help triage patients for TMD based on the RDC/TMD criteria.[16] The three-step screening procedure is outlined in **Box 3**.

Physical examination should include inspection and palpation of mandibular motion, muscles of mastication, and cervical musculature as well as the salivary glands and cervical lymph nodes. Evaluation of the ear, external auditory canal, and tympanic membrane with otoscopy can rule out an otologic cause. Auscultation of the TMJ and the carotid arteries is also important to assess for crepitus and bruits, respectively.

Box 3
TMD checklist

Questionnaire
1. Do you have pain in the face, jaw, temple, in front of ear, or in the ear in the past month? (if yes, score 4; if no, score 0)
2. Are you older than 36 years? (if yes, score 3; if no, score 0)
3. During the last 6 months have you had a problem with headache or migraine? (if yes, score −1; if no, score 0)
4. Does your present jaw problem prevent or limit you from chewing or yawning or having your usual facial appearance? (if yes, score 1; if no, score 0)
5. Does your jaw click or pop when you open or close your mouth or when chewing? (if yes, score 1; if no, score 0)

If the total score is <3, the prediction is TMD negative. If the total score is ≥3, the patient needs the following examination.

Examination
1. Joint pain on mouth opening
2. Muscle pain on protrusive jaw movement
3. Joint sound on mouth closing
4. Joint pain on palpation

If none of the aforementioned examination items is positive, prediction is TMD negative. Otherwise, TMD is predicted.

Examination of the cranial nerves with emphasis on the trigeminal branches (V1, V2, V3) is helpful in ruling out other serious causes of facial pain. Other diagnostic studies helpful in the workup include blood work (eg, serum inflammatory markers), imaging (eg, CT, MRI), diagnostic nerve blocks and injections (eg, corticosteroid, hyaluronic acid), and surgery (eg, diagnostic arthroscopy).[8]

MANAGEMENT

There are several therapeutic options for the treatment of TMD. Conservative measures should be tried before escalation to more invasive modalities. Literature indicates that successful treatment of TMD leads to the resolution of otolaryngologic symptoms.[12] Treatment is determined by symptomatology and can be targeted to either intra-articular or extra-articular etiology, although both tend to occur concurrently.[13] Approximately 80% to 95% of TMDs, whether articular or muscular, can be treated with noninvasive, reversible interventions, while up to 40% of patients may experience spontaneous resolution of symptoms without interventions.[8]

It is essential that patients first be counseled on the disease process of TMD and known triggers. These include jaw clenching, eating or chewing hard foods, engaging in extremes of jaw mechanical movements (eg, yawning), and certain habits such as chewing gum or biting nails. Patients should adhere to a soft food diet and engage in relaxation techniques and passive jaw movements. The application of a heating pad, hot towel, or warm water bottle may provide symptomatic relief of muscular pain. More vigorous treatments (eg, ultrasound, short-wave diathermy heat treatments) can be pursued with physical medicine providers.[8]

Medical management of TMDs aims at alleviating pain and inflammation. Nonsteroidal anti-inflammatory drugs (NSAIDs) provide symptomatic relief in the acute stages.[8] A 7- to 14-day course of NSAIDs with concurrent lifestyle modifications as described earlier has been shown to be effective in reducing intra-articular inflammation and pain. Patients who do not respond to NSAIDs may be offered a short course of steroids.[12,17] Opioids analgesics should be avoided, given the long-term risk of dependence. Patients with chronic neuropathic pain may be trialed on a course of gabapentin or antidepressants. Tricyclic antidepressants are the most commonly used and should be taken at bedtime with an expected effect noted within 2 to 4 weeks. Antidepressants offer great treatment value especially when there are signs of depression in addition to generalized muscular pain. Furthermore, appropriate referral to mental health providers should be pursued in patients who express emotional distress and signs of depression.[8,12]

Patients may further benefit from a referral to a dentist for evaluation of jaw splints and other intraoral occlusive devices which can improve mobility while reducing abnormal muscle function and protecting teeth from oral parafunctional habits. These modalities in addition to adjuvant therapies as described earlier have shown to reduce pain and temporomandibular dysfunction in 70% to 90% of patients, though, no benefit has been proven when used as a single modality.[8,18] However, a recent systematic review did not find a major role for dental occlusion in the pathophysiology of TMD and encourages dental clinicians to move forward from old traditions.[19]

Additional referral to physical therapy has demonstrated positive effects while using other conservative modalities. These therapies are focused on decreasing neck and jaw pain, improving range of motion, and promoting exercise.[20] Therapeutic exercises involve passive and active stretching of muscles aimed to increase mouth range of motion and postural exercises to improve head and neck posture. Manual therapy centered around joint mobilization, manipulation, and treatment of soft tissues can reduce local ischemia, stimulate proprioception, break fibrous adhesions, stimulate synovial fluid production, and reduce orofacial pain. Manual therapy targeted at the mobilization of the cervical spine also results in decreased pain intensity and reduced pain sensitivity. It is suggested to have an influence on orofacial pain and mouth range of motion through the shared connections of these 2 systems in the trigeminocervical nucleus.[20] Exercises and manual therapy are safe and simple interventions that serve as adjuvant treatment for TMDs.

If conservative options fail, it is unlikely that symptoms will resolve with nonsurgical interventions and therefore a referral to an oral maxillofacial surgeon is appropriate for further evaluation of intra-articular joint derangements. These result from displacement of the TMJ disk from its normal position or from deformation of the disk, leading to pain, synovitis, and limited motion. This may be evaluated with MRI and diagnostic and/or therapeutic arthroscopy. Initial treatment of derangement disorders begins with the same conservative measures established earlier but may require further invasive interventions such as intra-articular injection with steroids, arthrocentesis, or arthroscopy.[8,13]

DISCUSSION

TMDs remain a prominent reason for visits to medical providers. TMD prevalence estimates vary, with up to 40% of the general population affected, more commonly in women than men.[1,8] Common symptoms include HAs, facial pain, and jaw clicking or popping; however, it can also present with otologic symptoms, such as otalgia, tinnitus, and subjective hearing loss. Referrals to otolaryngologists are common and given the overlap with otologic symptoms due to anatomic proximity of shared neural pathways, a thorough history and physical examination is an essential first step. Temporomandibular pain can essentially be classified as myofascial pain or joint pain. This is synonymous within the literature to articular or nonarticular, intracapsular or extracapsular. The broad range of clinical problems are centered around the TMJ and the muscles of mastication (masseter, temporalis, medial and lateral pterygoids). The cause is thought to be multifactorial spanning from biological, behavioral, emotional, environmental, social, and cognitive. The workup and treatment can be started by a single provider but often necessitates a multidisciplinary approach including primary care providers, otolaryngologists, dentists, oral maxillofacial surgeons, psychiatrists, psychologists, and physical therapists. The most widely used diagnostic tool for TMD is the RDC/TMD. It allows for standardized evaluation and classification of patients with TMD containing both measurements for physical disorder and psychosocial illness impact factors.

Patients diagnosed with HAs and TMDs share a similar set of symptoms including pain in the face, head, and cervical area. HAs reported by TMD patients are frequently described in the literature and can often mimic TTHs or migraines.[21] Hoffman and colleagues surveyed 1511 participants with TMD and found a higher likelihood of HAs in the TMD patients compared with case-controls. Caspersen and colleagues reported a higher prevalence of temporomandibular pain in a TTH population compared with the general population.[5] Goncalves and colleagues found in a population with at least one TMD symptom there was a significant overrepresentation of HAs compared with TMD-free individuals (56.5% vs 31.9%) with the HA group reporting significantly more myofascial pain and tooth clenching.[22] Further studies have demonstrated a diagnosis of TMD within a HA population to be 56%, 67%, and 70%.[4,23,24] Notably, the peak age group for HAs is between 20 and 40 years.[4,25] The HAs present in the TMD population are more likely due to myogenic TMD versus arthrogenous TMD.[1,24–26] Current literature suggests there is a close relationship between primary HAs and TMDs, possibly due to an underlying common pain pathway; however, further research is needed to investigate underlying pathophysiological mechanisms. Special attention should be given to patients aged 20 to 40 years, as HA prevalence is higher in this population. It is imperative for the otolaryngologist to recognize the prevalence of primary HAs in the TMD patient population and consider a broad treatment strategy with referrals to HA specialists as appropriate to ensure comprehensive HA management.

The International Classification of Headache Disorder (ICHD-II) has created a helpful framework to help classify primary and secondary HAs that is now in its third edition.[27] HATMD is a secondary HA characterized by unilateral or bilateral temporal HAs caused by a disorder involving structures in the temporomandibular region (see **Box 1**). Before the third edition, several studies sought to improve the diagnostic criteria of HAs attributed to TMD.[10,28] The revised criteria had higher sensitivity and specificity than the ICD-II criteria (89% and 87% vs 84% and 33%, respectively). The evolving literature on improving diagnostic criteria suggests further research is required to elucidate the relationship between primary HAs, TMD, and secondary HAs attributed to TMD. Shiffman argues that previous literature of TMD association with primary HAs may be partially explained by the fact that some of these primary HAs could be more correctly diagnosed as secondary HAs attributed to TMD. Although it is difficult to discern the root behind HAs, the ICHD-III classification provides the best diagnostic criteria for secondary HAs attributed to TMD and should be used by the otolaryngologist when evaluating this patient population.

Once a diagnosis of TMD and HA is established, it is imperative to begin treatment as literature shows that symptoms of TMD, including HAs, are often resolved after treatment.[8,12,18,20] Noninvasive, conservative treatments are the recommended modality of initial management. Notably, Hoffman and colleagues found the most effective relief in his study of 1511 TMD patients was thermal therapy (74%) followed by jaw exercises (49%). Hara and colleagues investigated in a HATMD population the temporal association between TMD-related symptoms and HA during noninvasive TMD treatment. Patients received instructions on how to perform muscle-stretching exercises 5 times a day and were instructed to refrain from taking new drugs or receiving other treatments. The exercises for massaging targeted temporal and masseter at specific tender points while muscle stretching targeted temporal, master, medial pterygoid muscles. HA intensity and frequency, rest pain in masticatory muscles, and pain intensity during palpation all significantly decreased after the intervention while an increase in pressure pain thresholds of all peri-cranial muscles was noted. Hara and colleagues also found an inverse correlation between involuntary nonfunctional tooth contact and pressure pain thresholds in both masseter and trapezius muscles, demonstrating a possible contributing role of oral parafunctional behavior; however, further research on the use of intraoral occlusion devices is needed.[8,19] This study highlights the potential beneficial effects of home physical therapy to alleviate TMD HAs and provides a simple treatment plan that can be carried out by the otolaryngologist.

SUMMARY

TMDs are a prominent reason for visits to medical providers. The presentation of HAs within this population remains a challenging diagnosis, given the prevalence and overlap of symptomatology of both conditions. Although the most recent ICHD-III provides a strong foundation of diagnostic criteria to correctly identify a HA attributed to TMD, there is still an undeniable association between primary HAs and TMD. This queries whether patients are misdiagnosed and untreated for TMD within the primary HA population. Regardless of causality and etiology, the literature supports that prompt diagnosis and treatment results in improvement or resolution of symptoms, including HAs. Treatment of TMD HAs should begin with conservative measures including medical management with NSAIDs, heat therapy, and muscle-stretching exercises. If conservative measures fail and there is high suspicion for nonfunctional tooth contact, oral parafunctional behaviors, or functional joint derangements, referrals to dentists and oral maxillofacial surgeons may be indicated. It is best practice to involve a multidisciplinary team including primary care providers, otolaryngologists, dentists, oral maxillofacial surgeons, psychiatrists, phycologists, and physical therapists for comprehensive TMD HA management.

CLINICS CARE POINTS

- When evaluating a patient with a suspected temporomandibular disorder with/without headache, a thorough history and physical, including a detailed otologic examination, is imperative to rule out otolaryngologic causes.

- There is a higher prevalence of headaches within the TMD population, which can manifest as primary headache disorders (tension-type headaches and migraines) or secondary headache disorders (headache attributed to TMD).

- TMD symptoms tend to improve with treatment, and therefore prompt recognition and initiation of treatment are essential. The RDC/TMD and ICHD are valuable resources to use when evaluating this patient population and should be readily available to the otolaryngologist.

- Favorable conservative treatments include NSAIDs, heat therapy, and muscle-stretching exercises. There is mixed literature regarding intraoral occlusive devices but the decision to refer to a specialist should be made on a case-by-case basis.

- The cause of TMD is thought to be multifactorial spanning from biological, behavioral, emotional, environmental, social, and cognitive. Given its complex etiology, it is best practice to involve a multidisciplinary team including primary care providers, otolaryngologists, dentists, oral maxillofacial surgeons, psychiatrists, psychologists, and physical therapists for comprehensive TMD headache management.

DISCLOSURE

The authors have nothing to disclose.

REFERENCES

1. Graff-Radford SB, Bassiur JP. Temporomandibular disorders and headaches. Neurol Clin 2014;32(2):525–37.
2. Jensen R, Stovner LJ. Epidemiology and comorbidity of headache. Lancet Neurol 2008;7(4):354–61.
3. Anderson GC, John MT, Ohrbach R, et al. Influence of headache frequency on clinical signs and symptoms of TMD in subjects with temple headache and TMD pain. PAIN 2011;152(4):765–71.
4. Di Paolo C, D'Urso A, Papi P, et al. Temporomandibular disorders and headache: a retrospective analysis of 1198 patients. Pain Res Manag 2017;2017.
5. Caspersen N, Hirsvang JR, Kroell L, et al. Is there a relation between tension-type headache, temporomandibular disorders and sleep? Pain Res Treat 2013;2013.
6. Glaros AG, Urban D, Locke J. Headache and temporomandibular disorders: evidence for diagnostic and behavioural overlap. Cephalalgia 2007;27(6):542–9.

7. Lupoli TA, Lockey RF. Temporomandibular dysfunction: an often overlooked cause of chronic headaches. Ann Allergy Asthma Immunol 2007;99(4):314–8.

8. Scrivani SJ, Keith DA, Kaban LB. Temporomandibular disorders. New Engl J Med 2008;359(25):2693–705.

9. Schiffman E, Ohrbach R, Truelove E, et al. Diagnostic criteria for temporomandibular disorders (DC/TMD) for clinical and research applications: recommendations of the International RDC/TMD Consortium Network and Orofacial Pain Special Interest Group. J Oral Facial pain headache 2014;28(1):6.

10. Schiffman E, Ohrbach R, List T, et al. Diagnostic criteria for headache attributed to temporomandibular disorders. Cephalalgia: An Int J Headache 2012;32(9): 683–92.

11. Lee E, Crowder HR, Tummala N, et al. Temporomandibular disorder treatment algorithm for otolaryngologists. Am J Otolaryngol 2021;103155.

12. Stepan L, Shaw CL, Oue S. Temporomandibular disorder in otolaryngology: a systematic review. The J Laryngol Otology 2017;131(S1):S50–6.

13. Israel HA, Davila LJ. The essential role of the otolaryngologist in the diagnosis and management of temporomandibular joint and chronic oral, head, and facial pain disorders. Otolaryngologic Clin North America 2014;47(2):301–31.

14. Costen JB. I. A syndrome of ear and sinus symptoms dependent upon disturbed function of the temporomandibular joint. Ann Otology, Rhinology Laryngol 1934; 43(1):1–15.

15. Cooper BC, Kleinberg I. Examination of a large patient population for the presence of symptoms and signs of temporomandibular disorders. CRANIO 2007; 25(2):114–26.

16. Zhao NN, Evans RW, Byth K, et al. Development and validation of a screening checklist for temporomandibular disorders. J orofacial pain 2011;25(3).

17. Dionne RA. Pharmacologic treatments for temporomandibular disorders. Oral Surg Oral Med Oral Pathol Oral Radiol Endodontics 1997;83(1):134–42.

18. Wassell RW, Adams N, Kelly PJ. The treatment of temporomandibular disorders with stabilizing splints in general dental practice: One-year follow-up. J Am Dental Assoc (1939) 2006;137(8):1089, 9.

19. Manfredini D, Lombardo L, Siciliani G. Temporomandibular disorders and dental occlusion. A systematic review of association studies: End of an era? J Oral Rehabil 2017;44(11):908–23.

20. Armijo-Olivo S, Pitance L, Singh V, et al. Effectiveness of manual therapy and therapeutic exercise for temporomandibular disorders: Systematic review and meta-analysis. Phys Ther 2016;96(1):9–25.

21. Glaros AG, Hanson AH, Ryen CC. Headache and oral parafunctional behaviors. Appl psychophysiology biofeedback 2014;39(1):59–66.

22. Goncalves DA, Bigal ME, Jales LC, et al. Headache and symptoms of temporomandibular disorder: An epidemiological study. Headache 2010;50(2):231–41.

23. Ballegaard V, Thede-Schmidt-Hansen P, Svensson P, et al. Are headache and temporomandibular disorders related? A blinded study. Cephalalgia: An Int J Headache 2008;28(8):832–41.

24. Ciancaglini R, Radaelli G. The relationship between headache and symptoms of temporomandibular disorder in the general population. J Dentistry 2001; 29(2):93–8.

25. Manfredini D, Chiappe G, Bosco M. Research diagnostic criteria for temporomandibular disorders (RDC/TMD) axis I diagnoses in an Italian patient population. J Oral Rehabil 2006;33(8):551–8.

26. Hara K, Shinozaki T, Okada-Ogawa A, et al. Headache attributed to temporoman-dibular disorders and masticatory myofascial pain. J Oral Sci 2016;58(2): 195–204.
27. Headache classification committee of the international headache society (IHS) the international classification of headache disorders, 3rd edition. Cephalalgia: An Int J Headache 2018;38(1):1–211.
28. Olesen J, Steiner T, Bousser MG, et al. Proposals for new standardized general diagnostic criteria for the secondary headaches. Cephalalgia: An Int J Headache 2009;29(12):1331–6.

Masticatory/Temporomandibular Disorders

Practical Assessment and Care Concepts for the Otolaryngologist

Donald R. Tanenbaum, DDS, MPH[a,b,c,d,*],
Matthew R. Lark, DDS, FAGD[a,e,f,g]

KEYWORDS

• Temporomandibular joint • Temporomandibular disorder • Ear symptoms

KEY POINTS

- To appreciate the relationship of temporomandibular disorders to the emergence of ear-related symptoms, it is essential to understand (1) normal anatomy/orthopedic function of the TM joint and associated muscles, and (2) the consequences of tissue injury.
- To define the examination findings and symptoms that are essential to support the diagnosis of a temporomandibular disorder.
- To define the broad range of causal and common risk factors that are associated with the onset, perpetuation, and progression of TM disorders.
- To outline basic treatment concepts and options that can be used to address common temporomandibular problems and the associated ear symptoms.

Other than consultation with general dentists or oral surgeons, the emergence of jaw/orofacial pain and/or limitations of jaw function prompt consultations with physicians specifically otolaryngologists. This pattern of care-seeking is common as jaw symptoms are often accompanied by a variety of ear and sinus symptoms, which may include a description of fullness, clogging, or pain in the ears, pressure, or headache pain in the sinuses, tinnitus, or other disturbing sound sensations. If a thorough clinical examination, diagnostic tests, and scans do not reveal objective pathology in the

[a] Diplomate, American Board of Orofacial Pain; [b] Clinical Assistant Professor, Department of Oral & Maxillofacial Surgery, School of Dental Medicine at Stony Brook University; [c] Section Head, Facial Pain and Dental Sleep Medicine, Department of Dental Medicine, Long Island Jewish Medical Center; [d] Clinical Assistant Professor, Hofstra Northwell School of Medicine; [e] Faculty, Univ of Toledo Medical College; [f] Faculty, Univ of Michigan School of Dentistry; [g] Scientific Advisor Orofacial Pain Kois Center
* Corresponding author: 630 5th Avenue, Suite 1857, New York, NY 10111.
E-mail addresses: drdonaldt@gmail.com (D.R.T.); Abiento@aol.com (M.R.L.)

Otolaryngol Clin N Am 55 (2022) 659–679
https://doi.org/10.1016/j.otc.2022.02.012
0030-6665/22/© 2022 Elsevier Inc. All rights reserved.

sinus, ear, nose, or throat, a tentative diagnosis of a temporomandibular disorder (TMD) may be made.

Certainly, a judgment made by an otolaryngologist when confronted by a patient with jaw/ear symptoms, that a disorder exists within the temporomandibular (TM) system may be considered accurate particularly if jaw motion is viewed as compromised, joint noises are present or crowding of the teeth or a "bad bite" is noted. However, these findings upon further exploration may not be indicative of a primary jaw disorder but rather deviations from the norm and with a history of occurrence/presence long before symptoms emerged. In addition, just the presence of pain in the jaw muscles and orofacial region is often insufficient to make a diagnosis of a TMD. Specifically, as with other pain complaints throughout the body, the location of a pain complaint can have little to do with its origin, and in the orofacial arena, the potential for what is called heterotopic pain is common; when the location of the pain is not the origin of the pain.[1] Therefore, unless adequate time is spent to fully consider the full spectrum of biological, biomechanical, and psychosocial factors that may be initiating and perpetuating the alleged jaw disorder, misjudgments can be made.

In addition, although TM problems are commonly associated with multiple otologic symptoms such as ear pain, tinnitus, and vertigo,[2,3] as a result of both jaw muscle and temporomandibular joint (TMJ) pathology, and embryonic origins shared between the ear and jaw structures, symptoms without detail or a supporting history and examination may have little to do with jaw structures. As a result, a diagnosis of a TMD may be made, care initiated and disappointment realized by the patient when symptoms do not resolve.

BEFORE MAKING A TEMPOROMANDIBULAR DISORDER DIAGNOSIS REGIONAL PATHOLOGY MUST BE CONSIDERED

First and foremost, it is vital to have a diagnosis before commencing treatment protocols, and sometimes this is difficult. As inflammatory crosstalk between the ear and TMJ is common, it is essential that an ear infection for instance is ruled out before concluding the presence of a primary TMD. And an abnormal tympanogram in the absence of demonstrable swelling and fever can be a result of inflammation of the TMJ. Concerning pharyngeal and parotid gland pathology particularly in their incipient state can lead to trigeminal nerve excitation and the onset of pain and/or jaw motion limitations, mimicking a TMD problem, as muscles splint and guard. Conversely, a benign problem such as Masseter Parotid Hypertrophy Syndrome can lead to facial and jaw swelling and concern about aggressive regional pathology though not present.

THE CROSSOVER BETWEEN MEDICAL DISORDERS, OTOLARYNGOLOGY, AND DENTISTRY

The emergence of pain in the head and face often drives patients into the offices of dentists and otolaryngologists. Developing odontogenic problems, tension and migraine headaches, true cranial neuralgias, neuropathic pain problems, cervicogenic headaches, and pathology in the ear, sinus, throat, and nose must all be considered when a working diagnosis is being considered for a set of pain complaints that may be vague, confusing in their presentation and widespread in location.

Symptoms of primary headache disorders such as migraine, and tension-type headaches present with midface and temporalis pain, respectively, and can be interpreted as a jaw problem. Sinus contact headaches can prompt the emergence of convergent TMD midface pain and tension-type muscle overuse headaches can refer pain to the sinuses. Therefore, care seeking by the patient can be solely driven by the location of their symptoms (not the origin), resulting in the delay of appropriate care being put into place.

Beyond these crossovers, the term Otomandibular Syndrome coined in the 1970s by Harold Arlen MD, a practicing otolaryngologist in NY City, provides insights into why countless patients often complain of pain in and around the ears, fullness in the ears, hearing loss, tinnitus, and loss of balance with no evidence of pathology during an ENT examination.[4] On examination of the TM complex, however, there was often evidence of jaw muscle hyperactivity, soreness, and guarding. Arlen pointed to human embryology to make the connection between the ear and the TM complex. His postulations focused on the fact that the trigeminal nerve, derived from the mandibular arch, innervated not only the muscles of mastication, the mylohyoid, and the anterior belly of the digastric but also the tensor tympani and the tensor veli palatini muscles, thus establishing neural patterns early on embedded in the brainstem.

With the knowledge that the tensor tympani upon its contraction influences the position of the tympanic membrane (and therefore influences the way that sound vibrations from the outer air transmit to the auditory ossicles), and that the tensor veli palati functions to open the eustachian tube, a disturbance in neuromuscular function in the trigeminal system would have the potential to give rise to ear symptoms in the absence of pathology. As such, Arlen theorized that a malfunctioning of the tensor veli palati could reduce the patency of the eustachian tube leading to symptoms of fullness in the ears, hearing loss, and disequilibrium. And tonic contractions of the tensor tympani muscles would have the potential to be associated with otalgia, disequilibrium, and tension headache. Although research over the last 50 years has led to variable conclusions about whether these muscles in the presence of a TMD become dysfunctional and responsible for ear symptoms in the absence of disease, a nod to embryology must be considered when assessing patients with challenging symptoms.

CHAPTER GOALS

As a result of these complexities, this article will be designed to help the otolaryngologist understand:

1. What TMDs are, and what they are not?
2. What is the best terminology to use when diagnosing these problems and what are the most common diagnostic categories encountered?
3. What line of questioning and examination findings can most predictably lead to an accurate diagnosis of a TMD?
4. What are the most likely origins of a TM problem?
5. Beyond an examination, what diagnostic tests are most relevant?
6. What are the most appropriate first-line therapies?
7. When a referral to a specialist is in order
8. How to distinguish jaw disorders from other painful conditions in the orofacial and head regions?
9. Airway assessment and relationship to TMDs.

WHAT ARE TEMPOROMANDIBULAR DISORDERS?

During a routine day, most people never give a second thought to the function of their jaw; how far it opens, the presence or absence of joint noises during jaw movement, and/or the way their teeth function when chewing. Although a healthy functioning jaw is necessary to speak, eat, smile, kiss, and laugh, its complex function is never thought about until movement limitations and/or pain emerge. It is fully understandable that the general public never thinks twice about jaw function until problems arise.

Presently, the definition of TMDs that came about as a result of the American Dental Association's Consensus Conference in 1983 still guides the research community.[5] In their words, TMDs are a set of diseases or disorders that are related to alterations in structure, function, or physiology of the masticatory system and that may be associated with other systemic and comorbid medical conditions. TMDs can be usefully separated into 2 groups: the common TMDs with validated diagnostic criteria and the uncommon TMDS that do not yet have validated diagnostic criteria because of the challenges of conducting research on rare conditions. An individual may have more than one TMD and may also have comorbid conditions.

Through the years, additional research efforts led to a 2014 publication of the diagnostic criteria for TMDs,[6] which outlined the full spectrum of muscle, joint, headache, and other disorders that are considered TMDs. These diagnoses reflect that some jaw disorders are accompanied by pain. In contrast, others are best defined by anatomic changes in the joint itself, leading to motion restrictions, joint noises, and bite changes often without associated pain. When pain is present, these diagnoses also provide recognition that central pain mechanisms and not just tissue injury may be responsible for persistent pain. In addition, as this classification system recognized that these disorders are complex, having multiple diagnoses coexist was not only possible but common. As a result, specific TMJ disorders, masticatory muscle disorders, and headache disorders could be diagnosed in the same individual presenting for care.

THE MASTICATORY SYSTEM

Before considering the most common diagnostic categories associated with TM problems, a brief review of the anatomy and neuroanatomy of this region is essential.[7]

The primary skeletal framework that supports the masticatory system includes the maxilla, the mandible, and the temporal bone. Although it does not attach directly to the mandible, the hyoid bone acts as a stabilizer during swallowing and breathing due to attachments to the muscles of the tongue, the floor of the mouth, and the anterior neck.

Jaw motion is accomplished primarily by 4 paired muscles. The masseter and temporalis muscles are jaw elevators responsible for bringing the teeth into contact. The medial pterygoid is also a closing muscle and participates in mandibular protrusion. However, when there is only unilateral contraction of the medial pterygoid, it influences the lateral shift of the jaw to the opposite side. The lateral pterygoid is a jaw depressor and jaw protruder when muscle contraction is bilateral. Lateral shift to the opposite side occurs with unilateral lateral pterygoid contraction. The masticatory muscles are innervated by motor and sensory branches of the trigeminal nerve.

The anterior and posterior digastric muscles and the hyoid muscles directly assist mandibular function as the jaw opens. Neck muscles that stabilize the skull are essential in supporting mandibular posture at rest and during function. These muscles have been called the accessory muscles of mastication (**Fig. 1**).

THE TEMPOROMANDIBULAR JOINT

The TMJ, or jaw joint, is a synovial joint involving the condylar head of the mandible and the mandibular fossa of the temporal bone. The condyle, the mandibular fossa, and articular eminence are covered with highly adaptive fibrocartilage, and the joint is divided into upper and lower spaces by an articular disc. This biconcave collagenous disc is interposed between the condyle and fossa. The disc position is stabilized

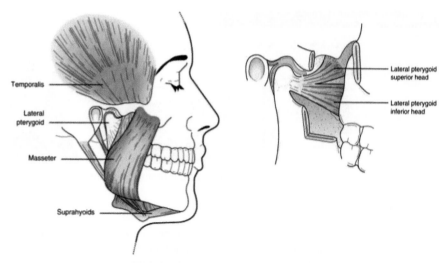

Fig. 1. The masticatory system.

by lateral and medial collateral ligaments and a posterior elastic ligament which allows the disc to slide anteriorly during translatory movements, which occur during chewing and opening of the jaw. The disc serves as a moving shock absorber and stabilizer between the condyle and fossa. As the jaw opens, the condyle first rotates and then slides forward within the fossa with the disc between the condyle and fossa. The TMJ capsule, which is fibrous in nature, surrounds the joint and helps define the inferior and superior joint spaces in conjunction with the articular disc.

The articular disc is stabilized in its orientation on the mandibular condyle by ligaments, attachment to the joint capsule itself, the posterior retrodiscal tissues, and tone of the lateral pterygoid muscles. Although the articular disc is avascular and non-innervated, the retrodiscal loose connective tissue at the rear end of the articular disc is highly innervated and vascular. These tissues act to restrict movement of the disc and retract the disc when the mouth is open wide. The retrodiscal tissue is surfaced by a synovial membrane, which releases synovial fluid into the joint, which is the primary source of joint nutrition. The synovial fluid also provides wetting lubrication and, most importantly, helps maintain the shape of the articular disc. The trigeminal nerve provides sensory innervation to the TMJ, facial dermatomes, and both motor and sensory innervation to the muscles of mastication.[8]

It should therefore be recognized that pain in the joint and/or mechanical impairments of joint motion are the end result of many factors, including compromise in synovial fluid volume or quality, ligament elongation or sprain, adhesive phenomena, a shift in the position of the articular disc, muscle hyperactivity, injury to the retrodiscal tissues, and/or structural changes in the shape of the mandibular condyle, fossa or articular eminence. Obtaining a history and clinical examination findings and imaging are therefore critical in determining where tissue injury exists and why it has likely occurred (**Fig. 2**).

The retrodiscal laminae, normally situated posterior to the condyle, is highly innervated and vascular. If ligament injury occurs, this retrodiscal tissue can be drawn over the condyle, potentially giving rise to pain and mechanical compromises of jaw motion.

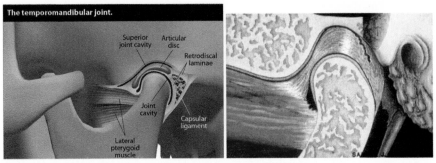

Fig. 2. The temporomandibular joint. (Permission to use granted by Samuel Higdon, DDS)

TISSUE INJURY

As with all orthopedic systems, injuries occur, leading to pain and compromises in function. Muscle problems are more common regarding the TM complex, but when present joint compromises lead to more profound symptoms. When tissue injury occurs, the pain is due to inflammation, which can lead to allodynia and hyperalgesia in the acute phase. If the source of acute tissue injury is identified early on and removed, healing is predictable. If, however, the initial injury is excessively traumatic and/or if a new injury cannot be avoided, peripheral sensitization associated with inflammation continues, and symptoms linger and often get bigger and broader. With time, the pain from lingering somatic tissue injury can become centralized, and heterotopic pain emerges, leading to new and often confusing symptoms. As a result, the earlier a diagnosis is made, the better the chance for a successful outcome once treatment is initiated. In the presence of central sensitization, a chronic and persistent pain condition may result ,though the somatic tissues may appear normal.

CLUES LEADING TO A WORKING DIAGNOSIS

Although there are common and specific muscle and joint problems associated with the TM complex, it is more than likely that more than one specific diagnosis characterizes the patient's symptoms and clinical examination. As TM problems can be acute, chronic, and/or progressive in nature, obtaining a careful history often helps establish the origin of the problem and better understand why symptoms may have persisted and /or gotten worse over time.

Although there are a variety of questioning strategies that can be taken to obtain the history of present illness, starting with a listing of current symptoms can very quickly define not only if they have a jaw problem but whether that problem is more dominated by functional limitations and/or pain. If a TM problem is to be diagnosed, one or a combination of symptoms are likely present.[9,10]

1. Pain over the TMJs/jaw muscles commonly increases with jaw function. Pain in these structures at rest is less common but reported. Morning pain if present ,is often associated with sleep bruxism.
2. Ear pain that is associated with jaw function
3. Dietary limitations prompted by jaw pain and/or jaw motion restrictions.
4. Limitation of jaw function, most often defined as limited jaw opening, "lockjaw."
5. The presence of joint noises that are likely new in origin or of a changed character that concerns the patient.
6. A change in the way the teeth come together.

7. A sense that their jaw position has changed and/or is off balance
8. Fear that their jaw will lock in open position if they open their mouth too widely.
9. A sense by the patient that their breathing efficiency, particularly while sleeping, may have changed. (As degenerative TMJ changes can decrease the condyle ramus vertical dimension negatively impacting the pharyngeal airway, there can be an increased risk for sleep-related breathing disorders.)

As these symptoms alone are not diagnostic of a primary TMD and could be present as a result of pathology in the head and neck or other pain orofacial pain disorders, the following categorizations should be remembered about the most common problems.[11]

1. Musculoskeletal disorders (like true TMD problems) are characterized by pain that is provocable with function and manipulation.
2. Neurovascular pain is episodic with pain-free periods between attacks, and the pain is typically not related to or provoked by jaw function.
3. Neuropathic pain is either continuous and may be aggravated by light touch or episodic and characterized by brief periods of excruciating pain that come on spontaneously or triggered by stimulation of trigger zones, and then ease markedly or disappear until the next episode.

Therefore, ask the patient how the pain initially presented and whether the character of the pain has changed over time. The history provided will also determine if the condition is acute, chronic, or progressive in nature. The keys to making a diagnosis are therefore dependent on:

1. Onset of symptoms
2. Location of the pain
3. Duration of the pain
4. Timing of the pain
5. The nature of the pain: (heavy pressure, sharp, stabbing, lancinating, dull ache, burning, tingling, numbing.)
6. Has the pain character changed?

To gather additional clues, Pain Mapping is a valuable tool to assess the perceived location of pain onset and distinguishing spreading pain fields and regions of dysesthesia or anesthesia.[12] Localized unilateral problems tend to be more somatic in nature, and more extensive regions of pain involvement may indicate central pain involvement.

EXAMINATION OF THE TEMPOROMANDIBULAR COMPLEX

If one keeps in mind that common TM problems are essentially orthopedic problems, then the clinical examination is straightforward and should take no longer than 5 minutes. The clinical examination consists of joint and muscle palpation, jaw range of motion measurements, and a superficial assessment to determine if the patient can bring their teeth together consistently and in a familiar position. As you move through your examination, the patient will likely identify what hurts and/or what is stiff and tight, joint noises, and/or if the jaw does not move in a free and easy way. The patient will also likely show you an altered bite relationship if it exists and/or a change in jaw position if it is present.

Although common jaw problems are often due to inflammation which will lead to pain symptoms (dolor) and reduced function/motion (function lasea), it is rare that the inflammation associated with these common problems will be associated with visible redness (rubor), swelling (tumor), and superficial heat (calor). In the presence of these findings, other regional pathology inclusive of that relating to the teeth, salivary glands, nose, sinuses, and oropharyngeal region should be suspected.

The examination should be inclusive of measuring jaw motion. Typically, jaw motion should be 40 to 45 mm with a straight pathway identified in the absence of pain. Three fingers stacked on top of each other and placed between the upper and lower incisor teeth typically represents normal motion capacity. Unless the patient tells you that they never could open their mouth widely, deviations less than 3 fingers may represent a hypomobile condition. The presence of joint noises, a hesitant pattern of jaw opening, a skewed pathway of jaw opening/closing, and/or evidence of joint locking and jamming all represent structural changes within the joint itself. Auscultating the joints with a stethoscope or a Doppler ultrasound may be helpful to discern the presence of clicks, pops, or crepitation-like noises. These findings and their relative importance will be defined and discussed later in this article. An inability to move the jaw forward and back or to the right or left with or without pain also likely indicates some form of structural incapacity within the joints. With the jaw at rest with the teeth apart, if palpation of the lateral pole of the condyle and posterior aspect of the joint prompts pain, this will indicate the presence of inflammation in one or multiple parts of the joint. Head range of motion should be noted in flexion, extension, side bend, and rotation.

Palpating the muscles of mastication and neck muscles is also an essential part of the examination. The goal is to identify taut muscle bands, painful myoneuronal trigger points, generalized muscle soreness, and overuse hypertrophy. Palpation of a jaw/neck muscle trigger point might set off a pain response in another site, which is called heterotopic pain. Muscle trigger points can refer pain to intraoral structures, inclusive of the teeth/gums, the ears, scalp, eyes, and sinuses. Myofibrotic contracture feels very stiff and unrelenting.

Most importantly, have the patient clench their teeth. If the masseter and temporalis muscles bulge outward and are sore to palpation, these 2 jaw elevator muscles are likely being overworked, and this requires investigation.[12]

COMMON JAW-RELATED MUSCLE DISORDERS

The terms myalgia and myofascial pain are often used to describe pain that originates from muscles. Within the TM complex, muscle pain is often experienced in the jaw elevators, which bring the teeth together from an open mouth position (masseters, temporalis, and medial pterygoid) and in the jaw depressors, which are primarily responsible for jaw opening and jaw protrusion (lateral pterygoids). Pain in these muscles often remains in a well-circumscribed area, is often elicited by examiner palpation, and commonly increases as the muscle is brought into function. Limited jaw motion in all directions, inability to bring the teeth together in a consistent fashion, and pain with eating and/or yawning, for instance, are all signs and symptoms of painful muscle disorders. At times, jaw function deviations and limitations due to muscles can also occur without pain but are less common.

All muscle disorders are not the same, and it should be appreciated that there likely is a continuum of disorders that can coexist if muscle pain becomes persistent.[13,14] If muscle pain is not brought on by a specific traumatic event, its origin is likely the result of persistent influences (see the section on causality/risk factors) that initially lead to what is termed protective cocontraction or muscle splinting/guarding. This is essentially a central nervous system (CNS) reflex in response to multiple factors that can include a change in jaw use, jaw overuse, nerve excitation, an activated autonomic nervous system, emotional upset, and/or chronic neck pain, as just a few examples. As a result, jaw muscles shorten, and motion becomes limited with reported muscle stiffness. If the reasons why muscle guarding occurred in the first place continue, a second muscle-related problem develops called delayed onset muscle soreness. This noninflammatory condition[15] is characterized by the emergence of pain as energy reserves are depleted as muscles stay shortened, and blood flow delivering oxygen and nutrients is slowed. The resulting muscle soreness is essentially the byproduct of a changing chemical environment in the muscle. Lactic acid, neuroactive substrates such as calcitonin gene-related peptide, substance-P, and tumor necrosis factor will irritate nerve fibers and lead to pain. Patients may describe muscle weakness and sensations of tingling, which occur as a result of tissue hypoxia. At times true muscle spasm occurs with associated limited jaw motion and/or a positional change of the jaw preventing a patient's teeth from coming together in their normal way. This is a rare occurrence.[16]

With persistence, spreading pain may develop or heterotopic pain (site of pain may not be the source of the pain) may develop as a result of central mediated mechanisms driven by chemically driven peripheral nerve sensitization. Pain in teeth, sinuses, or the ears may be the result of this phenomenon called myofascial pain. At times these referred symptoms can be prompted by maintained digital pressure on tender points in the involved muscles. This concept of heterotopic pain in the orofacial region due to striated muscles being in a state of overexcitation is analogous to cardiac referred pain and therefore must be considered when making a differential diagnosis.

Beyond these categories of muscle pain, there is another entity termed centrally mediated myalgia or chronic myositis. This is not an acute muscle pain condition but rather occurs as a result of chronic continuous muscle pain and its impact on the CNS. Peripheral muscle nociceptors are activated due to neurogenic inflammation and glutamate receptor neuroplasticity in the CNS. This condition is characterized by continuous pain, increases with function, but is not accompanied by reddening, swelling, or other cardinal signs of inflammation.

A true inflammatory condition that can be considered in a patient who presents with longstanding jaw pain that increases with function would be tendonitis in either the masseter where it attaches on the zygoma or the temporalis where it attaches to the coronoid process. These muscle insertion sites can become chronically inflamed and unresponsive to many traditional care efforts inclusive of oral anti-inflammatory medication. Diagnostic injections with local anesthesia if relieving pain, can provide a definitive diagnosis and then lead to treatment as will be discussed.[17]

Before leaving this section on common orofacial muscle disorders, it is important to remember that cervical spine injury and structural compromises[18] can give rise to pain symptoms in the jaw, sore jaw muscles on palpation, and limitations of jaw motion. These phenomena occur as a result of constant deep pain input originating in the cervical spine leading to referred pain (sensory disturbance) and/or shortening of the masticatory muscles (motor disturbance). As the dermatomes for C-2 and C-3 provide sensory innervation to much of the lower third of the face, it is critical when evaluating patients with orofacial/jaw pain and motion limitations, to obtain a thorough medical history inclusive of past traumas. This information may provide critical insights particularly if the initial assessment has left some gaps in understanding why the patient is suffering. The intimate relationship that the cervical spine has to masticatory comfort and function has made evaluation of this anatomic region mandatory during the initial examination[19] (**Fig. 3**).

The neck muscles have an anatomically intimate relationship to the TM complex and the cross-talk between the trigeminal and cervical nerves can create diagnostic confusion.

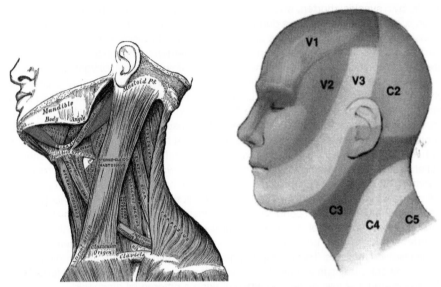

Fig. 3. Anatomy and Neuroanatomy link the trigeminal and peripheral cervical nerves

COMMON JOINT DISORDERS

As with muscles, there are both painful and nonpainful conditions that are common in the overall population. In fact, upwards of 6% to 48% of the population have been shown to have some sort of joint noise when their jaw is in function.[20] The vast majority of these people, however, do not seek care, many do not even know they have a disorder and most of the joint noises do not progress to a more problematic state. Joint noises, however, are not always benign, can be accompanied by pain, and therefore represent one of several symptoms that define a specific orthopedic problem in the TMJs.

When pain is present in the TMJ, it is referred to as "Arthralgia." The pain is typically inflammatory in nature and can be associated with the joint capsule, the supportive ligaments, the synovium, the retrodiscal tissues, and associated soft tissue structures of the joint. Painful arthritic conditions can also afflict the TMJ when the protective fibrocartilage covering the osseous structures become compromised. When viewed from an orthopedic perspective, the diagnoses associated with these inflamed tissues are no different from other joints in the body and arise for many of the same reasons as will be discussed in a later part of this article.

As with many painful muscle conditions, most joint pains experienced by the patient are often directly related to jaw function and the intensity of the pain is proportionate to the amount of function. In fact, if a patient can open and close their mouth, and/or move their jaw rigorously to the right and left or forward without pain or pain intensification, it is unlikely that profound joint inflammation is present. Rather, if there is minor pain or discomfort expressed during jaw motion and noted to be forward of the TMJ articulation, it may be of masseter origin due to protective muscle guarding.

For the purpose of this article distinguishing whether the arthralgia when present is due to ligamentous pain, retrodiscal pain, or capsular pain is not viewed as overly critical. Rather it is more critical that myalgia be distinguished from arthralgia.

The TMJ capsule, which is fibrous in nature, surrounds the joint and in conjunction with the articular disc, helps define the inferior and superior joint spaces. The capsule is lined by a synovial membrane and therefore pain directly over the TMJ condyle may emerge as a result of synovitis or capsulitis. Once the capsule is inflamed even subtle movements of the lower jaw can prompt pain. As a result, a complaint of continuous pain and joint stiffness even at a low level described as achiness may suggest the presence of joint capsulitis. This low level of continuous pain may recruit the jaw muscles to assume a guarded posture limiting jaw motion. From an examination perspective, there is palpable tenderness directly over the TMJ condyle, pain is increased by jaw motion, and jaw motion may be restricted. Inflamed synovial tissues, called synovitis, can produce acute pain, and an inability to bring the teeth together fully as redundant synovial tissue occupies space ,preventing full condyle seating in the fossa. Any accululation of fluid within the joint, called an effusion, or a swelling of the retrodiscal tissues can also lead to acute pain and chnages in the way the teeth come together.

The ligament structures of the TMJ are innervated for proprioceptive function (they are part of the GPs system of jaw function), are designed to maintain joint stability, and most importantly their integrity is essential to keep the shock-absorbing articular disc positioned securely on the condyle at rest and during function. If the ligaments that attach the articular disc to the condyle elongate, the articular disc can then begin to slide asynchronously, leading to joint noises and what has been termed a disc interference disorder. These noises are often described by the patient as a clicking or popping sound, which may or may not be audible. What may start out as a nonpainful condition, can over time progress within a continuum of potential structural compromises. From an orthopedic perspective then, patients commonly sprain their TMJs leading to pain and restricted motion due to protective muscle guarding. Sprains occur due to a multitude of factors including food injuries, grinding and clenching of the teeth, excessive wide jaw opening, vomiting, intubation during general anesthesia, long dental appointments, intimacy, and countless jaw overuse behaviors during the day. This line of questioning is therefore critical when a patient initially presents for a consultation visit.

Clinical findings associated with ligament compromise may include any of the following: pain mainly accompanying jaw motion, joint noises during jaw motion which may be audible or only discerned while palpating the joint or via auscultation, restricted jaw motion, or an altered pathway of jaw motion due to a disc interference. An 'S' pattern of jaw motion is often seen with early-stage disc unilateral interference disorders. When both joints have disc displacement problems, then arthrokinetics are variable.

A common presentation of a TMD problem is a clicking disc signifying compromise of the collateral ligaments, which partially or completely displaces the TMJ disc into a medial anterior posture. During jaw opening, the condyle reduces itself under the displaced disc causing a clicking sound. The click is the disc moving back into a normal position relative to the condyle but in a more anterior orientation. This repositioning is known as reduction, a posture that may be helpful while treating retrodiscal arthralgia. On closure, the condyle positions itself back off the distal aspect of the disc as the disc orients into the dislocated posture and the condyle retrudes against the posterior aspect of the glenoid fossa resting on the retrodiscal bilaminar zone. The retrodiscal tissues are composed of highly vascularized and innervated loose connective tissue and normally act to restrict movement of the disc and retract the disc when the mouth is open wide. As the retrodiscal tissues are surfaced by a synovial membrane, they also play a critical role in releasing synovial fluid into the joint, which is the primary source of joint nutrition. Fortunately, despite ligament instability, which can lead to a clicking joint and loading to the retrodiscal tissues, progression to a painful state is not predictable and the clicking related to these structural problems can continue for years without escalation and/or the emergence of inflammation.[21] In fact, when subject to excessive loading overtime, the retrodiscal tissues can scar and form callous, limiting the potential for inflammation down the line. Clinical findings, however, that help identify retrodiscal injury (inflammation and swelling) include a marked increase of pain when the teeth are fully brought together, and an inability to bring the teeth together fully, particularly on the symptomatic side. If a tongue blade was inserted between the teeth on the symptomatic side before biting, the pain experienced would be markedly reduced.

The next stage of disc displacement occurs when there is a complete tear and stretch of collateral and retro discal ligaments, which causes a complete anterior medial dislocation of the disc, which does not reduce on opening. This results in a closed locked disc where the jaw opening is reduced to about 25 to 30 mm, or about one knuckle, and deflected in a 'C' path to the injured side. It is not uncommon that despite these profound structural compromises (the retrodiscal tissues are located where the disc used to be) that healing can occur with the formation of a pseudo disc that becomes an adequate substitute for the displaced disc. However, in the presence of persistent pain, dietary limitations, and overconsumption of analgesics/anti-inflammatory medication, this condition may require a lysis and lavage procedure, called arthrocentesis or arthroscopy to help free up adhesions associated with the locked joint, and reduce inflammation giving nature a chance to initiate an adaptive response.

Degenerative joint disease or osteoarthritis can also develop in the TMJs as a result of single past traumas or the impact of long-term risk factors that can lead to the degeneration of the protective fibrocartilage that covers the articular surfaces of the joint as a result of a displacement of the articular disc. With the articular disc no longer protecting the condyle, the job is left to the retrodiscal tissues. Over time, perforations in the displaced retro discal ligament can occur leaving the articular surface of the condyle and eminence at risk for degenerative change due to functional physiologic degradation, and lack of proper synovial nourishment, leading to the breakdown of the condylar cortical bone. Ultimately the underlying osseous tissue can become inflamed leading to symptoms of dull aching pain commonly increased during function.[22] The presence of joint noise in an arthritic joint is variable and can have a characteristic coarse dry gravel-like sound particularly if there is radiographic evidence of alteration of the osseous surfaces. If degenerative changes associated with the TMJ

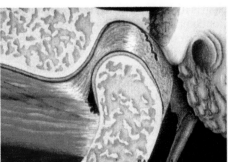 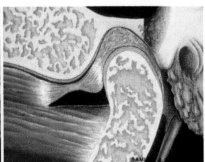

Normal joint   Anterior disc displacement

Fig. 4. An anterior disc displacement can lead to pain and symptoms of joint noise or restriction of motion. (Permisssion to use granted by Samuel J. Higdon ,DDS)

condyle or fossa persist, the way a patient's teeth come together may change. If changes in condylar form are profound, changes in mandibular posture particularly when sleeping can lead to airway constriction (**Fig. 4**).

An anterior disc displacement can lead to pain and symptoms of joint noise or restriction of motion.

IMAGING FOR TEMPOROMANDIBULAR DISORDERS

Although a great deal of diagnostic information when evaluating a TMD case can be gathered by a thorough history and examination, clinical assessment is unreliable for determining the status of the joint. Therefore, when indicated, imaging can play a vital role in establishing a diagnosis and uncovering other comorbid conditions that may impact the diagnosis. The commonly used radiograph is the panoramic radiograph. Although helpful to provide a screening view of the TMJs, it has limited value for complete evaluation as it offers merely a narrow trough of radiologic survey and may miss vital details (**Fig. 5**).

As an alternative, a high-resolution TMJ computed tomography (CT) and even cone beam CT contain a volume of diagnostic information which can be evaluated in several ways.

1. Three-dimensional volumetric imaging of the skull and cervical vertebrae. Cysts, tumors, impacted teeth, ear cerumen, enlarged tonsils and adenoids, infectious tracts, salivary stones, disordered nasal anatomy, and sinus pathology.
2. Cephalometrically corrected slice views of the condyles in sagittal, axial, and coronal planes. This allows interpolation of the condyle/fossa relationship, measurement of condyle vertical dimension, and allows inspection of the surface changes in the condyle and fossa.
3. Three dimensional panoramic with a specific field of view enables pinpointing and direct measurement of lesions and identification of the location of the inferior alveolar nerve as it courses through the mandible.
4. Volumetric data measuring the airway dimensions and observing skeletal or soft tissue elements which can cause airway impingement.

MRI is useful in diagnosing soft tissue pathology in the TMJ and surrounding structures. The disc position and morphology as well as the bone structure/status are clearly visualized on closed mouth images and the relationship of the disc and condyle can be assessed on open mouth images (**Figs. 6–8**).

It is the clinician's choice as to which study offers the best diagnostic information based on the presentation.

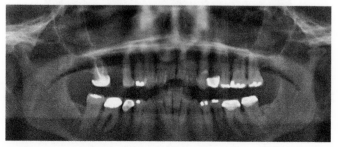

Fig. 5. Panoramic x-ray revealing a shape change of the left condyle.

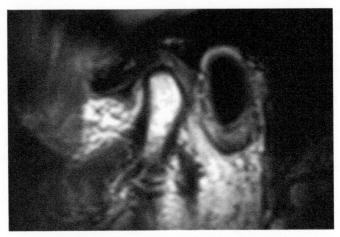

Fig. 6. Normal TMJ MRI showing disc in its normal orientation.

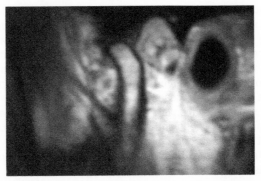

Fig. 7. Normal MRI of TMJ in an open mouth position. The disc assumes a bowtie-like appearance on top of the condyle.

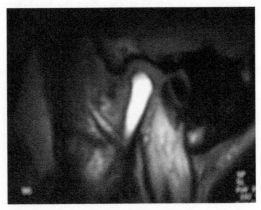

Fig. 8. MRI showing disc out of place in forward position.

WHY TEMPOROMANDIBULAR DISORDERS OCCUR

With the understanding that common and classifiable TMDs are essentially orthopedic problems, then it should become easier to appreciate that the true and predictable origins of these problems are finite. In fact, other than traumatic events impacting the somatic and neural tissues that make up and serve the TM complex, respectively, most all other influences that are commonly talked about should be classified as potential risk factors. Among the risk factors worth exploring when trying to determine why a patient's jaw symptoms have emerged, consideration should be given to:

- Daytime jaw overuse behaviors such as awake bruxism (tooth contact), nail and cuticle biting, pen biting, jaw muscle bracing, gum chewing, and/or any activity that overworks the jaw leading to muscle fatigue and soreness along with joint inflammation and ligamentous sprain. Though these behaviors are seemingly benign, when persistent they have the potential to create and then perpetuate tissue injury.
- Postural fatigue of the neck muscles supporting the head: Though only a risk factor, the intimate relationship of the trigeminal and cervical nerve systems can lead to jaw symptoms inclusive of pain and motion restrictions. Hours on the computer and/or handheld mobile devices on a consistent basis, along with driving in daily traffic to and from work, is all it takes to trigger neck muscle fatigue/inflammation and subsequent excitation of the trigeminal nerve.
- Persistent neck inflammation secondary to trauma or an underlying medical disorder. The intimate relationship between the trigeminal and cervical neural systems can lead to jaw pain, and/or jaw muscle guarding resulting from a primary neck-related problem.
- Food choices that overwork the jaw: At times patients alter their diet and begin to eat foods that require increased levels of muscle effort and joint stability. Nuts, energy bars, chewing gum, dried fruit, bagels, hard crusty pieces of bread, uncooked vegetables, Bavarian pretzels, beef jerky, popcorn, and so forth, can all have consequences over time.
- Excessive tongue movements: Since the tongue is attached to the floor of the mouth and therefore the lower jaw, excessive tongue movements that may accompany the presence of intraoral piercing and efforts to clean food impacted between teeth after meals can be a source of muscle fatigue and potential sprain to TMJ ligaments.
- Excessive yawning and vomiting: Wide yawns that are at times enjoyed by patients and that occur frequently can be a source of ligament injury. In a similar fashion, violent and/or frequent vomiting that may accompany an eating disorder can prompt tissue injury.
- Intimacy: Though asking questions along these lines is sometimes uncomfortable, consideration is important.
- Sleep bruxism: Clenching or grinding of the teeth at night is considered by some researchers as normal behavior, while it is also primarily categorized as a movement disorder. Despite a great deal of study, the origin of sleep bruxism remains unclear. There, however, appears to be a consensus that transient cortical arousals in the brain may be the triggering factor. It must be understood, however, that though sleep bruxism can be directly responsible for jaw symptoms inclusive of pain, joint noises, and mechanical compromises, no direct causal relationship has been established between the presence of sleep bruxism and the emergence of symptoms. In fact, many nighttime grinders and clenchers

deny the presence of bruxism despite evidence of tooth wear and well-developed muscles.

- Specific medical disorders: Systemic inflammatory/Autoimmune disorders that compromise the integrity of connective tissue and increase inflammation put the TM complex at risk. Juvenile idiopathic arthritis, rheumatoid arthritis, psoriatic arthritis, Ehlers-Danlos syndrome, seronegative arthritis, and so forth. These medical problems and their associated inflammation can create both peripheral and central sensitization and associated pain. In addition, joint hypermobility and ligament laxity, preadolescent growth disorders (Juvenile Osteochondrosis), retrognathia resulting in a long face syndrome often associated with a narrow nasal cavity, adenoidal presentation, high palatal vault, and nasal and pharyngeal airway constriction can all be potential risk factors predisposing to TMD problems.
- Medications: When viewed as risk factors, there are a few medications that have commonly been associated with either the onset and/or aggravation of a preexisting set of jaw complaints. Specifically, the medications used to treat ADD/ADHD inclusive of Adderal, Strattera, Concerta, Vyvanse, and Ritalin have been part of patient medical histories. Among teen and adolescent populations, the use of these medications has become more prevalent and used beyond days of test-taking. Rather when used on a regular schedule, these medications have the potential to upregulate the sympathetic drive of the patient, leading to changes in muscle tone, breathing dynamics, and sleep quality. As a result of this triad, musculoskeletal pain may emerge. It is also not uncommon for patients on these medications to report jaw muscle tension and increased tendencies toward awake bruxism and jaw muscle bracing.
- Other medications such as a number of the selective serotonin reuptake inhibitors (SSRIs) have been shown to not only increase the likelihood of sleep bruxism but also influence the outcome of sleep bruxism on the jaw muscles and TMJs. If the history provided suggests that a newly prescribed SSRI coincides with concerns about a jaw problem, collaboration with the prescribing physician will be important.
- Primary anxiety disorders and posttraumatic stress disorder (PTSD): To broadly discuss the impact of these 2 specific medical diagnoses on orofacial/TMD pain and suffering is well beyond the scope of this article. However, it is important to understand that as patients with primary anxiety disorders are often in a hypervigilant state, the resultant imbalance between an overactive sympathetic state and insufficient parasympathetic response, sets the table for a muscle-based pain experience.
- Similarly, a diagnosis of PTSD is commonly associated with pain problems as an HPA axis dysregulation which occurs in the presence of a "brain under siege" increases the risk for chronic pain. It is important therefore to remember that there is considerable indirect evidence that a prior history of anxiety, and physical and psychological trauma, are significantly predictive of the onset of chronic pain later in life.
- Daily stress/Loss of control in life. With evidence mounting that prolonged exposure to unavoidable stress produces a reduction of dopamine output and the development of persistent hyperalgesia, it is common for patients to present with TMD symptoms during periods of persistent life stress. These life stresses also most assuredly lead to changes in breathing, postures, and sleep hygiene with unfavorable pain outcomes.
- Insomnia/Airway insufficiency and other sleep-related disorders. Anything that persistently fragments sleep will over time likely lead to some form of

neurotransmitter dysregulation increasing the risk for both somatic and neuro-pathic pain. Questions relating to sleep are therefore critical in assessing patients with TMD problems.

- A bad bite (malocclusion). Over the years this has been the most contentious issue when debating the origins of TMDs. All relevant studies, however, have come to the same conclusion. A person's bite in isolation of other factors likely has little or nothing to do with the emergence of a jaw problem. An uneven bite, deep bites, crossbites, crowded dentitions, shifting teeth, and so forth, are no more than a risk factor that has the potential when coupled with other fac-tors to contribute to the emergence and perpetuation of jaw symptoms. With the appreciation that close to 70% of all patients seeking care for jaw symptoms are women, even strong advocates of the "bite as cause" need to take pause as they consult with and plan treatment for patients who seek care in their office. In re-ality, it is more likely that what a patient does with their teeth and bite is more important than how their teeth actually come together. From this perspective, identification of daytime behaviors that bring the teeth together becomes even more relevant. This discussion is not meant to discard the teeth and what we call the dental occlusion (The bite) from the conversation, but to rather place them alongside other possible risk factors. Therefore, although it is appropriate for an examining physician to note a malocclusion, they should not suggest to the patient that their symptoms are a direct result of tooth arrangements and that corrections should be part of first-line treatment efforts.
- Jaw posture and other structural considerations. Here too, there remains debate about whether or not the relationship of the maxilla to mandible can be impactful to the TMJ and jaw muscles in a way that prompts tissue injury and the onset of symptoms. Analysis of populations of patients who have been evaluated for corrective jaw surgery to address imbalances between the maxilla and mandible and the consequent way the teeth come together have revealed that pain was not the most dominant factor prompting patients to seek care. Chewing consider-ations and esthetics were the primary reasons why consults were sought. Over the last 20 years, however, there has been a subset of patients who when as-sessed for corrective jaw surgery have been found to have significant airway compromises due to the structure and relationship of the maxilla, mandible, and nasal complex. These patients are often compromised by excessive fatigue and daytime sleepiness due to poor oxygen saturation when sleeping and many present with a diagnosis of obstructive sleep apnea. Remarkably, although some of these patients are also headache sufferers (may or may not relate to the airway issues), the vast majority do not seek care because of the presence of persistent jaw pain and mechanical failings during jaw function. In addition, though sleep bruxism may at times be associated with airway problems, jaw symptoms asso-ciated with the postulated airway initiated bruxism do not appear any more likely or acute. The take-home message: airway problems due to jaw asymmetries and imbalances need to be recognized and potentially addressed, but should not be looked at as anything more than a risk factor for TMJ disorders.
- Airway patency. Sleep airway disorders have their origin as either nasal, velopa-latal, retroglossal, or hypopharyngeal impingement. Deviated septa, concha bul-losa, sinus disease, anterior nasal valve insufficiency, tonsillar and adenoid hypertrophy, and hyoid positional disorders can all impact the airway. Though worth mentioning as a risk factor, it remains unclear as to whether airway com-promises drive the onset of jaw symptoms.

- The patient as a person. The bottom line is that TMDs are driven by a multitude of potential risk factors. Other than the factors listed, medical comorbidities need to be considered, as the conditions themselves may directly or indirectly excite the trigeminal system (ie, migraines, chronic gastrointestinal disease, past chemotherapy) giving rise to peripheral and central sensitization and the emergence of pain in the face. In addition, just the stress of medical disorders that are impactful to life may be enough to trigger TM complaints. Ultimately, if there are enough risk factors that light up the trigeminal/cervical nerves, and impair the body's endogenous descending pain modulation systems, then TMD and other orofacial pain symptoms can emerge as a result of central pain phenomena.

What should be clear from this extensive list is that TMDs have multiple physical, psychological, and social factors that play a role in the onset and progression of the experienced condition.[23] Only this biopsychosocial approach,[24] which focuses on the whole person, has strong evidence and strong theory relating clinical findings to symptoms and approaches to treatment that are consistent with what is known about chronic pain elsewhere in the body.[25]

APPROPRIATE FIRST-LINE TREATMENT FOR A TEMPOROMANDIBULAR DISORDER

If a diagnosis of a TMD has been made and the location of the tissue injury identified, care must be designed to accomplish 2 goals: stop new tissue injury and promote tissue healing. To this end, the following will serve as a guide to direct "do no harm" treatment and/or buy time until an appropriate referral.

1. Identify daytime overuse jaw behaviors and require patient participation to make changes. Introduce breathing techniques as a way to calm the nervous system and reduce the likelihood of tension-relieving oral behaviors.
2. Talk about dietary modifications and leaning toward a softer diet.
3. Identify head posture concerns relating to computer and handheld device use and try to limit this source of neck muscle fatigue
4. Determine if sleep bruxism may be playing a role based on the presence of morning jaw symptoms. If so, for the short term, an over-the-counter bruxism guard could be purchased but follow-up with a dentist would be highly recommended.
5. Encourage the use of an anti-inflammatory medication if not contraindicated from a medical perspective. The timeframe and dosage would be determined based on whether there was a muscle or joint injury to be addressed and whether the problem was acute or chronic.
6. Encourage the use of home remedies for muscle pain. For instance, the application of moist heat several times a day on the jaw and neck muscles for 20 minutes. Topical menthol-based rubs or creams containing anti-inflammatory medication if not medically contraindicated. For pain specifically over the TMJs, ice would be preferred for 5 to 7 minutes 3 to 4 times a day.
7. Provide the patient with simple muscle massage techniques and/or jaw/neck exercises for muscle problems. If the problem is primarily in the joint, referral to a specialist is likely the best course of action.
8. Prescribe a muscle relaxant primarily before bedtime to help diminish the impact of sleep bruxism and/or to promote sedation. The use of medications such as Trazadone, valium, Xanax, or clonazepam at bedtime can also be useful for 1 to 2 weeks.
9. During the day, muscle relaxants can also be used in patients who experience symptom escalation as the day progresses. Sedation must be monitored.

10. Some patients with TMD problems also have symptoms that seem to have a neuropathic character due to the chronicity of their problem. To confront these symptoms, the use of medications to control and/or dampen nerve discharge can be used at bedtime.
11. If there appears to be a dominant neck problem driving jaw symptoms, referral to a physical therapist, osteopath, and/or chiropractor should be considered.
12. In the presence of evidence pointing to anxiety-driven symptoms referral to a psychologist and/or psychiatrist with expertise in pain should be considered.

A significant reduction in symptoms with these efforts would confirm the presence of a TMD. Partial improvement would also lend support to an accurate diagnosis; however, if symptoms persist, muscle or joint pathology would likely require additional care best directed by a specialist. This care could include alternative medications, muscle/joint/tendon injections, Botox, physical therapy, custom oral appliances, and at times surgery. No improvement on the other hand would likely force a reconsideration of a TMD diagnosis.

For a broader discussion of what has been termed evidence-based care for TMD problems, a review of the Chapter entitled "Caring for Individuals with a TMD" in the Consensus Study Report for Temporomandibular Disorders, 2020 should be considered, along with an article by Charles Greene DDS, JADA, 2020.[26]

SUMMARY

As a variety of ear symptoms commonly accompany TM problems, patients will continue to seek care in the office of otolaryngologists. Therefore, a fuller appreciation of the signs, symptoms, and origins of these problems will facilitate the assessment of these patients, and a prompt determination as to whether or not a primary jaw problem is present.

CLINICS CARE POINTS

1. Disorders in the masticatory system inclusive of those in the temporomandibular joints are orthopedic problems and should be assessed and managed accordingly.

2. If a problem within the masticatory system inclusive of the temporomandibular joints and associated musculoskeletal structures is identified and seemingly responsible for ear symptoms, the identification and modification of daytime jaw overuse behaviors and fatiguing neck postures is often key to achieving symptom relief.

3. The majority of TM disorders can be managed nonsurgically and do not require reshaping of the teeth or treatment designed to change a patient's bite.

4. Understanding who the patient is from a medical and psychosocial perspective is essential to determine whether comorbidities may be partly responsible for symptom onset.

5. Do not assume that if a patient has a bad bite and crowded teeth, that these are the primary reason why a jaw problem is present.

6. If TMJ noises are noted and associated with progression inclusive of locking and pain referral to a specialist is advised

7. The use of NSAIDs and muscle relaxants have a place in the management of masticatory disorders, but may fall short if the causal or risk factors driving the onset are not identified.

DISCLOSURE

The authors have nothing to disclose.

REFERENCES

1. Murray GM. Referred Pain, Allodynia, and Hyperalgesia. J Am Dent Assoc 2009; 140:1121–4.
2. Manfredini D. Tinnitus in temporomandibular disorders patients: any clinical implications from research findings? Evid Based Dent 2019;20(1):30–1.
3. Porto De Toledo I, et al. Prevalence of otologic signs and symptoms in adult patients with temporomandibular disorders: A systemic review and meta-analysis. Clini Oral Investig 2017;21(2):597–605.
4. Arlen H. The otomandibular syndrome: clinical management of head, neck and TMJ pain and dysfunction. New York: W. B. Saunders Company; 1977.
5. Laskin DW, Greenfield W, Gale E, et al, editors. President conference on examination , diagnosis and management of TMD. Chicago (IL) American Dental Association; 1983.
6. Schiffman E, Ohrbach R, et al, International RDC/TMD Consortium Network, International Association for Dental Research, Orofacial Pain Special Interest Group, International Association for the Study of Pain. Diagnostic Criteria for Temporomandibular Disorders (DC/TMD) for clinical and research applications. J Oral Facial Pain Headache 2014;28(1):6–27.
7. Laskin D, Greene C, Hylander W. Temporomandibular Disorders, an evidence based approach to diagnosis and management. Quintessence Publishing Company, Inc; 2006.
8. Pertes R, Gross S. Clinical management of temporomandibular disorders and orofacial pain. Chicago (IL): Quintessence Publishing Company; 1995.
9. De Leeuw R, Glasser G. Orofacial pain, guidelines for classification, assessment and management, ed 5. Chicago: Quintessence; 2013.
10. Laskin D, Greene C, Hylander W. Temporomandibular disorders, an evidence based approach to diagnosis and management. Chicago (IL): Quintessence Publishing Co, Inc; 2006.
11. Robert L. Merrill, orofacial pain mechanisms and their clinical application. Philadelphia: Dental Clinics of North America; 1997. p. 185.
12. Wright E. Manuel of temporomandibular disorders. 2nd edition. Chicago (IL): Wiley -Blackwell; 2010.
13. Bell WE. Temporomandibular disorders, ed 3. Chicago Year Book Medical; 1990.
14. Stohler CS. Clinical perspectives on masticatory and related muscle disorders. In: Sessle BJ, Bryant PS, Dionne RA, editors. Temporomandibular disorders and related pain conditions. Seattle: IASP; 1995. p. 3–29.
15. Okeson J. Bell's oral and facial pain. 7th edition. Pains of Muscle Origin, Quintessence Publishing Company, Inc; 2014. p. 293.
16. Okeson J. Bell's oral and facial pain. 7th edition. Pains of Muscle Origin, Quintessence Publishing Company, Inc; 2014. p. 295.
17. Okeson J. Bell's oral and facial pain. 7th edition. Pains of Muscle Origin, Quintessence Publishing Company, Inc; 2014. p. 308.
18. Okeson J. Bell's oral and facial pain. 7th edition. Pains of Muscle Origin, Quintessence Publishing Company, Inc; 2014. p. 339.
19. Sharav Y, Benoliel R. Orofacial pain and headache. Mosby Elsevier; 2008.
20. Locker D, Slade G. Prevalence of symptoms associated with temporomandibular disorders in a Canadian Population. Community Dent Oral Epidemiol 1988;16(5): 310–3.

21. Tanaka E, Kawai N, et al. The frictional coefficient of the temporomandibular joint and its dependency on the magnitude and duration of joint loading. J Dent Res 2004;83(5):404–7.
22. Stegenga B. Osteoarthritis of the temporomandibular joint organ and its relationship to disc displacement. J Orofac Pain 2001;15(3):193–205.
23. Scrivani, Steven DDS. Temporomandibular Disorders. N Engl J Med 2008; 359(25):2693–705.
24. Fricton J. Temporomandibular disorders: a human systems approach. J Calif Dent Assoc 2014;42(8):523–35.
25. Consensus Study Report, Temporomandibular Disorders, Priorities for Research and Care, The national academies of sciences. Engineering.Medicine. The National Academies Press; 2020.
26. Greene CS. Managing the care of patients with temporomandibular joint disorders, a new guideline for care. J Am Dent Assoc 2010;14(9):1086–8.

Headache in Pregnancy

Isabelle Magro, MD, MS, Margaret Nurimba, MD*,
Joni K. Doherty, MD, PhD

KEYWORDS

- Pregnancy • Breastfeeding • Primary headache • Secondary headache

KEY POINTS

- Most headaches in pregnancy are migraine or tension-type headaches.
- Pregnant women presenting with headaches should be screened for red flag symptoms.
- Though nonpharmacologic therapies are preferred in the management of headaches, pharmacologic treatments, when necessary, should be chosen while considering possible adverse effects to the pregnancy and fetus.

INTRODUCTION

Headache disorders are common with an estimated prevalence of 50% worldwide.[1] The International Classification of Headache Disorders (ICHD) classifies headache disorders as primary or secondary.[2] Primary headaches are disorders characterized by head pain that cannot be attributed to another underlying disorder. In contrast, secondary headaches are characterized by head pain that is attributed to another underlying disorder.

Primary headache disorders, including tension-type headaches (TTHs), migraine headaches, and trigeminal autonomic cephalalgias (TACs), are the most common cause of headaches. Primary headache disorders are benign but can impose a significant burden on quality of life.[3] Secondary headache disorders such as temporomandibular joint (TMJ) dysfunction and sinusitis can also be benign. However, other causes including those of vascular etiology such as a cerebrovascular event, intracranial hemorrhage, cerebral venous thrombosis (CVT), or those of neoplastic etiology such as benign and malignant brain tumors, can be life-threatening.[4] These life-threatening disease processes should always be considered in patients presenting with headaches and particularly in pregnant women who are at an increased risk of vascular events due to hormone changes and hypercoagulability associated with pregnancy.

Women in pregnancy can present with a history of primary headache and report their usual headache, present with a history of primary headache and report

Caruso Department of Otolaryngology-Head and Neck Surgery, Keck School of Medicine of the University of Southern California, 1537 Norfolk Street, Suite 5800, Los Angeles, CA 90033, USA
* Corresponding author.
E-mail address: margaret.nurimba@med.usc.edu

a headache that differs in quality, intensity, duration, and associated symptoms compared with their usual headache, or present without a history of primary headache and with their first severe headache during pregnancy.[4] Pregnant women presenting with red flag symptoms, particularly in their second and third trimesters, should be evaluated for causes of secondary headache.[4,5] The following review will discuss the clinical presentation of primary and secondary headaches and their treatment in pregnancy.

CLINICAL PRESENTATION AND DIAGNOSIS OF PRIMARY HEADACHE
Primary Headaches

Primary headaches, namely migraine and TTH, are the most common cause of headaches in pregnant women.[4,5] The diagnosis of primary headaches is determined according to the criteria outlined by the ICDH. In the absence of red flag symptoms, which are outlined in **Table 1**, no further diagnostic workup is indicated for primary headache.

Observational studies have shown that primary headaches in pregnancy can change in intensity and character. Both migraine and TTH have been shown to decrease in intensity and frequency during pregnancy.[4]

Migraine

Migraine is the most common cause of headaches in pregnant women.[5,6] Migraines can be classified into 2 major times: migraine without aura (MO) and migraine with aura (MA).[2] Vestibular migraine should also be considered in a patient with headaches and vertigo. The ICHD-3 diagnostic criteria for these diagnoses are included in **Table 2**.

Most pregnant women with preexisting migraine tend to experience a decrease or complete resolution of migraine symptoms during pregnancy.[4,6,7] This effect may be attributed to an increase in the pain threshold secondary to elevated estrogen and endogenous opioid levels and the absence of fluctuating hormone levels during pregnancy.[8] Women with MO are more likely to experience an improvement in their symptoms during pregnancy than women with MA, which may be attributed to increased endothelial vasoreactivity in patients with MA.[4,8,9] Pregnant women with preexisting migraine who continue to experience symptoms can experience a change in their migraine from MA to MO and vice versa.[4] There are no studies in the literature that

Table 1 Red flags for headache in pregnancy		
Clinical Presentation	**History**	**Inciting Factors**
Change in headache from a previously stable headache pattern	History of malignancy	Changes with posture (eg, standing up)
Peaks in severity in <5 min	History of HIV or active infections	Precipitated by physical activity or Valsalva
New headache type	History of pituitary disorders	
Awakens the patient	History of recent travel at risk for infectious disease	
Any associated:	Recent trauma	
Thrombophilia		
Neurologic symptoms		
Fever		
Seizures		
Elevated blood pressure		

Data from Negro A, Delaruelle Z, Ivanova TA, et al. Headache and pregnancy: a systematic review. *J Headache Pain.* 2017;18(1). https://doi.org/10.1186/s10194-017-0816-0.

Table 2
Diagnostic criteria for migraine with and without aura and vestibular migraine as defined by the ICHD-3

A. Migraine Without Aura	B. Migraine with Aura	C. Vestibular Migraine
At least 5 episodes of headache that meet criteria 1–3	At least 2 episodes of headache that meet criteria 1–3	A current or past history of migraine with or without aura
1. Lasting 4–72 h	1. At least one of the following fully reversible aura symptoms: visual, sensory, speech and/or language/motor, brainstem, retinal	At least 5 episodes that meet criteria 1–2
2. At least 2 of the following characteristics: unilateral location, pulsating quality, moderate or severe pain intensity, causing avoidance of routine physical activity 3. At least one of the following associated symptoms: nausea and/or vomiting, photophobia and phonophobia	2. At least 3 of the following characteristics: • At least one aura symptom occurs gradually over 5 min or more • Two or more aura symptoms occur in succession • Each aural symptom lasts 5–60 min • At least one aura symptom is unilateral • At least one aura symptom is positive • The aura is accompanied or followed within 60 min by headache	1. Vestibular symptoms of moderate or severe intensity, lasting between 5 minutes and 72 h 2. At least half of episodes are associated with at least one of the following characteristics • Headache with at least 2 of the following: unilateral location, pulsating quality, moderate or severe intensity, aggravation by routine physical activity • Photophobia and phonophobia • Visual aura

Data from Olesen J. Headache Classification Committee of the International Headache Society (IHS) The International Classification of Headache Disorders, 3rd edition. *Cephalalgia*. 2018;38(1):1-211. https://doi.org/10.1177/0333102417738202.

characterize vestibular migraine in pregnancy, although an improvement in symptomatology may also be expected, given the overall clinical course of migraine observed in pregnancy.

Pregnant women without preexisting migraine can also have their first episode of migraine. Women without preexisting migraine are more likely to develop MA in pregnancy than in MO. Pregnant women without preexisting migraine who develop migraine symptoms should undergo an MRI and/or computed tomography (CT) to rule out secondary causes of headache as new-onset headache is a red flag symptom.[4]

Women tend to have an increase in migraine symptoms in the postpartum period.[10] This change is attributed to falling estrogen levels after childbirth and the increase in stress, sleep deprivation, and anxiety of caring for a newborn.[8] Studies suggest that breastfeeding may have a protective effect on the recurrence of migraine symptoms in the postpartum period due to the secretion of oxytocin, which increases the pain threshold, and prolactin, which inhibits ovulation and fluctuating estrogen levels.[8,10,11]

Although migraine headaches do not cause adverse outcomes in pregnancy, women with migraine are at an increased risk of cardiovascular events.[12] Pregnancy results in a hypercoagulable state whereby elevated estrogen levels stimulate the production of coagulation factors, circulating cholesterol levels and elevated progesterone levels cause increased venous dilation and stasis of blood flow.[4,8] Migraines, particularly MA, are also associated with hypercoagulability secondary to thrombocytosis and platelet hyperactivity, erythrocytosis, and increased levels of von Willebrand factor, fibrinogen, and t-PA.[8] Given that hypercoagulability is associated with conditions that can manifest as secondary headaches, health care providers should be aware of this association when caring for pregnant patients with migraine who are presenting with headaches.

Tension headaches

TTH is the second most common cause of headaches during pregnancy.[4] The ICHD-3 diagnostic criteria for TTH are included in **Box 1**. TTH also improves in intensity and quality in pregnancy though not to the same degree as is MO.[4] TTH can also change in characteristics to resemble MA/MO and vice versa.[4,13] TTH are not associated with adverse effects in pregnancy, nor are they associated with an increased risk of other conditions.[13]

Trigeminal autonomic cephalalgias

TACs are a rare cause of headache that occurs more frequently in men than in women. TACs, the most common of which is cluster headache (CH), are seen in less than 0.3% of pregnancies.[4,14] The ICHD-3 diagnostic criteria for CH are included in **Table 3**. Pregnant women with a history of CHs often do not experience a change in the

---

Box 1
Diagnostic criteria for tension-type and cluster headaches as defined by the ICHD-3

Tension-Type Headaches
  Subdivided into various subtypes depending on the frequency of episodes
  Episode of headache that meets criteria 1 to 3
1. Lasting 30 minutes to 7 days
2. At least 2 of the following characteristics:
  • Bilateral location
  • Pressing or tightening quality
  • Mild or moderate intensity
  • Not aggravated by routine physical activity
3. Are not associated with nausea or vomiting
4. Are not associated with both photophobia and phonophobia

Cluster Headaches
  At least 5 episodes of headache that meet criteria 1 to 3
1. Severe unilateral orbital, supraorbital, and/or temporal pain lasting 15 to 180 minutes
2. At least one of the following:
  • At least one of the following autonomic symptoms ipsilateral to the headache: conjunctival injection and/or lacrimation, nasal congestion and/or rhinorrhea, eyelid edema, forehead and facial sweating, miosis and/or ptosis
  • A sense of agitation or restlessness
3. Occurs between once every other day up to 8 times per day

Data from Olesen J. Headache Classification Committee of the International Headache Society (IHS) The International Classification of Headache Disorders, 3rd edition. *Cephalalgia.* 2018;38(1):1-211. https://doi.org/10.1177/03331024177382.

Table 3
Safety profile of commonly used medications for the treatment of primary headache and temporomandibular joint in pregnancy

Medications	Notes
Over-The-Counter Analgesics	
Acetaminophen	Considered first-line Possible increased risk of behavioral disorders such as ADHD
Aspirin	Safe to use in low doses in the first and second trimester Risk of postpartum bleeding, neonatal bleeding, premature closure of the ductus arteriosus in the third trimester Risk of Reye syndrome in the infant during breastfeeding
NSAIDS	Safe to use in the second trimester Risk of miscarriage in the first trimester Risk of premature closure of the ductus arteriosus, cerebral palsy, impaired renal function, and neonatal intraventricular hemorrhage in the third trimester
Abortive Therapies for Primary Headache	
Triptans	Risk of atonic uterus and postpartum hemorrhage when used in the third trimester
Ergots and ergots alkaloids	Fetal distress and malformation secondary to a uterotonic and vasoconstrictive effect during pregnancy
Lidocaine	Transnasal formulation of lidocaine is preferred as it is considered to be safer than systemic formulations
Corticosteroids	Risk of early lung maturation and cleft palate
Dietary Supplements	
Magnesium	Maximum dose of 350 mg/d; higher doses associated with transient neurologic symptoms in newborns and hypotonia IV Magnesium for >5 d may be associated with fetal bone abnormalities
Coenzyme 10	Safe in low doses
Preventative Therapies for Primary Headache	
Beta-blockers	Metoprolol is the first line for migraine prophylaxis Should be tapered in the third trimester to avoid bradycardia hypotension and hypoglycemia in the infant
Calcium channel blockers	Verapamil is first line for CH prophylaxis
Antidepressants	Amitriptyline is the second line for migraine prophylaxis in pregnancy Possible risk of TCAs includes fetal cardiovascular or limb difference, but causal evidence is lacking
Antiepileptics	Lamotrigine is the first line with a good safety profile Valproate is associated with craniofacial, cardiac, and urologic defects Topiramate is associated with low birth weight and craniofacial abnormalities Gabapentin is associated with osteological abnormalities

Data from Negro A, Delaruelle Z, Ivanova TA, et al. Headache and pregnancy: a systematic review. J Headache Pain. 2017;18(1). https://doi.org/10.1186/s10194-017-0816-0 and MacGregor EA. Migraine in pregnancy and lactation. *Neurol Sci.* 2014;35(SUPPL. 1):83-93. https://doi.org/10.1007/s10072-014-1744-2.

intensity or frequency of their symptoms.[4] Pregnant women are unlikely to experience their first CH during pregnancy, but a small percentage experience their first episode after pregnancy.[15]

CLINICAL PRESENTATION AND DIAGNOSIS OF SECONDARY HEADACHES OF OTOLARYNGOLOGIC ETIOLOGY
Sinusitis

Rhinitis and infectious sinusitis are reported at increased incidence during pregnancy and should be considered in pregnant women presenting with chronic headaches with nasal symptoms.[16,17] Diagnosis of sinusitis in the pregnant patient should focus on a careful physical examination, and nasal cytology may be considered a noninvasive approach to differentiating infectious versus allergic sinusitis.

Temporomandibular Joint Dysfunction

Temporomandibular joint dysfunction (TMD) is another cause of chronic headache during pregnancy that may be associated with pain in the masticatory muscles, TMJ, and limitation of jaw function and sounds in the TMJ. Estrogen signaling has been implicated in alveolar bone remodeling and TMD, which is reported to have an increased incidence in females compared with their male counterparts.[18,19] Some studies report increased incidence of TMD, especially during pregnancy,[20] whereas other studies report improvement of TMD symptoms during pregnancy.[21] Diagnosis of TMD is typically clinical. However, diagnostic imaging may be beneficial in patients with malocclusion or intra-articular abnormalities.

TREATMENT OF PRIMARY AND SECONDARY HEADACHES OF OTOLARYNGOLOGIC ETIOLOGY
Nonpharmacologic Treatment and Prevention of Headaches

The preferred treatment of primary and secondary headaches of ENT etiology is preferred to be nonpharmacologic in pregnancy, given the potential for adverse effects on the developing fetus. Lifestyle modifications and the avoidance of triggers such as sleep deprivation, skipping meals, and emotional stress are essential to the prevention of primary headaches and TMJ.[4,5,22–24] Nonpharmacologic therapies such as acupuncture, yoga, massage therapy, and behavioral therapies like biofeedback are also useful in the prevention and treatment of primary headaches and TMJ.[22,25,26] TMJ can also be treated with occlusal devices and physical therapy.[26]

High flow oxygen therapy can be used in CHs with no known effects on the pregnancy or fetus.[24] Nasal saline irrigation may be used to treat chronic sinusitis if symptoms are mild.

Pharmacologic Therapies in Pregnancy

Pharmacologic therapies should be considered if nonpharmacologic therapies are insufficient in managing headaches. An undertreated headache can lead to stress, sleep deprivation, depression, and poor nutritional intake, which negatively affect the pregnancy and the developing fetus.[4,5] There is limited information regarding dietary supplementation and medication safety during pregnancy. The safety of a few medications has been tested in pregnancy, and current recommendations are based primarily on observational studies. The US Food and Drug Administration (FDA) previously classified medications in pregnancy into risk letter categories. However, the FDA discontinued this classification in 2014 in favor of health care providers weighing the risk and benefits of taking medication during pregnancy.

In general, if pharmacologic therapies are deemed necessary in pregnancy and breastfeeding, women should be given medications with the least amount of risk at the lowest therapeutic dose and for the shortest duration of treatment.[4] The safety profile of these medications is discussed in the following sections and is detailed in **Table 4**.

Over-the-Counter Analgesics

Over-the-counter medications are commonly used in headaches include acetaminophen, aspirin, caffeine, and nonsteroidal anti-inflammatory drugs. Acetaminophen has historically been considered the safest pharmacologic agent to treat acute headaches in pregnancy.[4,5] However, newer studies may suggest an association between acetaminophen exposure during pregnancy with an increased risk of behavioral disorders such as attention-deficit disorder.[27] Caffeine and aspirin are considered safe in low doses but may be associated with adverse effects in moderate to high doses. Aspirin exposure at high and low doses in the third trimester is associated with adverse fetal and maternal outcomes.[9] NSAIDs appear to be safe to use in the second trimester but are associated with adverse fetal outcomes in the first and third trimesters.[4,9] Over-the-counter analgesics may be used safely in breastfeeding with the exception of aspirin, which may lead to Reye syndrome in the infant.[9]

Abortive Therapies for Primary Headache

If over-the-counter medications are insufficient in managing headaches, other medications specific to the treatment of migraines and CHs may be considered. Triptans are not associated with adverse outcomes in the fetus when taken during pregnancy or breastfeeding. However, the use of triptans in the third trimester has been associated with an increased risk of atonic uterus and postpartum hemorrhage.[9] Ergots and ergots alkaloids are contraindicated during pregnancy or breastfeeding because of their teratogenicity.[9]

Lidocaine may be used in pregnancy and breastfeeding to treat CH when high flow oxygen therapy is insufficient.[24] Corticosteroids such as prednisone and prednisolone should be avoided if possible during pregnancy, given the potential risk of early lung maturation and cleft palate, particularly in the first trimester. However, these medications may be considered in disabling CH and status migrainous. Prednisone and prednisolone are generally safe in breastfeeding, but prolonged high-dose therapy should be avoided.[4]

Preventative Therapies for Primary Headache

Dietary supplements have been used in the prevention of primary headaches. Magnesium was previously considered to be safe in pregnancy but doses greater than 350 mg/d may be associated with adverse effects on the fetus.[4] Furthermore, treatment with intravenous magnesium for a period longer than 5 days has been associated with fetal bone abnormalities.[5] The use of Coenzyme Q10 during pregnancy has not been associated with adverse outcomes to date, although there are limited data available.[4,5] Feverfew, butterbur, and high dosed riboflavin are not recommended during pregnancy.[4]

Antihypertensives, antidepressants, and antiepileptics may be used for headache prophylaxis. Beta-blockers, preferably metoprolol, are the first-line therapy for migraine prophylaxis in pregnant and breastfeeding women.[4] Beta-blockers should be tapered off before labor if possible to avoid bradycardia hypotension, and hypoglycemia in the newborn.[9] Tricyclic antidepressants, preferably amitriptyline, are considered second-line therapy for migraine prophylaxis in pregnant women. Serotonin-norepinephrine reuptake inhibitors should be avoided in pregnancy.

Table 4
Safety profile of commonly used medications for treatment of rhinitis and sinusitis

Class	Adverse Effects	Notes
Antihistamines, oral and intranasal		
First Generation		Preferred to withdraw at least 3d prior to delivery
Tripelennamine, chlorpheniramine Hydroxyzine		Safe in pregnancy per ACOG, AAAAI
Diphenhydramine	Fetal development of cleft palate during TR1; oxytocin-like effect at high doses	
Second Generation		Preferred to withdraw at least 3d prior to delivery
Cetirizine, loratadine		Generally safe in pregnancy, use if refractory to tripelennamine and chlorpheniramine
Fenofexadine	Associated with low birth weight	
Azelastine	Associated with minor adverse effects on fetal animals; absorbed systematically with sedative effects	Intranasal steroids preferred over intranasal antihistamines
Corticosteroids		
Oral	Increased risk of cleft lip with or without cleft palate during TR1	
Intranasal		
Budesonide		Preferred agent, more extensive safety data is available for pregnant patients
Fluticasone, mometasone	Increased risk of orofacial, neural tube defects, congenital malformations, premature birth, low birth weight during TR1	
Triamcinolone	Increased risk of respiratory system defects, cleft palate abnormalities on fetal animals	
Decongestants		
Topical agents		
Phenylephrine, naphazoline, tetrahydrozoline, oxymetazoline Xylometazoline	Absorbed systemically after topical use	Topical agents are preferred over systematic agents during TR1, however women should be cautioned regarding rebound effects during pregnancy

(continued on next page)

Table 4 (continued)		
Class	**Adverse Effects**	**Notes**
Oral		
Pseudoephedrine	Risk of gastroschisis, small intestinal atresia during TR1	Recommend use sparingly (<3 day course) after TR1
Cromolyn Sodium		Safe in pregnancy per AAAAI
Antibiotics		
First-line		
Amoxicillin, amoxicillin-clavulanic acid		Increased doses recommended in pregnancy due to decreased serum levels, safe for use through all trimesters
B-lactam allergy		
Azithromycin TMP-SMX Clarithromycin	Risk of neural tube, cleft palate, cardiac, urinary defects in TR1 Increased risk of miscarriage	Preferred for use in patients with B-lactam allergy

Acronyms: AAAAI, American Academy of Allergy, Asthma, Immunology; ACOG, American College of Obstetricians and Gynecologists; TMP-SMX, trimethoprim-sulfamethoxazole; TR1, trimester 1.

Lamotrigine may be used in pregnancy and breastfeeding as it has not been associated with adverse fetal or infant outcomes. However, other antiepileptics such as valproate, topiramate, and gabapentin should be generally avoided during pregnancy and breastfeeding.[4] Verapamil is the first-line treatment for CH prophylaxis in pregnant and breastfeeding women.

Peripheral nerve blocks, preferably with lidocaine, may be used for the treatment of primary headaches and are generally considered safe in pregnancy and breastfeeding because of their local effect.[4]

Treatment of Rhinitis and Sinusitis

First-line treatment of rhinitis in pregnancy should focus on nasal saline rinses and first-line antihistamines, which are considered safer than second-generation antihistamines and topical decongestants in pregnancy (**Table 4**).[16,17] Although previous FDA safety data regarding intranasal corticosteroids suggest that budesonide is safer in pregnancy than other intranasal corticosteroids, more recent reviews suggest that beclomethasone, budesonide, fluticasone, and mometasone are safe for use in pregnancy.[28,29]

The drugs of choice for treating bacterial sinusitis in pregnancy are ampicillin or amoxicillin. For pregnant women with β-lactam allergies, azithromycin is preferred over trimethoprim-sulfamethoxazole, clarithromycin, or fluoroquinolones because of its relative safety in pregnancy (see Table 4).

SECONDARY HEADACHES OF VASCULAR ETIOLOGY: CLINICAL PRESENTATION, DIAGNOSTICS, AND TREATMENT

Pregnancy is associated with hypercoagulability, which increases the risk of vascular causes of headaches. Pregnant patients presenting with headaches should be

Table 5
Clinical presentation in the diagnosis of secondary headache disorders in pregnant women

Clinical Presentation	Differential Diagnosis	Initial Diagnostics
Relapsing thunderclap headaches	RCVS Primary cerebral vasculitis	CT or diagnostic angiogram, MRI, LP CT or diagnostic angiogram, MRI, LP
Single thunderclap headache	Aneurysmal subarachnoid hemorrhage RCVS CVT Pituitary apoplexy Cervical artery dissection	CTH without contrast CT or diagnostic angiogram, MRI, CSF MRV or CTV MRI CTA or MRA
Hypertension	Preeclampsia/eclampsia PRES RCVS	Blood pressure, ophthalmoscopy, urine protein MRI/MRA/CT CT or diagnostic angiogram, MRI, LP
Visual loss	Preeclampsia/eclampsia PRES Pituitary apoplexy IIH CVT	Blood pressure, ophthalmoscopy, urine protein MRI/MRA/CT MRI Ophthalmoscopy, MRI, LP MRV
Seizures	Eclampsia CVT PRES RCVS	Blood pressure, ophthalmoscopy, urine protein MRV MRI/MRA/CT CT or diagnostic angiogram, MRI, LP
Horner syndrome	Cervical artery dissection	CTA or MRA
Papilledema	CVT IIH Space-occupying lesion	MRV ophthalmoscopy, MRI, LP MRI or CTH without contrast
Focal neurologic deficits	Ischemic stroke Intracranial hemorrhage CVT PRES RCVS	CTH without contrast CTH without contrast MRV MRI/MRA/CT CT or diagnostic angiogram, MRI, LP

Abbreviations: CSF, cerebrospinal fluid; IIH, idiopathic intracranial hypertension; MRA, magnetic resonance angiography; PRES, posterior reversible encephalopathy syndrome; RCVS, reversible cerebral vasoconstriction syndrome; LP, lumbar puncture; CTH, computed tomography of the head; MRV, magnetic resonance venography; CTV, computed tomography venography; CTA, computed tomography andgiography

Data from Anderson A, Singh J, Bove R. Neuroimaging and radiation exposure in pregnancy. In: Handbook of Clinical Neurology. ; 2020. https://doi.org/10.1016/B978-0-444-64239-4.00009-6 and Martin SR, Foley MR. Approach to the Pregnant Patient With Headache. Clin Obstet Gynecol. 2005;48(1). https://doi.org/10.1097/01.grf.0000153208.93620.39.

evaluated for "red flag symptoms" (Table 1) to avoid missing life-threatening causes of secondary headaches (**Table 5**).

The mainstay of diagnostics for secondary headaches relies on imaging, including CT and MRI. Although intravenous contrast agents for CT and MRI are used to provide a better structural definition for assessing abnormalities, noncontrast studies are generally preferred in pregnant patients because of the risk of exposure to the infant. MRI is preferred over CT for its structural resolution and diminished radiation to the fetus. CT of the head exposes a limited amount of radiation to the fetus, but shielding is still recommended. If indicated, arterial studies with iodinated contrast (CT) or gadolinium (MRI) may be performed if the clinical suspicion for vascular-associated secondary headache is high.[30] Highlighted below are "do not miss" diagnoses for causes of secondary headache in pregnancy.

Preeclampsia and Eclampsia

Headaches are often a herald sign of preeclampsia, occurring in 5% of pregnancies.[14] Women who develop headaches between the 20th week of pregnancy and the postpartum period should be evaluated for preeclampsia, which is diagnosed in patients with hypertension and signs of end-organ damage, most commonly proteinuria in the early stages. Eclampsia occurs when preeclampsia progresses to cause seizures. Headaches associated with these conditions are often diffuse, pulsating, aggravated by physical activity, and refractory to over-the-counter remedies. They may be associated with visual changes similar to an aura.[2] Definitive treatment of preeclampsia is delivery of the fetus, while antihypertensives and magnesium sulfate are used as adjunctive measures.

Posterior Reversible Encephalopathy Syndrome

Insidious onset of dull bilateral occipital headache, associated visual changes (scotomas, diplopia, blurry vision, hemianopia), and altered mental status should raise suspicion for increased cerebral posterior reversible encephalopathy syndrome (PRES).[31] It is often associated with hypertension or preeclampsia and may be concurrent with reversible cerebral vasoconstriction syndrome (RCVS). MRI/magnetic resonance angiography (MRA)/CT imaging is significant for multilobar/hemispheric edema, often involving the parietal and occipital lobes. Treatment includes magnesium, antihypertensives, and treatment for concurrent preeclampsia/eclampsia.

Cerebrovascular Accidents (Hemorrhagic or Ischemic Stroke)

Cerebrovascular accidents (CVAs) are the sixth leading cause of maternal death in the United States, accounting for 4.7% of maternal deaths.[32] Headaches associated with CVAs are bilateral or ipsilateral to the stroke, tension-like, and typically accompanied by focal neurologic signs and/or alterations in consciousness.[33] Headache alone rarely presents as a sole symptom of CVAs, and diagnostics can be made with noncontrast CT. Management of ischemic stroke in the pregnant patient focuses on thrombolysis versus mechanical thrombectomy, whereas management of hemorrhagic stroke focuses on prevention of rebleeding and expansion of hematoma.[34]

Subarachnoid Hemorrhage

Headache is a prominent symptom of subarachnoid hemorrhage (SAH), typically described as thunderclap headaches with a sudden, severe intensity that peaks in seconds to minutes and is followed by vomiting and loss of consciousness.[35] These headaches are sudden in onset and may be distinguished from primary thunderclap headaches, which may be associated with physical exercise or sexual activity. Noncontrast CT is used as the imaging modality of choice for diagnosis of SAH; however, if negative or equivocal, lumbar puncture can be used to analyze for xanthochromia.

Cerebral Venous Thrombosis

CVT is a rare disease that complicates an estimated 0.004% to 0.01% of pregnancies. CVT causes about 2% of pregnancy-associated strokes, with increasing incidence during the third trimester and puerperium.[36] Headache is present in 80% to 90% of cases and has no specific signs. Often headaches associated with CVT can be diffuse, progressive, and severe, but can also be unilateral and acute, or migraine-like. Focal neurologic signs (neurologic deficits or seizures) and/or signs of increased intracranial pressure (nausea, papilledema) may be present.[37] CVT can be diagnosed on MR venography, which is preferred over CT venography. Anticoagulation is the therapeutic modality of choice.

Arterial Dissection

Cervicocephalic dissections in pregnancy are rare causes of intracranial hemorrhage, including subarachnoid or intracerebral hemorrhage, and may be associated with pre-eclampsia[38] or hypertensive disorders of pregnancy.[39] Headaches associated with arterial dissection may be associated with nausea, vomiting, and neurologic deficits, including Horner syndrome, tinnitus, or hypoglossal nerve palsy. Arterial dissection is diagnosed with MRA or CTA of the head and neck, and treatment consists of antithrombotics, thrombolysis, or endovascular therapy.[40]

Reversible Cerebral Vasoconstriction Syndrome and Cerebral Vasculitis

Headaches caused by RCVS are often recurring severe, diffuse thunderclap headaches that are triggered by physical or sexual activity, Valsalva, or emotion.[41] These headaches may be associated with fluctuating neurologic deficits and are usually self-limited and relapse in days to weeks. In rare cases, RCVS may be complicated by ischemic or hemorrhagic strokes. It may also occur concurrently with PRES.

Another clinical entity that must be ruled out in the diagnosis of RCVS is primary cerebral vasculitis, which presents with subacute to chronic dull, aching headache. Both RCVS and primary cerebral vasculitis have similar imaging features on neurovascular imaging, with multifocal narrowing of the cerebral vasculature. Unlike the normal brain parenchyma visualized on CT or MRI imaging with RCVS, primary cerebral vasculitis is characterized by irreversible microangiopathic changes of the grey- or white matter.[41] Treatment for RCVS has been poorly studied, including calcium-channel blockers, glucocorticoids, magnesium sulfate, or observation. Unlike RCVS, immunosuppression is a primary treatment for primary cerebral vasculitis.

Idiopathic Intracranial Hypertension

Headaches associated with visual changes and nausea that worsen with the Valsalva maneuver should raise suspicion for idiopathic intracranial hypertension (IIH), especially in pregnant women with elevated body mass index.[42,43] Visual changes may progress from unnoticed peripheral vision loss to obscuration of vision. As a result, patients may not present until advanced disease, leading to delayed presentation and irreversible vision loss. Patients who present with symptoms of IIH should be expeditiously assessed by ophthalmoscopy for papilledema. If confirmed, secondary causes of intracranial hypertension should be excluded with neuroimaging to rule out space-occupying lesions or CVT, which can cause secondary intracranial hypertension.[42] A lumbar puncture should also be performed to evaluate cerebrospinal fluid (CSF) opening pressure and to rule out meningitis or malignancy. A lumbar puncture can also be therapeutic. Conservative management includes weight management and dietary modification, and treatment with a carbonic anhydrase inhibitor, acetazolamide, is the mainstay of medical management of IIH.[44] CSF diversion with lumboperitoneal shunts or ventriculoperitoneal shunts are reserved for cases refractory to medical therapy.[44]

Pituitary Apoplexy

Pituitary apoplexy is a rare endocrinologic emergency that presents with sudden onset retro-orbital headache, nausea, vomiting with visual changes including visual field defects or cranial nerve palsies, and hypopituitarism.[45] Pituitary apoplexy can be associated with pituitary tumors or physiologic enlargement during pregnancy secondary to hyperplasia and hypertrophy of lactotroph cells by estrogen. Enlargement of the pituitary gland increases intracapsular pressure in the sella turcica, which can lead to infarction or hemorrhage of the pituitary gland.[46,47] MRI is the diagnostic modality of choice to confirm pituitary apoplexy. Initial treatment consists of stabilization with preservation of electrolyte and fluid balance and replacement of deficient hormones. Conservative management with dopamine agonists such as bromocriptine or cabergoline can be used for prolactin-secreting pituitary adenomas. Surgical decompression is preferred for patients with severe neuro-ophthalmic signs.[45]

SUMMARY

Headache is a common complaint in the general population and pregnancy. Similar to the general population, migraine constitutes the majority of headaches in pregnant women. Increased hypercoagulability, hemodynamic changes, and hormonal changes in pregnancy place the pregnant patient at risk of life-threatening causes of secondary headaches, which require urgent evaluation. Care should be taken to assess the risks and benefits of pharmacologic treatment of headache in pregnancy, as many medications can cause adverse effects to the fetus and mother.

CLINICS CARE POINTS

- The majority of headaches in pregnancy are migraine or tension type headaches.
- Migraine headaches place women at greater risk of vascular events during pregnancy.
- Consideration of red flag symptoms is critical when evaluating pregnant women presenting with headaches.
- Pregnant women with suspected secondary headaches due to a vascular or neoplastic etiology should be evaluated promptly with the appropriate diagnostic workup.
- Nonpharmacologic treatments are preferred in the treatment of primary headaches and secondary headaches such as sinus headaches or temporomandibular joint disorder.
- If nonpharmacologic treatments are insufficient, the selection of pharmacologic treatments should be made with attention to possible adverse effects to the pregnancy and fetus.

DISCLOSURE

The authors have nothing to disclose.

REFERENCES

1. Organization WH. Headache Disorders. 2016. Available at: https://www.who.int/news-room/fact-sheets/detail/headache-disorders. Accessed October 5, 2021.
2. Olesen J. Headache Classification Committee of the International Headache Society (IHS) The International Classification of Headache Disorders, 3rd edition. Cephalalgia 2018;38(1):1–211.

3. James SL, Abate D, Abate KH, et al. Global, regional, and national incidence, prevalence, and years lived with disability for 354 Diseases and Injuries for 195 countries and territories, 1990-2017: A systematic analysis for the Global Burden of Disease Study 2017. Lancet 2018. https://doi.org/10.1016/S0140-6736(18) 32279-7.

4. Negro A, Delaruelle Z, Ivanova TA, et al. Headache and pregnancy: a systematic review. J Headache Pain 2017;18(1). https://doi.org/10.1186/s10194-017-0816-0.

5. Burch R. Headache in Pregnancy and the Puerperium. Neurol Clin 2019;37(1): 31–51.

6. MacGregor EA. Headache in Pregnancy. Neurol Clin 2012;30(3):835–66.

7. Sances G, Granella F, Nappi RE, et al. Course of migraine during pregnancy and postpartum: A prospective study. Cephalalgia 2003;23(3):197–205.

8. Allais G, Chiarle G, Sinigaglia S, et al. Migraine during pregnancy and in the puerperium. Neurol Sci 2019;40. https://doi.org/10.1007/s10072-019-03792-9.

9. MacGregor EA. Migraine in pregnancy and lactation. Neurol Sci 2014;35(SUPPL. 1):83–93.

10. Kvisvik EV, Stovner LJ, Helde G, et al. Headache and migraine during pregnancy and puerperium: The MIGRA-study. J Headache Pain 2011. https://doi.org/10. 1007/s10194-011-0329-1.

11. Hoshiyama E, Tatsumoto M, Iwanami H, et al. Postpartum migraines: A long-term prospective study. Intern Med 2012. https://doi.org/10.2169/internalmedicine.51. 8542.

12. Schürks M, Rist PM, Bigal ME, et al. Migraine and cardiovascular disease: Systematic review and meta-analysis. BMJ 2009. https://doi.org/10.1136/bmj.b3914.

13. Maggioni F, Alessi C, Maggino T, et al. Headache during pregnancy. Cephalalgia 1997. https://doi.org/10.1046/j.1468-2982.1997.1707765.x.

14. Christy F P, Wendy F H. Headache and neurological disease in pregnancy. Clin Obstet Gynecol 2012;55(3):810–28. https://doi.org/10.1097/GRF. 0b013e31825d7b68.

15. Van Vliet JA, Favier I, Helmerhorst FM, et al. Cluster headache in women: Relation with menstruation, use of oral contraceptives, pregnancy, and menopause. J Neurol Neurosurg Psychiatry 2006. https://doi.org/10.1136/jnnp.2005.081158.

16. Lal D, Jategaonkar AA, Borish L, et al. Management of rhinosinusitis during pregnancy: systematic review and expert panel recommendations. Rhinol J 2016; 54(2). https://doi.org/10.4193/Rhino15.228.

17. Incaudo GA. Diagnosis and Treatment of Allergic Rhinitis and Sinusitis During Pregnancy and Lactation. Clin Rev Allergy Immunol 2004;27(2). https://doi.org/ 10.1385/CRIAI:27:2:159.

18. Warren MP, Fried JL. Temporomandibular Disorders and Hormones in Women. Cells Tissues Organs 2001;169(3). https://doi.org/10.1159/000047881.

19. Robinson JL, Johnson PM, Kister K, et al. Estrogen signaling impacts temporomandibular joint and periodontal disease pathology. Odontology 2020;108(2). https://doi.org/10.1007/s10266-019-00439-1.

20. Fichera G, Polizzi A, Scapellato S, et al. Craniomandibular Disorders in Pregnant Women: An Epidemiological Survey. J Funct Morphol Kinesiol 2020;5(2). https:// doi.org/10.3390/jfmk5020036.

21. LeResche L, Sherman JJ, Huggins K, et al. Musculoskeletal orofacial pain and other signs and symptoms of temporomandibular disorders during pregnancy: a prospective study. J Orofac Pain 2005;19(3).

22. Wells RE, Turner DP, Lee M, et al. Managing Migraine During Pregnancy and Lactation. Curr Neurol Neurosci Rep 2016. https://doi.org/10.1007/s11910-016-0634-9.

23. Airola G, Allais G, Gabellari IC, et al. Non-pharmacological management of migraine during pregnancy. Neurol Sci 2010. https://doi.org/10.1007/s10072-010-0276-7.

24. Calhoun AH, Peterlin BL. Treatment of cluster headache in pregnancy and lactation. Curr Pain Headache Rep 2010. https://doi.org/10.1007/s11916-010-0102-1.

25. Tepper D. Pregnancy and lactation - Migraine management. Headache 2015. https://doi.org/10.1111/head.12540.

26. Gauer RL, Semidey MJ. Diagnosis and treatment of temporomandibular disorders. Am Fam Physician 2015;91(6).

27. Liew Z, Ritz B, Rebordosa C, et al. Acetaminophen use during pregnancy, behavioral problems, and hyperkinetic disorders. JAMA Pediatr 2014. https://doi.org/10.1001/jamapediatrics.2013.4914.

28. Alhussien AH, Alhedaithy RA, Alsaleh SA. Safety of intranasal corticosteroid sprays during pregnancy: an updated review. Eur Arch Oto-rhino-laryngology 2018;275(2). https://doi.org/10.1007/s00405-017-4785-3.

29. Ellegard EK, Hellgren M, Karlsson NG. Fluticasone propionate aqueous nasal spray in pregnancy rhinitis. Clin Otolaryngol Allied Sci 2001;26(5). https://doi.org/10.1046/j.1365-2273.2001.00491.x.

30. Anderson A, Singh J, Bove R. Neuroimaging and radiation exposure in pregnancy. In: Handbook of clinical Neurology. 2020. https://doi.org/10.1016/B978-0-444-64239-4.00009-6.

31. Brewer J, Owens MY, Wallace K, et al. Posterior reversible encephalopathy syndrome in 46 of 47 patients with eclampsia. Am J Obstet Gynecol 2013;208(6). https://doi.org/10.1016/j.ajog.2013.02.015.

32. Berg CJ, Callaghan WM, Syverson C, et al. Pregnancy-Related Mortality in the United States, 1998 to 2005. Obstet Gynecol 2010;116(6). https://doi.org/10.1097/AOG.0b013e3181fdfb11.

33. Verdelho A, Ferro JM, Melo T, et al. Headache in Acute Stroke. A Prospective Study in the First 8 Days. Cephalalgia 2008;28(4). https://doi.org/10.1111/j.1468-2982.2007.01514.x.

34. Zambrano MD, Miller EC. Maternal Stroke: an Update. Curr Atheroscler Rep 2019;21(9). https://doi.org/10.1007/s11883-019-0798-2.

35. Linn FHH, Rinkel GJE, Algra A, et al. Headache characteristics in subarachnoid haemorrhage and benign thunderclap headache. J Neurol Neurosurg Psychiatry 1998;65(5). https://doi.org/10.1136/jnnp.65.5.791.

36. Saposnik G, Barinagarrementeria F, Brown RD, et al. Diagnosis and Management of Cerebral Venous Thrombosis. Stroke 2011;42(4). https://doi.org/10.1161/STR.0b013e31820a8364.

37. Kashkoush AI, Ma H, Agarwal N, et al. Cerebral venous sinus thrombosis in pregnancy and puerperium: A pooled, systematic review. J Clin Neurosci 2017;39:9–15. https://doi.org/10.1016/J.JOCN.2017.02.046.

38. Manasewitsch NT, Hanfy AA, Beutler BD, et al. Postpartum vertebral artery dissection: case report and review of the literature. Thromb J 2020;18(1). https://doi.org/10.1186/s12959-020-00243-w.

39. Shanmugalingam R, Reza Pour N, Chuah SC, et al. Vertebral artery dissection in hypertensive disorders of pregnancy: a case series and literature review. BMC Pregnancy Childbirth 2016;16(1). https://doi.org/10.1186/s12884-016-0953-5.

40. Peng J, Liu Z, Luo C, et al. Treatment of Cervical Artery Dissection: Antithrombotics, Thrombolysis, and Endovascular Therapy. Biomed Res Int 2017;2017. https://doi.org/10.1155/2017/3072098.

41. Calabrese LH, Dodick DW, Schwedt TJ, et al. Narrative Review: Reversible Cerebral Vasoconstriction Syndromes. Ann Intern Med 2007;146(1). https://doi.org/10.7326/0003-4819-146-1-200701020-00007.

42. Park DSJ, Park JSY, Sharma S, et al. Idiopathic Intracranial Hypertension in Pregnancy. J Obstet Gynaecol Can 2021. https://doi.org/10.1016/j.jogc.2020.12.019.

43. KESLER A, KUPFERMINC M. Idiopathic Intracranial Hypertension and Pregnancy. Clin Obstet Gynecol 2013;56(2). https://doi.org/10.1097/GRF.0b013e31828f2701.

44. Tang RA, Dorotheo EU, Schiffman JS, et al. Medical and surgical management of idiopathic intracranial hypertension in pregnancy. Curr Neurol Neurosci Rep 2004;4(5). https://doi.org/10.1007/s11910-004-0087-4.

45. Piantanida E, Gallo D, Lombardi V, et al. Pituitary apoplexy during pregnancy: a rare, but dangerous headache. J Endocrinol Invest 2014;37(9). https://doi.org/10.1007/s40618-014-0095-4.

46. Grand' S, Weber F, Bédard MJ, et al. Pituitary apoplexy in pregnancy: A case series and literature review. Obstet Med 2015. https://doi.org/10.1177/1753495X15598917.

47. Martin SR, Foley MR. Approach to the Pregnant Patient With Headache. Clin Obstet Gynecol 2005;48(1). https://doi.org/10.1097/01.grf.0000153208.93620.39.

Nummular and Side-locked Headaches for the Otolaryngologist

Sheng Zhou, MD[a,*], Ido Badash, MD[a], Joni K. Doherty, MD, PhD[b]

KEYWORDS

• Nummular • Side-locked • Headaches • Hemifacial pain

KEY POINTS

- Nummular headache is a primary headache that presents as a coin-shaped area of pain that does not change location.
- Side-locked headaches are unilateral secondary headaches that have a wide-ranging differential including neuralgias, trigeminal autonomic cephalgias, ophthalmologic disorders, otolaryngologic disorders, and vascular disorders.
- Loss of cranial nerves in the setting of nummular or side-locked headache is a red flag symptom that warrants further workup for cervical artery dissection, skull base osteomyelitis, or malignancy.
- Vision changes concurrent with nummular or side-locked headache necessitates further evaluation of changes in visual acuity and may represent an ophthalmic emergency.
- Otolaryngologists are centrally positioned to assist in assessing patients with nummular or side-locked headaches for therapeutic consideration or referral to other subspecialists.

INTRODUCTION

Side-locked and nummular headaches are named based on the size and distribution of the headaches. Side-locked headaches refer to unilateral headaches that do not shift sides; they are a symptomatic description that is used to aid in diagnosis. Nummular headaches refer to the size of a headache and were first described by Pareja and colleagues[1] in 2002. In contrast to side-locked headaches, they are considered a primary headache. According to the international classification of headache disorders, nummular headaches are sharply contoured, fixed in size and shape, and roughly 1 to 6 cm in size.[2]

[a] LAC+USC Medical Center Otolaryngology Department, 1200 North State Street, Suite A2E, Los Angeles, CA 90033, USA; [b] USC Caruso Department of Otolaryngology Head and Neck Surgery, 1450 San Pablo Street #5100, Los Angeles, CA 90033, USA
* Corresponding author.
E-mail address: sheng.Zhou@med.usc.edu

Otolaryngol Clin N Am 55 (2022) 697–706
https://doi.org/10.1016/j.otc.2022.02.008
0030-6665/22/© 2022 Elsevier Inc. All rights reserved.

Nummular headaches commonly affect the parietal region and can have various qualities of pain. These sensations can include pressurelike sensation or a sharp, stabbing pain. Concurrent with the localized sensation, they may also have perturbation in sensation.[3] True nummular headaches are thought to evolve from a peripheral neuropathy of terminal branches of the scalp.[4] However, the mechanism has not been confirmed in mechanistic studies.

There is relatively little literature regarding the true prevalence of nummular headache. Nummular headache is considered a rare headache, with Pareja and colleagues[5] finding its incidence to be 6.4/100,000/y in their hospital. In the largest published case series of patients with nummular headaches, Guerrero and colleagues[6] found that nummular headache made up 4.6% of all headaches over close to a 4-year time period. The review by Schwartz and colleagues[3] of 250 cases of nummular headache in the literature finds a 1.8:1 female to male ratio with 45.4 years being the average age of onset. Notably, 46.7% of patients with nummular headaches also have other concurrent headaches.

Side-locked headaches affect a far greater proportion of patients. Ramón and colleagues[7] observed that side-locked headaches accounted for ~20% of patients who presented to a headache clinic. Although many of these patients present primarily to a primary care physician or neurologist, they also present to otolaryngology offices. In fact, many primary causes to secondary side-locked headaches have a therapeutic role for otolaryngology. As such, it is important for practicing otolaryngologists to have a broad understanding of the differential for unilateral hemifacial cephalgia in addition to the salient clinical features and workup for these symptoms. This description of side-locked and nummular headaches is focused on a clinically orientated review of their relevant findings for an otolaryngologist.

EVALUATION

An otolaryngologist's examination includes a cranial nerve examination by necessity. In the setting of side-locked and nummular headaches, workup should further include palpation and inspection of the scalp, the pericranial muscles, nerves, and arteries[8]; this is especially important because the review of 250 published cases of nummular headaches by Schwartz and colleagues[3] suggested that 49.7% of patients with nummular headache have concurrent allodynia. Nummular headache can further present with trophic changes. A brief neurologic examination should also be performed focused on gait, muscle tone, and peripheral neurologic deficits. This examination is especially important because the differential for unilateral neuralgias also includes systemic disorders such as multiple sclerosis. Laboratory workup should include complete blood count (CBC), basic metabolic panel (BMP), liver function tests (LFT), thyroid function test (TFT), erythrocyte sedimentation rate (ESR), alkaline phosphatase (ALP), antinuclear antibody (ANA), and rheumatoid factor (RF).. The multitude of laboratory tests is important because patients with nummular and side-locked headaches are found to have a high prevalence of autoimmune disease.[9] Computed tomography (CT) of the head and MRI of the brain should be performed to exclude any structural abnormality.[8] These are discussed further in the differential diagnosis section.

DIFFERENTIAL DIAGNOSIS AND THERAPEUTIC OPTIONS

Nummular headache is considered a primary headache. There is no consensus of treatment. However, primary treatment is often initiated with nonsteroidal antiinflammatory drugs, triptans, gabapentin, or tricyclic antidepressants.[8,10] None of these modalities have been shown to completely resolve patient symptoms. Despite its proposed peripheral etiology, peripheral nerve blocks have not been shown to be successful.[3]

Nummular headaches, however, can also be a secondary headache. The differential diagnosis of side-locked headaches and secondary nummular headache is broad. This breadth creates a challenge in assigning an accurate diagnosis because of the often overlapping symptoms of patients. The discussion focuses on the following categories: neuralgias, trigeminal autonomic cephalgias (TACs), ophthalmologic disorders, otolaryngologic disorders, and vascular disorders. Following elaboration of these categories, there is also a discussion of other rare entities that can mimic nummular headache or cause side-locked headaches.

NEURALGIAS

Neuralgias are an important consideration in the differential diagnosis because they have the potential to cause poorer health status and significantly impair quality of life.[11,12] In the case of trigeminal neuralgia, a retrospective cohort study performed by Zakrezewska and colleagues[13] found that nearly 80% of their 225 patients had been to one specialist center, which did not provide appropriate first-line management.

Neuralgias can be divided into trigeminal and occipital neuralgias. Trigeminal neuralgias can further be divided into specific distributions of pain, which can include supraorbital[14,15] and auriculotemporal neuralgias.[16] In order for a neuralgia to be diagnosed, there needs to be an absence of other neurologic deficits.

When diagnosing neuralgias, it is important to perform a full dental examination and avoid treatment with opioids. Commonly, patients with trigeminal neuralgia often receive dental overtreatment[17–19] and are first treated with opioids[19] as a first-line treatment instead of carbamazepine.

The recognized cranial neuralgias can be differentiated from nummular headache by their distribution; they commonly do not have a round or elliptical boundary consistent with nummular headaches.[4,14,20–22] Instead, their spatial organization presents with severe stabbing pain that is more localized to the distribution of the nerve.[10] These cranial neuralgias further are responsive to anesthetic blockade.[14,22]

There is, however, one peripheral phenomenon that also presents in a well-delineated round or oval shape, epicranial fugax. This entity exists frequently in concert with symptoms of nummular headache. This syndrome presents as a short electrical pain that cannot be attributed to a single epicranial nerve.[23,24] The similarities of this entity to nummular headache further include its propensity to target the same area. However, epicranial fugax tends to radiate posteriorly, whereas nummular headache does not radiate. Epicranial fugax can be one of the causes of side-locked headache because the pain only affects one hemicranium. The pathophysiology for epicranial fugax, like nummular headache, is uncertain. Like nummular headache, it is also thought to be due to peripheral terminal branches of the occipital and trigeminal nerves.[25] The classic radiation of pain, though, is thought to possibly be the result of more central connections between trigeminal and cervical afferents.[26,27] In contrast to nummular headache, gabapentin and lamotrigine have been effective in treating epicranial fugax. Occipital nerve blockages have also been successful.[24,28]

Taken together, neuralgias are an important consideration in the etiology of side-locked headaches. Neuralgias all have key distinguishing characteristics from nummular headaches. Further elaboration regarding neuralgias is performed in the article by Cutri and colleagues' article, "Neuralgia and Atypical Facial, Ear, and Head Pain," in this issue.

TRIGEMINAL AUTONOMIC CEPHALGIAS

Separate from peripheral nerve sensory aberrations is the grouping of unilateral cephalgias known as TACs. Like nummular headache, this is also a grouping of primary headache disorders. According to the International Classification of Headache Disorders, they can be subdivided into cluster headaches, short-lasting unilateral neuralgiform headache attacks (SUNCT), and hemicrania continua.[2] TACs are characterized by unilateral pain in the distribution of the first division of the trigeminal nerve with overwhelming parasympathetic activation.[29] The category of primary headache disorders affects ~0.05% of the population.[30]

Cluster headaches are the most common TAC. Cluster headaches have a male predominance and result in severe unilateral pain lasting for up to 3 hours; they are acutely treated with high-flow oxygen and subcutaneous sumatriptan.[31] Chronic, nonremitting cluster headaches may require daily therapy with calcium channel blockers, lithium, or biologics.[31,32]

SUNCT contrasts with cluster headaches in that its attacks last for seconds to minutes. Also unlike cluster headaches, they can result in repeated exacerbations averaging 59 episodes in a day.[33] SUNCT further differ from nummular headache in their distribution of pain. In contrast to localized pain in nummular headaches, SUNCT like other TACs will radiate often to the orbital and periorbital areas.[11] In cases of SUNCT, first-line treatment consists of lamotrigine, but can also include other anticonvulsants or corticosteroids.[34,35]

Hemicrania continua is differentiated from the previous TACs by its response to indomethacin. Similar to migraines, it can last hours to days with pain intensity far less severe than that of cluster headaches or SUNCT. Hemicrania continua is included in the same family because of functional MRI study showing activation of identical brain structures leading to a disinhibition of the trigeminal autonomic reflex.[36]

OPHTHALMOLOGIC CONSIDERATIONS

Unilateral side-locked pain can also present in the form of ophthalmologic emergencies. In the case of temporal arteritis, patients can often present with sudden-onset unilateral pain focused on the temporal region.[37,38] Similar to nummular headaches, they can have hyperesthesia over the scalp or temporal artery on palpation. Also, similar to the previous discussion of TACs, they can have visual disturbances. However, in TAC, these are commonly parasympathetic symptoms such as increased tearing. In temporal arteritis, diplopia can occur[39] and may precede visual loss.[40]

For an otolaryngologist, temporal arteritis can also be confused with temporomandibular joint disorder. However, this can be distinguished by the onset of pain with mastication. Temporal arteritis commonly presents with jaw claudication meaning that the pain sets in only after repetitive chewing of food. It is not immediate.[41]

Owing to its nonspecific symptoms, temporal arteritis can be confused for a trigeminal autonomic cephalagia.[42,43] As such, it is important to enquire regarding the quality of the pain and whether there has been an acute change in onset especially in women older than 50 years.[39] Furthermore, it is important to palpate the temporal artery in addition to assessing the scalp or tongue for ischemic changes.[44,45] It is further prudent to obtain urgent laboratory and ophthalmologic consultation. In cases of temporal arteritis, the ESR is often greater than 50/h and the C-reactive protein (CRP) is greater than 50 mg/L.[46] The gold standard of diagnosis is temporal artery biopsy.[47]

Another consideration for acute visual changes and side-locked headache is acute angle-closure glaucoma. In this case, patients will commonly present with photophobia, nausea, and vomiting. The presentation can mimic that of a migraine. However, acute angle-closure glaucoma can present with worsening visual acuity in contrast to classic migrainous presentations. Acute angle-closure glaucoma further will have an unresponsive middilated pupil with a firm eyeball on palpation, and intraorbital pressures should be measured by an ophthalmologist.[48]

OTOLARYNGOLOGY CONSIDERATIONS

Focusing on secondary side-locked headaches, they can also arise from many conditions that commonly present at an otolaryngologist's office; these can commonly be divided by anatomic site. From an otologic standpoint, acute otitis externa and acute otitis media can cause side-locked headaches. These conditions typically do not get confused for nummular headaches because they will not result in a coin-shaped pain distribution. Instead, they are localized to the ear canal or external ear with possible radiation to the mastoid area in the case of acute otitis media.

In cases of more diffuse, radiating headache, it is also important to consider skull base osteomyelitis,[49] which is particularly important in diabetic or immunocompromised patients with persistent headache and/or unilateral otalgia, for which imaging workup should be initiated even in the absence of otologic sequelae or cranial nerve deficits.[50] Cranial neuropathies tend to only occur in advanced disease.[51]

Another consideration of unilateral side-locked headache and otalgia is temporomandibular joint disorder. This disorder can present with concurrent worsening with mastication and/or feelings of malocclusion.[52–54] Furthermore, it can worsen headache severity and often presents concurrently with a unilateral headache.[53,55–57] Further elaboration of the salient features in this consideration is done by Garcia and colleagues' article, "Temporomandibular Joint Syndrome from an Ear versus Dental-Related Standpoint," in this issue.

Aside from otologic and mandibular causes, Eagle syndrome is also an important consideration that can be confounded with neuralgia, migraine, and temporomandibular joint disorder.[58,59] Eagle syndrome commonly presents with dysphagia and continuous pain in the temporal or retromandibular area worsened by mastication.[60,61] Workup with CT imaging is the most useful tool in diagnosis.[62–64] Nonsurgical treatment can be offered with steroid injection, analgesic medication, and anticonvulsants.[64] Surgical treatment involving styloidectomy can also be pursued.[65] Other aberrations in skull architecture that can also result in side-locked headache include craniosynostosis,[66] Paget disease,[39,67] and fibrous dysplasia.[68]

Side-locked headaches that present further anteriorly should raise suspicion for sinus disease or migraine. This pain often worsens with barometric or pressure changes.[69] Depending on the time course of the headache, they can either be classified as acute or chronic rhinosinusitis. Acute rhinosinusitis commonly resolves with medical management.[70] Chronic rhinosinusitis requires further workup that is beyond the scope of this article. Sinus headaches are elaborated in greater detail in Henna D. Murthy and Sarah E. Mowry's article, "The Role of the Otolaryngologist in the Evaluation and Management of Headache" and Nathalia Velasquez and John M. Del-Gaudio's article, "The Role of the Otolaryngologist in the Evaluation and Management of "Sinus Headache"" in this issue.

VASCULAR

Vascular causes of side-locked headache represent an important consideration in nummular and side-locked headache. As previously mentioned regarding evaluation, careful palpation and localization of the pain is important to diagnosis, and this is especially important in cases of superficial fusiform aneurysms that have been demonstrated to be a secondary cause of nummular headache.[71] This is a particularly relevant consideration in patients with Marfan syndrome in which fibrillin-1 coding defects can result in predisposition to fusiform aneurysms.[72]

In the case of acute and persistent side-locked headache in the setting of Horner syndrome, it is important to consider cervical artery dissection.[73,74] In this setting, it is crucial to enquire about a history of neck trauma or cervical manipulation. Initial evaluation is often performed with a CT angiography, but MRI will most accurately identify a mural hematoma.[75]

OTHER CONSIDERATIONS

In addition to all the previous primary disorders mentioned, there are 2 major body systems that are worth considering: central nervous system and dermatologic. Central nervous system causes of side-locked or nummular headache will often be noted on imaging. Important disorders to consider include meningiomas or arachnoid cysts.

Dermatologic phenomenon that may result in nummular headache include Langerhans cell histiocytosis,[76] nummular dermatitis,[77] and trichodynia.[78] In the case of Langerhans cell histiocytosis, complete excision of the lesion was found to resolve the nummular headache. Nummular eczema presents as a coin-shaped lesion with well-defined borders. Finally, trichodynia is known as "burning scalp syndrome" and often presents with alopecia.[79,80] The mechanism is unknown but thought to be the result of depression, stress, anxiety, and autoimmune disorders.[81] Dermatologic lesions found in the setting of side-locked or nummular headache warrant biopsy for further workup.[82]

Finally, malignancy is always a differential in head and neck pain. In the case of side-locked headache, lung malignancy is an occult yet important diagnosis. In this case, referred pain often is confused with temporal arteritis, hemicrania continua, or other primary headaches.[74,83] The triad of smoking history, elevated ESR, and periauricular pain has been suggested to indicate possible lung carcinoma.[83]

RED FLAGS

Red flag findings have been previously discussed in the preceding article. Relevant to nummular and side-locked headaches are findings of acute initiation of pain in the setting of cranial neuropathies. Of the many disorders mentioned, temporal arteritis, acute angle-closure glaucoma, and cervical dissection are the most emergent. These disorders all present with vision changes and acute onset of pain. Furthermore, they have distinct characteristics in their history as previously described.

SUMMARY

Taken in concert, unilateral headache can have many different causes. Although nummular headache is a primary headache, side-locked headache is the result of many secondary diagnoses. Otolaryngologists are uniquely positioned to address many of the therapeutic considerations behind side-locked headache. Furthermore, a careful otolaryngology examination of the patient may help expedite accurate diagnosis for this pervasive patient population.

CLINICS CARE POINTS

- Vascular and ophthalmologic disorders represent the red flag diagnoses of side-locked headache; they require careful assessment of changes in vision and sudden cranial nerve deficits.

- Temporal arteritis can masquerade as temporomandibular joint disorder and requires an astute clinician to palpate the temporal region and assess for any diplopia.
- The presence of nummular or side-locked headache may not indicate a primary headache disorder and requires further workup to determine an otolaryngologist's therapeutic role.

DISCLOSURES

The authors have nothing to disclose.

REFERENCES

1. Pareja JA, Caminero AB, Serra J, et al. Nummular headache: a coin-shaped cephalgia. Neurology 2002;58(11):1678–9.
2. Headache classification committee of the international headache society (IHS) the international classification of headache disorders. 3rd edition. Cephalalgia 2018;38(1):1–211.
3. Schwartz DP, Robbins MS, Grosberg BM. Nummular headache update. Curr Pain Headache Rep 2013;17(6):340.
4. Pareja JA, Montojo T, Alvarez M. Nummular headache update. Curr Neurol Neurosci Rep 2012;12(2):118–24.
5. Pareja JA, Pareja J, Barriga FJ, et al. Nummular headache: a prospective series of 14 new cases. Headache 2004;44(6):611–4.
6. Guerrero ÁL, Cortijo E, Herrero-Velázquez S, et al. Nummular headache with and without exacerbations: comparative characteristics in a series of 72 patients. Cephalalgia 2012;32(8):649–53.
7. Ramón C, Mauri G, Vega J, et al. Diagnostic distribution of 100 unilateral, side-locked headaches consulting a specialized clinic. Eur Neurol 2013;69(5):289–91.
8. Grosberg BM, Solomon S, Lipton RB. Nummular headache. Curr Pain Headache Rep 2007;11(4):310–2.
9. Chen W-H, Chen Y-T, Lin C-S, et al. A high prevalence of autoimmune indices and disorders in primary nummular headache. J Neurol Sci 2012;320(1–2):127–30.
10. Wilhour D, Ceriani CEJ, Nahas SJ. Nummular headache. Curr Neurol Neurosci Rep 2019;19(6):26.
11. Melek LN, Devine M, Renton T. The psychosocial impact of orofacial pain in trigeminal neuralgia patients: a systematic review. Int J Oral Maxillofac Surg 2018;47(7):869–78.
12. Zakrzewska JM, Wu N, Lee JYK, et al. Characterizing treatment utilization patterns for trigeminal neuralgia in the United States. Clin J Pain 2018;34(8):691–9.
13. Zakrzewska JM, Wu J, Mon-Williams M, et al. Evaluating the impact of trigeminal neuralgia. Pain 2017;158(6):1166–74.
14. Pareja JA, Caminero AB. Supraorbital neuralgia. Curr Pain Headache Rep 2006; 10(4):302–5.
15. Mulero P, Guerrero ÁL, Pedraza M, et al. Non-traumatic supraorbital neuralgia: a clinical study of 13 cases. Cephalalgia 2012;32(15):1150–3.
16. Ruiz M, Porta-Etessam J, Garcia-Ptacek S, et al. Auriculotemporal neuralgia: eight new cases report: table 1. Pain Med 2016;17(9):1744–8.
17. von Eckardstein KL, Keil M, Rohde V. Unnecessary dental procedures as a consequence of trigeminal neuralgia. Neurosurg Rev 2015;38(2):355–60.
18. Tripathi M, Sadashiva N, Gupta A, et al. Please spare my teeth! dental procedures and trigeminal neuralgia. Surg Neurol Int 2020;11:455.

19. Antonaci F, Arceri S, Rakusa M, et al. Pitfalls in recognition and management of trigeminal neuralgia. J Headache Pain 2020;21(1):82.

20. Sjaastad O, Pareja JA, Zukerman E, et al. Trigeminal neuralgia. clinical manifestations of first division involvement. Headache J Head Face Pain 1997;37(6): 346–57.

21. Pareja J, Cuadrado M, Caminero A, et al. Duration of attacks of first division trigeminal neuralgia. Cephalalgia 2005;25(4):305–8.

22. Cuadrado ML, López-Ruiz P, Guerrero ÁL. Nummular headache: an update and future prospects. Expert Rev Neurother 2018;18(1):9–19.

23. Cuadrado ML, Guerrero AL, Pareja JA. Epicrania Fugax. Curr Pain Headache Rep 2016;20(4):21.

24. Pareja JA, Cuadrado ML, Fernández-de-las-Peñas C, et al. Epicrania fugax: an ultrabrief paroxysmal epicranial pain. Cephalalgia 2008;28(3):257–63.

25. McMahon SB, editor. Wall and Melzack's textbook of pain. 6th edition. Elsevier/Saunders; 2013.

26. Bartsch T, Goadsby PJ. The trigeminocervical complex and migraine: current concepts and synthesis. Curr Pain Headache Rep 2003;7(5):371–6.

27. Kerr FW. Structural relation of the trigeminal spinal tract to upper cervical roots and the solitary nucleus in the cat. Exp Neurol 1961;4:134–48.

28. Cuadrado ML, Ordás CM, Sánchez-Lizcano M, et al. Epicrania fugax: 19 cases of an emerging headache. Headache 2013;53(5):764–74.

29. Robbins MS. Diagnosis and management of headache: a review. JAMA 2021; 325(18):1874.

30. Robbins M, Lipton R. The epidemiology of primary headache disorders. Semin Neurol 2010;30(02):107–19.

31. Robbins MS, Starling AJ, Pringsheim TM, et al. Treatment of cluster headache: the american headache society evidence-based guidelines: headache. Headache J Head Face Pain 2016;56(7):1093–106.

32. Goadsby PJ, Dodick DW, Leone M, et al. Trial of galcanezumab in prevention of episodic cluster headache. N Engl J Med 2019;381(2):132–41.

33. Giani L, Proietti Cecchini A, Leone M. Cluster headache and TACs: state of the art. Neurol Sci 2020;41(S2):367–75.

34. Wei DY, Jensen RH. Therapeutic approaches for the management of trigeminal autonomic cephalalgias. Neurotherapeutics 2018;15(2):346–60.

35. Groenke BR, Daline IH, Nixdorf DR. SUNCT/SUNA: case series presenting in an orofacial pain clinic. Cephalalgia Int J Headache 2021;41(6):665–76.

36. Matharu MS, Cohen AS, McGonigle DJ, et al. Posterior hypothalamic and brainstem activation in hemicrania continua. Headache J Head Face Pain 2004;44(8): 747–61.

37. Pradeep S, Smith JH. Giant cell arteritis: practical pearls and updates. Curr Pain Headache Rep 2018;22(1):2.

38. Ling ML, Yosar J, Lee BW, et al. The diagnosis and management of temporal arteritis. Clin Exp Optom 2020;103(5):572–82.

39. Caselli RJ, Hunder GG, Whisnant JP. Neurologic disease in biopsy-proven giant cell (temporal) arteritis. Neurology 1988;38(3):352.

40. Miller NR. visual manifestations of temporal arteritis. Rheum Dis Clin North Am 2001;27(4):781–97.

41. Smetana GW. Does this patient have temporal arteritis? JAMA 2002;287(1):92.

42. Jimenez-Jimenez FJ, Garcia-Albea E, Zurdo M, et al. Giant cell arteritis presenting as cluster headache. Neurology 1998;51(6):1767–8.

43. Rozen TD. Brief sharp stabs of head pain and giant cell arteritis. Headache J Head Face Pain 2010;50(9):1516–9.

44. Tsianakas A, Ehrchen JM, Presser D, et al. Scalp necrosis in giant cell arteritis: case report and review of the relevance of this cutaneous sign of large-vessel vasculitis. J Am Acad Dermatol 2009;61(4):701–6.

45. Husein-ElAhmed H, Callejas-Rubio J-L, Rios-Fernández R, et al. Tongue infarction as first symptom of temporal arteritis. Rheumatol Int 2012;32(3):799–800.

46. Kermani TA, Schmidt J, Crowson CS, et al. Utility of erythrocyte sedimentation rate and c-reactive protein for the diagnosis of giant cell arteritis. Semin Arthritis Rheum 2012;41(6):866–71.

47. Mahr A. Temporal artery biopsy for diagnosing giant cell arteritis: the longer, the better? Ann Rheum Dis 2006;65(6):826–8.

48. Dietze J, Blair K, Havens SJ. Glaucoma. In: StatPearls. Treasure Island (FL): Stat-Pearls Publishing; 2021. Available at: http://www.ncbi.nlm.nih.gov/books/NBK538217/. Accessed October 2, 2021.

49. van der Valk J, Treurniet F, Koopman JP, et al. Severe daily headache as an uncommon manifestation of widespread skull base osteomyelitis. Case Rep Neurol 2019;11(2):178–82.

50. Muranjan SN, Khadilkar SV, Wagle SC, et al. Central skull base osteomyelitis: diagnostic dilemmas and management issues. Indian J Otolaryngol Head Neck Surg 2016;68(2):149–56.

51. Grobman LR, Ganz W, Casiano R, et al. Atypical osteomyelitis of the skull base. Laryngoscope 1989;99(7):671–6.

52. Scrivani SJ, Keith DA, Kaban LB. Temporomandibular disorders. N Engl J Med 2008;359(25):2693–705.

53. Ballegaard V, Thede-Schmidt-Hansen P, Svensson P, et al. Are headache and temporomandibular disorders related? A blinded study. Cephalalgia 2008; 28(8):832–41.

54. Look JO, Schiffman EL, Truelove EL, et al. Reliability and validity of Axis I of the Research Diagnostic Criteria for Temporomandibular Disorders (RDC/TMD) with proposed revisions*: RELIABILITY AND VALIDITY OF AXIS I OF THE RESEARCH DIAGNOSTIC CRITERIA. J Oral Rehabil 2010;37(10):744–59.

55. Schiffman E, Ohrbach R, Truelove E, et al. Diagnostic criteria for temporomandibular disorders (DC/TMD) for clinical and research applications: recommendations of the international RDC/TMD consortium network* and orofacial pain special interest group†. J Oral Facial Pain Headache 2014;28(1):6–27.

56. Ekberg E, Vallon D, Nilner M. Treatment outcome of headache after occlusal appliance therapy in a randomised controlled trial among patients with temporomandibular disorders of mainly arthrogenous origin. Swed Dent J 2002;26(3): 115–24.

57. Stepan L, Shaw C-KL, Oue S. Temporomandibular disorder in otolaryngology: systematic review. J Laryngol Otol 2017;131(S1):S50–6.

58. Fini G, Gasparini G, Filippini F, et al. The long styloid process syndrome or Eagle's syndrome. J Craniomaxillofac Surg 2000;28(2):123–7.

59. Prasad KC, Kamath MP, Reddy KJM, et al. Elongated styloid process (Eagle's syndrome): a clinical study. J Oral Maxillofac Surg 2002;60(2):171–5.

60. Omami G. Retromandibular pain associated with eagle syndrome. Headache J Head Face Pain 2019;59(6):915–6.

61. Michaud P-L, Gebril M. A prolonged time to diagnosis due to misdiagnoses: a case report of an atypical presentation of eagle syndrome. Am J Case Rep 2021;22.

62. Badhey A, Jategaonkar A, Anglin Kovacs AJ, et al. Eagle syndrome: a comprehensive review. Clin Neurol Neurosurg 2017;159:34–8.

63. Galletta K, Siniscalchi EN, Cicciù M, et al. Eagle syndrome: a wide spectrum of clinical and neuroradiological findings from cervico-facial pain to cerebral ischemia. J Craniofac Surg 2019;30(5):e424–8.

64. Piagkou M, Anagnostopoulou S, Kouladouros K, et al. Eagle's syndrome: a review of the literature. Clin Anat 2009;22(5):545–58.

65. Mortellaro C, Biancucci P, Picciolo G, et al. Eagle's syndrome: importance of a corrected diagnosis and adequate surgical treatment. J Craniofac Surg 2002; 13(6):755–8.

66. López-Mesonero L, Porta-Etessam J, Ordás CM, et al. Nummular Headache in a Patient with Craniosynostosis: One More Evidence for a Peripheral Mechanism. Pain Med 2014;15(4):714–6.

67. Poncelet A. The neurologic complications of paget's disease. J Bone Miner Res 1999;14(S2):88–91.

68. Álvaro L, Garcí J, Areitio E. Nummular headache: a series with symptomatic and primary cases. Cephalalgia 2009;29(3):379–83.

69. Patel ZM, Thamboo A, Rudmik L, et al. Surgical therapy vs continued medical therapy for medically refractory chronic rhinosinusitis: a systematic review and meta-analysis. Int Forum Allergy Rhinol 2017;7(2):119–27.

70. Hu S, Helman S, Filip P, et al. The role of the otolaryngologist in the evaluation and management of headaches. Am J Otolaryngol 2019;40(1):115–20.

71. López-Ruiz P, Cuadrado M-L, Aledo-Serrano A, et al. Superficial artery aneurysms underlying nummular headache–2 cases and proposed diagnostic work-up. Headache 2014;54(7):1217–21.

72. Garcia-Pastor A, Guillem-Mesado A, Salinero-Paniagua J, et al. Fusiform aneurysm of the scalp: an unusual cause of focal headache in marfan syndrome. Headache J Head Face Pain 2002;42(9):908–10.

73. Silbert PL, Mokri B, Schievink WI. Headache and neck pain in spontaneous internal carotid and vertebral artery dissections. Neurology 1995;45(8):1517–22.

74. Prakash S, Rathore C. Side-locked headaches: an algorithm-based approach. J Headache Pain 2016;17(1):95.

75. Engelter ST, Traenka C, Von Hessling A, et al. Diagnosis and treatment of cervical artery dissection. Neurol Clin 2015;33(2):421–41.

76. Silva Rosas C, Angus-Leppan H, Lemp MB, et al. Langerhans cell histiocytosis (eosinophilic granuloma) of the skull mimicking nummular headache. Report of two cases. Cephalalgia 2018;38(4):794–7.

77. Bonamonte D, Foti C, Vestita M, et al. Nummular eczema and contact allergy: a retrospective study. Dermatitis 2012;23(4):153–7.

78. Defrin R, Lurie R. Indications for peripheral and central sensitization in patients with chronic scalp pain (Trichodynia). Clin J Pain 2013;29(5):417–24.

79. Rebora A. Trichodynia: a review of the literature. Int J Dermatol 2016;55(4):382–4.

80. Willimann B, Trüeb RM. Hair pain (Trichodynia): frequency and relationship to hair loss and patient gender. Dermatology 2002;205(4):374–7.

81. Hoss D, Segal S. Scalp dysesthesia. Arch Dermatol 1998;134(3):327.

82. Camacho-Velasquez JL. Nummular headache associated with linear scleroderma: headache. Headache J Head Face Pain 2016;56(9):1492–3.

83. Eross EJ, Dodick DW, Swanson JW, et al. A review of intractable facial pain secondary to underlying lung neoplasms. Cephalalgia Int J Headache 2003; 23(1):2–5.

Printed and bound by CPI Group (UK) Ltd, Croydon, CR0 4YY

03/10/2024

01040476-0018